Patient Education
Nurses in Partnership with Other Health Professionals

Patient Education
Nurses in Partnership with Other Health Professionals

Edited by

Carol E. Smith, Ph.D., R.N.

Associate Professor
School of Nursing
College of Health Sciences
University of Kansas
Kansas City, Kansas

Grune & Stratton, Inc.

Harcourt Brace Jovanovich, Publishers

Orlando   New York   San Diego   London
San Francisco   Tokyo   Sydney   Toronto

Library of Congress Cataloging-in-Publication Data

Patient education

Includes bibliographies and index.
1. Patient education. 2. Nurse and patient. I. Smith, Carol E. [DNLM: 1. Nurse-Patient Relations. 2. Patient Education--methods. WY 87 P2983]
RT90.P3726 1987   610.73   86-27029
ISBN 0-8089-1833-8

Grune & Stratton, Inc.
Orlando, Florida 32887

Distributed in the United Kingdom by
Grune & Stratton, Ltd.
24/28 Oval Road, London NW 1

Library of Congress Catalog Number 86-27029
International Standard Book Number 0-8089-1833-8
Printed in the United States of America
86 87 88 89   10 9 8 7 6 5 4 3 2 1

For John

Contents

Foreword

Dr. Smith's book comes at a critical time in nursing because of the rapid changes and pressures in today's health care system. With the cost cutting/cost containment effort in full swing, the vital importance of patient teaching by nurses must be identified clearly and nurses themselves, as well as policy makers, must be aware of these aspects of patient care.

In the first section of the book each nurses's responsibility for patient teaching is spelled out, giving a historical background from Florence Nightingale to today. The challenge Dr. Smith gives us is that "teaching is a process assisting patients to learn and incorporate new behaviors into everyday life." Indeed the professional, and legal aspects of patient education are discussed as well as the ethical issues impacting directly on patient education. Dr. Smith continues in detail to spell out how to determine what to teach and how to evaluate learning. The chapter on distinguishing between counseling, discharge planning, and patient teaching is excellent and speaks clearly to the responsibilities of nurses in using these interventions. There is a teaching plan with each chapter that is an example of what the chapter has been about. Throughout the book various disease entities are covered: Uterine cancer, renal disease, stroke, diabetes, bronchitis, heart attack, cancer, arthritis, and potential nutritional deficiency.

In addition, the research that has been done in the area of patient teaching is included throughout the book and is most useful as we identify nursing science. The book includes information on how to assess knowledge deficit and establish behavioral objectives. The chapter on planning for patient teaching based on learning theory clearly identifies the principles of learning. Nurses in whatever setting will find them useful for their patient teaching. Technological aspects of teaching are covered from the typewriter to the computer and from the television to TV video conferences. The details will be useful for the patient educator in identifying all the factors involved in the preparation of patient teaching materials. The second section of the text conludes with details on evaluation.

In the last section of the text the role of the patient education coordinator is well defined, and concrete suggestions are given on how to proceed in such a position. The closing chapters address both nutrition and medication education as essential components of patient teaching. A review of the research literature and then the role of nutrition and medication education with patients, families, and communities is discussed.

The final chapter is written by a physician and the teaching plan has been developed by Dr. Smith. I found the materials written by the physician both exciting and thought-provoking. As he states "nurses in particular are especially well suited for the role of patient educators," he later writes "the physician cannot and should not assume primary responsibility for patient education that can be provided by a number of different agencies and professionals. Rather, as the primary contact for health services for most patients, the physician can facilitate and reinforce the work of others."

This text is a result of monumental effort on the part of the editor and her colleagues, who have put together a great deal of information, including reports of research in nursing to assist us in our responsibility for patient education. Dr. Smith has done a remarkable job for the nursing profession. She has brought together various professionals and molded a book that is comprehensive on patient teaching. She is to be commended.

Ida M. Martinson Ph.D., R.N., F.A.A.N.
Professor and Chair
Department of Family Health Care Nursing
School of Nursing
University of California-San Francisco

Preface

This text is intended to provide the information essential for providing health-related education to patients, their families, and communities at large. The first section of the text describes the steps of the teaching process: assessment, planning, implementation, and evaluation. Rationale for patient education is presented from the literature and issues related to the professional. Ethical and legal aspects of educating patients are addressed. Lastly, distinctions between patient education, counseling, and discharge planning are given.

The middle section of the text provides specific information about assessing for knowledge deficit, learning theories and domains, learning resources, behavioral objectives, and evaluation methods. The details in this section allow for development of well-grounded and cost effective patient education programs.

The last section of the text describes the use of the teaching process in developing patient education programs. A nurse, dietitian, pharmacist, and physician have contributed chapters that demonstrate patient teaching as a multidisciplinary process.

Teaching plans are presented at the end of each chapter. These teaching plans are used to illustrate the content in the chapter and are not meant to include all the material that might be taught a patient, family, or community on that particular topic.

The teaching plans, as well as the chapters themselves, were contributed by dedicated individuals who have accomplished much in the area of patient education. The philosophy shared by the contributors and undergirding the text is that patient education is essential to quality health care. Their writings will guide the reader through many rewarding teaching experiences with patients.

Acknowledgments

With heartfelt thanks to LaVonne Myers for her many contributions to this project, Gladys Franz for her encouragement, and the delightful smiles of Philip and Megan.

Contributors

Mary Jean Brown, B.S.N., R.N.
Infant Stimulation Certified Instructor
Head Nurse
Family Centered Care
St. Joseph Hospital
Kansas City, Missouri

Lucie McCallum Black, B.S.N., R.N.
Infant Stimulation Certified Instructor
Coordinator of Staff Development
Maternal Child
St. Joseph Hospital
Kansas City, Missouri

David W. Henry, M.S., R.Ph.
Assistant Professor of Pharmacy Practice
Department of Pharmacy
University of Kansas
College of Health Sciences and Hospital
Kansas City, Kansas

Sharon E. Hoffman, Ph.D., R.N.
Dean and Professor
College of Nursing
Medical University of South Carolina
Charleston, South Carolina

Brian H. Kaihoi
Assistant Director
Learning Resources Department
RMH Health Services, Inc.
Rochester, Minnesota

James W. Kleoppel, M.S., R.Ph.
Clinical Instructor Pharmacy Practice
Department of Pharmacy
University of Kansas
College of Health Sciences and Hospital
Kansas City, Kansas

Judith A. Kopper, M.S., R.N.
Associate Professor
Winona State University
Winona, Minnesota

Nancy R. Lackey, Ph.D., R.N.
Associate Professor and Chairman
Department of Medical-Surgical Nursing
School of Nursing
College of Health Sciences
University of Kansas
Kansas City, Kansas

Cheryl Ratliff, M.N., R.N.
Assistant Professor
Department of Pediatric Nursing
School of Nursing
College of Health Sciences
University of Kansas
Kansas City, Kansas

JoAnn B. Reckling, M.S., R.N.
Assistant Professor
Department of Medical-Surgical Nursing
School of Nursing
College of Health Sciences
University of Kansas
Kansas City, Kansas

John H. Renner, M.D.
Director
Sisters of Saint Mary's Regional Family
*   Practice Residency*
Family Practice Research and Devleopment
*   Center*
Kansas City, Missouri

Dorothy A. Ruzicki, Ph.D., R.N.
Patient Education Research Coordinator
Department of Educational Services
Sacred Heart Medical Center
Spokane, Washington

Sister Ann Schorfheide, Ph.D., R.N.
Assistant Professor
Department of Community Health Nursing
School of Nursing
College of Health Sciences
University of Kansas
Kansas City, Kansas
Barbara Schroeder, M.S., R.N.
Patient and Family Education Coordinator
Rochester Methodist Hospital
Rochester, Minnesota
Carol E. Smith, Ph.D., R.N.
Associate Professor
Department of Medical-Surgical Nursing

School of Nursing
College of Health Sciences
University of Kansas
Kansas City, Kansas

Linda Snetselaar, Ph.D., R.D.
Assistant Professor of Prevention and
*   Internal Medicine*
University of Iowa
Iowa City, Iowa

Bonnie L. Westra, M.S.N., R.N.
Assistant Professor
Luther College
Decorah, Iowa

Patient Education
Nurses in Partnership with Other Health Professionals

NURSES'S INCREASING RESPONSIBILITY FOR PATIENT EDUCATION

. . . the knowledge of nursing, or in other words, of how to put the constitution in such a state as that it will have no disease, or that it can recover from disease, takes a higher place.

Florence Nightingale (1932)

1

Nurses' Increasing Responsibility for Patient Education

Carol E. Smith

With Teaching Plan by
Nancy R. Lackey

OBJECTIVES

1. Discuss nurses' increasing responsibility for educating patients, families and communities.
2. Define the steps of the teaching process.
3. Predict the outcomes expected from patient education.
4. Develop a teaching plan for the patient and family that utilizes the steps of the teaching process to ensure positive expected outcomes after surgery.

Nurses have been teaching patients for decades. Nightingale, in her preface on Notes on Nursing (1932), speaks of nursing as putting the patients' constitution in such a state that will have no disease or that can recover from disease. Today's nurses speak in terms of supporting patients' abilities for self care, high-level wellness, adaptation to illness and compliance to health care regimens. Such terms can be aligned with Nightingale's early thoughts and nursing's present day goals for teaching patients.

Certainly preventions of or recovery from illness are key reasons for educating patients. People can be taught about nutrition, stress management, and early screening measures for detecting disease. Individuals and families who are provided with this type of guidance can anticipate health risks. In this way the public can be educated to recognize and eliminate risk factors that lead to disease. It is hoped that such knowledge would be incorporated into each person's everyday life so that high levels of wellness would be maintained and illnesses prevented.

When individuals are ill there are also many reasons for providing patient education. The person who is acutely ill and admitted to the hospital for diagnostic procedures or surgery needs information to help him adjust to the hospitalization. By the conclusion of the hospital stay the patient should have learned a variety of skills and attitudes that will ensure his ability to adapt and cope with his illness. This adaptation will allow the patient and his family to enjoy life while still managing the illness.

PATIENT EDUCATION: NURSES IN PARTNERSHIP
WITH OTHER HEALTH PROFESSIONALS

Patients who manage their illness have more positive long-range physiologic and health outcomes that allow them to be productive members of society. Fortunately, people with knowledge about their illnesses are less likely to be anxious or distressed about their situations. In addition, individuals who are engaged in patient teaching are likely to report positive perceptions of their health care.

Overall, the process of teaching adds to the patient's and family's sense of control over the situation. Patients and their significant others, whether they be family or friends, can use the information obtained from patient teaching to partake in the decisions with impact on their health. Patients as consumers of health care have been more active in seeking and using the knowledge they gain from health education since the early 1960s. In 1961 Henderson stated nursing was "to assist the individual, sick or well, in the performance of those activities contributing to health or its recovery (or to a peaceful death) that he would perform unaided if he had the necessary strength, will or knowledge." Virginia Henderson included in her definition of nursing the notion that patients would indeed benefit from health care information.

Almost two decades later the American Nurses Association indicated in the 1980 Social Policy Statement "nursing is the diagnoses and treatment of human responses to actual or potential health problems" (p. 9). Patient education is one of the major strategies for treating the multitude of human responses that nurses diagnose daily. Thus if nurses are to meet the overriding goals of their profession, respond to patients as consumers and support patients' progress in health or disease they must learn to teach.

DEFINING PATIENT TEACHING

Simply defined, teaching is the act of assisting another person to learn. However, when learning is considered to be "change in behavior" then this definition of teaching becomes more complicated. It may be simple to assist another to gain new information, skills, or attitudes. But to ensure that the person changes behavior based on the teaching is a continuing challenge. Teaching is a complex process involving a series of interactions between one or more persons that results in changes in behavior. Teaching basically is a process assisting patients to learn and incorporate the new behaviors into everyday life.

Overview of the Teaching Process

Like the nursing process the teaching process has a series of steps including assessment, planning, implementing and evaluating as illustrated in Table 1-1. These steps are to be used as guidelines that will ensure the patient and significant others are taught holistically in terms of their learning needs.

For a proper diagnosis of learning needs both the patient and his family must be assessed. As the teaching plan sample at the end of this chapter illustrates, the family, friends, or relatives of the patient can offer a great deal in terms of understanding patient concerns and identifying needed areas of information. The nurse will need to plan learning objectives or goals that will guide teaching for the patient as well as significant others. To carry out the third step of the teaching process nurses must be able to formulate, select, and employ basic instructional techniques. A variety of instructional strategies that can be used in patient teaching will be discussed in later chapters. Lastly, the nurse must evaluate patient teaching both with respect to the patient's ability to meet the learning objectives and the teaching strategies that were used. The last sections in

Table 1-1
Comparison of the Steps of the Teaching and the Nursing Process

Steps	Teaching process	Nursing process
Assessment	Learning needs identified	Biopsychosocial spiritual assessment
Planning	Learning objectives developed	Nursing diagnoses developed
Implementation	Learning methods and resources utilized	Nursing interventions utilized
Evaluation	Learning achievement judged	Biopsychosocial spiritual status judged

this chapter and the text illustrate several informal and research evaluations of patient teaching programs.

USING THE TEACHING PROCESS

The teaching process is basically a guideline similar to scientific problem-solving, which uses the steps of identifying problems, determining potential solutions, implementing solutions, and evaluating results (Knowles, 1980). Nurses use these four steps almost simultaneously once they have mastered the steps of the teaching process and tried some of the instructional techniques. For example, while admitting a patient to the hospital, the nurse can begin to assess and also plan for patient teaching needs. First, however, nurses need to become familiar with each step of the teaching process and the skills needed to carry these out. These steps are described individually and in detail below. Further examples of each step are given in the remaining chapters.

Assessment

Assessment is the first step in the patient teaching process (Lorig, 1977). Assessment is gathering data or information about the patient problem, in this case, what the patient needs to know to adjust to the illness. Assessment should also be done to determine what the patient needs to know to adjust to the illness. Assessment should also be done to determine what the patient or family already knows. Spending time teaching what patients and families have already learned is wasteful. Assessment also allows the nurse to determine what misinformation the patient may have. The assessment column of the teaching plan examples at the end of the chapters highlights the types of information nurses will want to gather prior to teaching. In addition, the chapters themselves describe specific information to be obtained about patients' learning style, level of knowledge, preferred teaching methods, chronic illness, and nutritional or pharmacological learning needs. The sections in the text on preventive teaching will describe methods for assessing groups or communities about their learning needs.

After the nurse, patient, family or community determine what needs to be learned the second step of the teaching process begins. Planning is the second step.

Planning

The most important part of the plan is the establishment of learning objectives. Objectives are similar to goals in that they stipulate what will be accomplished. Objectives are statements of patient outcomes that can be placed in the chart for all staff to use.

Objectives should also be discussed so that all health care personnel are aware of teaching plans. Two examples of objective/goal statements are: patient states the side effects of his heart medication; and the wife or patient demonstrates how they will change the bandages on the leg ulcer. Both statements are objectives that identify the goals and outcomes expected of the patient and family. Certainly, the patient and family should take an active role in determining what the objective or behavioral goals are. It is hoped that the objectives are comprehensive and address all areas of the patient and family learning needs.

Objectives in the patient' teaching plan should be written for the commonly used areas of learning. These areas of learning are knowledge, attitude, and psychomotor (manual) skills.

Knowledge area of learning encompasses the information or content a patient needs. A knowledge objective for a diabetic might read "patient explains what his insulin injection does for his blood sugar level." In addition to this knowledge, the diabetic must have a positive attitude about taking the medication. In other words, the patient must believe it is important to take the injection as scheduled each day. Accepting the need to incorporate the treatment into everyday life is an example of attitude learning. The objective that would set the goal for such attitude learning might read "patient and wife agree to delay breakfast each morning until urine testing." Manual or psychomotor skill learning is another important area to plan for teaching patients. In this example, a psychomotor objective might read "patient draws insulin dosage into syringe correctly." Thus, to really change the patient's behavior, the nurse should plan several objectives: some for knowledge, some for attitude, and some for manual skills. Figures 1-1, 1-2 and 1-3 reflect some of these learning needs assessed in a research project by registered nurses who teach family members to care for patients at home.

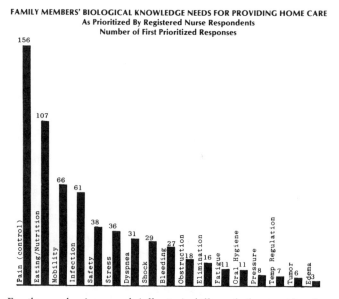

Figure 1-1. Family members' personal (affective) skill needs for providing home care. (From Quiring, J. D. R. N. Perspective of Home Health Care Needs of Family Members. *Kansas Nurse*, April 1985, p. 10. With permission.)

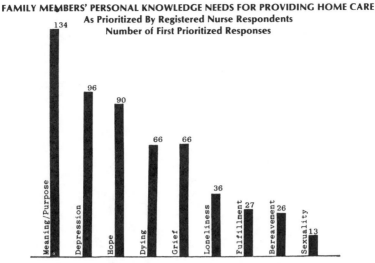

Figure 1-2. Family members' biological [cognitive] knowledge. Needs for providing home care. (From Quiring, J. D. R. N. perspective of Home Health Care Needs of Family Members. *Kansas Nurse,* April 1985, p. 9. With permission.)

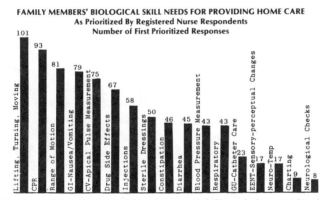

Figure 1-3. Family members' biological [psychomotor] skill needs for providing home care. (From Quiring, J. D. R. N. perspective of Home Health Care Needs of Family Members. *Kansas Nurse,* April 1985, p. 10. With permission.

Areas of learning will be discussed at length in Chapters 5 and 6 on Learning Domains and Learning Theories. Each area of learning should be addressed to plan a comprehensive approach for patient education (Hammer, 1977).

Implementing

After the learning objectives are established, the nurse must then implement the teaching plan with the patient and the family. The third step in the teaching process thus is instruction or actually doing the teaching. The sections in this text on teaching strategies, technologic innovations, and developing teaching materials describe the many alternatives nurses can use in providing instruction for patients. Techniques for providing health teaching to groups or communities are also described.

With many patient situations, instruction that is given the patient or family can be incorporated into everyday nursing care (McClurg, 1981). This, of course, is decided with the patient's needs, level of anxiety, and amount of time available for the learning. During home care treatments, while the patient is being admitted to the hospital or during the time the patient is being assisted with a bath, the nurse can do teaching.

Sometimes, though, the teaching interventions will be done separately. The nurse must decide if the learning objective requires a special time in which patient teaching is the only intervention being done. For example, when helping the patient learn how to take pills it's best to sit at the bedside and show the patient and family which pills are which, explain their purposes, and describe their side effects. For the nurse to sit and concentrate on this one task not only provides instruction but also indicates how very important the information is to learn.

Implementing patient teaching can be as simple as repeating information that other nurses and health care workers taught the patient (Smyth, 1971). A few minutes per shift to reinforce what has previously been taught is time well spent. Once nurses intervene with patient teaching they experience a sense of reward and accomplishment as the patient learns and as fellow workers commend their efforts.

Evaluation

The last step of the teaching process is evaluation. To evaluate if the patient has learned, the nurse must look for the behavior that was described in the objective. If the patient has not achieved the learning objective by changing behavior, then the evaluation must uncover the reasons. It may be that there has not been enough time for learning to take place. It may be that the information conveyed to the patient was overwhelming or that the patient was still denying that he or she has a health problem. The nurse must address any concerns that the patient has and then re-establish learning goals. The nurse may decide to use a different teaching intervention or to repeat the strategy used earlier (Ross and Mico, 1980). More often than not, however, the evaluation step will show that the patient has changed behavior or learned. Using the steps of the process and adhering to the principles of teaching help ensure a positive outcome.

Using the Teaching Process in Everyday Practice

The nurse must be ready to use the teaching process in a variety of situations. Many nurses find themselves asked to present health-related programs to large and small audiences. Nurses on television and radio provide weekly programs on health-related issues. Nurses provide health information to telephone callers on a 24-hour a day basis from some community hospitals. These examples are quite different from the everyday patient teaching interactions that occur between busy nurses and their patients.

There are multiple opportunities for teaching patients everyday (Redman, 1975). The public health nurse who, after taking a blood pressure can ask the patient to state their blood pressure medicine schedule, has assessed the need for patient teaching.

The school nurse who sets up an appointment with a group of teenagers to come and talk about establishing classes on sexuality begins the planning step of the teaching process. Staff nurses who explain and demonstrate aseptic technique while changing a dressing have implemented part of their teaching care plan. The gerontology nurse who conducts a research study to document the diet choices of the elderly after a nutrition class is evaluating her teaching.

As these examples illustrate, patient teaching ranges from informal on-the-spot interactions at the bedside to preplanned, formal community-oriented programs. In either case, the results expected from patient teaching are dependent upon an ability (a) to maintain the highest level of health possible, (b) to adjust to an illness and health care regimen and, (c) to prevent any complications from occurring. The nurse expects the results of teaching to benefit patients, families and communities in these ways.

EXPECTED OUTCOMES OF PATIENT EDUCATION

Patients who are educated partners in their care are able to adjust to the health care regimens used to treat illnesses today. Patients may even leave the hospital with complicated technical equipment or procedures they must perform. Individuals in the hospital thus need patient education programs that will enable them to care for themselves after discharge. In addition the patient teaching program will almost always include a referral to a community health nurse who can continue teaching the family posthospitalization. And in the reverse, the community health nurse who knows of patients to be hospitalized should teach these individuals what to expect when they are admitted for surgery, diagnositic tests, or therapy.

Patient teaching also makes a difference for individuals being admitted to a variety of health care agencies. For example, when elderly patients are moved into nursing homes they need introductions to the activities available, support services included, and any restrictions in their new living environment (Engle, 1985). Nurses have also been involved in teaching children who are being moved to a foster or adoptive home.

Patient teaching can be used to increase adaptation to new environments, as well as to new life styles. Community education programs can help families establish healthier life styles that include good nutrition, regular exercise, and use of health care screening services. In addition, today's nurse can help individuals adapt to normal life changes and to chronic illnesses by taking the role of patient educator.

Nurses Benefit by Taking the Role
of Patient Educator

In the realities of today's health care with shortened hospital stays, families managing increasingly complex home care and the growing awareness of the "wellness concept," nurses are key people sought to conduct patient teaching programs. The short length of many hospital stays makes it imperative that patients adjust rapidly. Another benefit is the economic value of patient education that nurses can provide the patient. For example, the mother who is taught to manage her child's colostomy or orthopedic prosthesis will require fewer costly doctor's office visits. The patient who is taught to manage his intravenous catheter at home (used for intravenous nutrition or chemotherapy) will reduce costly hospital stays. Nurses who teach gain a sense of accomplishment when they observe the positive attitudes and independence their patients display.

Health Care Systems and Providers Benefit
From Patient Education

The results of patient education significantly benefit those providing health care as well as the patients themselves. Patients who are educated are more cooperative because they recognize the reasons for their treatments, medications and/ or restrictions. Not only are educated patients more cooperative but they also adapt to change. The patient's adaptation will reduce the family's stress and decrease the tensions felt when individuals are ill. It's interesting too that patient education has contributed to a reduction in some types of medical emergencies. For example, diabetic patients who are taught to assess their urine for Ketones have fewer admissions to the emergency room for ketoadidosis.

Groups of healthy people also benefit from patient education. Communities that have nurses teach citizens to maintain their health and productivity will have a larger tax base from which to draw.

There are many fine patient education programs sponsored by the American Heart or Cancer Associations. These agencies provide models for teaching patients who are ill, yet there are also education programs available that encourage people to adjust to life cycle changes. For example, many women's associations are using nurses to teach programs on natural childbirth, parenting, returning to work, growing older, and even widowhood. The rapidity with which healthy individuals as well as patients must adapt to changes in everyday life and in their health status demands that nurses make educational opportunities available to them. It is essential that persons who have been diagnosed with heart disease, cancer, or arthritis learn to understand the disease and incorporate their treatments into their everyday life.

Families and Communities Benefit From Health Education

It is also important that the family or other significant persons in the patient's life avail themselves of health information. Families, and even communities, are being called upon increasingly to provide care for the ill person. The family who understands the psychological reactions to treatments and knows, for example, to expect the patient to be depressed, lonely, or withdrawn will be less frightened and better prepared to comfort the patient. Figure 1-4 identifies several reactions family members must learn to manage; thus nurses must teach about these.

Community groups also benefit from public health education programs. Programs describing lead poisoning from crib and wall paints can reduce the neurologic deficients that have been found in many children exposed to this toxin. In addition, the safety education programs, given by public health nurses for mothers of toddlers can reduce choking, scalding, and falling accidents in that age group. Industrial groups are also selling the benefits of health education for their employees that result in reduced absenteeism and accidents. Health insurance companies are hiring nurses to provide health promotion programs to industrial workers and executives alike. Nurses conduct on-the-job education programs to prevent back injuries, improve diet, and decrease stress.

Numerous media, newspaper, and television health-oriented programs are used to increase the public's health education. Such education programs benefit the public, specific communities, families, and ultimately individuals. It is in the area of individual patient teaching that detailed evaluation of education benefits has been documented.

DOCUMENTED OUTCOMES OF PATIENT TEACHING

Research has documented many positive results of patient education. Several studies will be reviewed in detail to illustrate the many benefits identified and the need for future patient education. Dr. Jean E. Johnson's work has served well as a model for developing

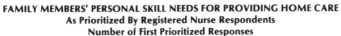

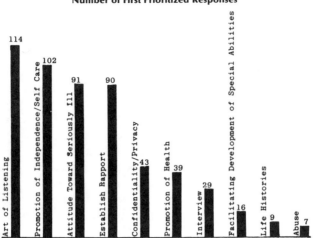

Figure 1-4. Family members' personal knowledge needs for providing home care. (From Quiring, J. D. R. N. perspective of home health care needs of family members. *Kansas Nurse,* April 1985, p. 10. With permission.)

and evaluating beneficial patient teaching programs (Horsley and Crane, 1981). Following discussion of Johnson's work, the landmark research supporting preoperative patient teaching is reviewed. Lastly, references to benefits of teaching the chronically and acutely ill are summarized.

A series of research studies based on the work done by Dr. Jean E. Johnson (1972) illustrates the positive benefits of teaching patients about uncomfortable or threatening events ranging from blood pressure measurement to surgery. The benefits from the instruction include reduced distress as well as decreased length of hospital stay. Dr. Johnson's research used the teaching process and determined through various assessment methods that people experiencing threatening procedures did indeed have distress. Plans and objectives were developed to provide patients with knowledge and skills to manage the distress. Teaching was implemented in a number of ways with a variety of patient groups, and rigorous research methods were used to evaluate the outcomes of the instruction.

Distress Reduction Through Patient Teaching

Dr. Johnson's research supports the teaching of several types of information including procedural, sensory, and coping instruction. Procedural instruction includes informing the patient and family about the events that may be new or threatening to them such as undergoing a pelvic examination or understanding the routine of the hospital itself. Procedural information increases the patient's understanding or knowledge of what is expected to occur. Specific information that should be provided about the procedure includes the time and place it will occur, the equipment that will be used, who will perform or be involved in the procedure, the sequence or steps involved, how the patient will be positioned and what the patient will be expected or asked to do prior to or during the event. For example, the patient may be required to have a special type of diet, medication, or skin cleansing prior to the procedure. During the procedure the patient may be expected to follow certain directions such as holding one's breath or maintaining a required position. It is expected that procedural instruction will enhance the patient's cooperation with the procedure and the confidence that they can manage throughout the event.

Sensory instruction includes informing the patient about the sensations to be expected during the procedure. Sensory information clearly describes the situation and may encourage the attitude that patients will manage what they experience. Any visual, tactile, auditory, olfactory, or taste sensations the procedure might create thus should be described. For example, specific sensory information for patients going for x-rays may include: they will be in a darkened room, the table they will lie on is flat and cold, the barium they must swallow has a chalky smell or taste, and they will hear a buzzing, whirring noise periodically as the x-rays are taken. It is expected that sensory instruction will reduce the anxiety and distress the patient experiences during these unfamiliar procedures.

Coping instruction involves teaching a psychomotor skill such as relaxation techniques or exercises. Such coping skills are expected to help the patient manage during the threatening procedure.

It is postulated that people who are well prepared with procedural and sensory information will know what to expect and can thus say to themselves, "This is the way the procedure is supposed to go," "I knew they would ask me to be on this uncomfortable table," "I'm feeling cold just as the nurse said I would," or "Now I can do my deep breathing to help me relax!" Patients taught should have expectations of the actual experience, and thus undergo less distress.

To test if procedure, sensory, and coping instruction does make a difference, several studies were conducted. Initially research was to determine if individuals prepared with sensation or with procedural information fared differently with their physical and emotional reactions to the ischemic pain created by a blood pressure cuff inflated to 250 mm. Those subjects prepared with sensation information or the typical sensations experienced (pressure, tingling, aching, and slight blueness of the fingernails) reported lower distress than subjects who received only a description of the procedure.

Additional experiments were undertaken to verify that less distress was indeed due to teaching sensation information and not to other extraneous causes. The additional blood pressure studies ascertained that sensation information did not lead subjects to believe the event was less dangerous or less painful. The sensation-informed subjects did not develop greater coping strategies, concentrate on the arm pain more closely, or become more susceptible to suggestion regarding the sensations they experienced. Further experiments revealed that subjects taught just two of the typically experienced sensations still had their distress reduced. Subjects informed of the sensations that infrequently occurred also were no more distressed than subjects given only explanations of the procedure. These were important findings that reassured the researchers that patients who knew only one or more sensations or who did not experience what they were taught would be no more distressed than those given procedural information only. The extensive blood pressure studies encouraged Dr. Johnson to continue her work educating patients for clinical procedures with both sensation and procedural information (Johnson and Rice, 1974; Johnson, Rice, Fuller, and Endress, 1978).

Clinical Studies

The first clinical study was undertaken with patients having endoscopic examinations. Patients undergoing endoscopy must swallow a pencil-thin flexible tube through which their gastrointestinal tract is viewed. Endoscopy patients were assessed to determine what sensations they should expect. Patients reported several sensations beginning with the drowsiness from preoperative medication, lowered room light in the x-ray area, throat tingling from swabbing, and a fullness in the stomach as the tube is inserted. Plans were made for teaching some endoscopy patients these sensations prior to their examination while some patients were taught procedural information only. In this study patients who heard the sensation description required smaller amounts of sedatives, gagged less frequently, and had more stable heart rates than control patients or those taught procedural information (Johnson and Leventhal, 1974; Johnson, Morrissey, and Leventhal, 1973). The results of this study were so beneficial that the endoscopy clinic personnel immediately began using sensation and procedure teaching prior to these procedures (RN, 1977).

This research with endoscopy preparation has been the basis for several creative patient teaching approaches. In a series of articles Beck (1981) describes the psychological and physical preparation necessary for esophagastroduodenoscopy preparation. Parker (1981) discusses the value of using movies as a preoperative teaching aid for patients undergoing a variety of endoscopic surgical procedures such as cystoscopic biopsy or transurethral prostatectomy. In using films of previous surgeries in the preoperative teaching program the patient obtains a clear view of the procedure, anatomical problem, and what is to be expected postoperatively. Pictures of the internal operations showing coagulation of bleeding vessels and removal of kidney stones are used to reinforce teaching before discharge. Parker (1981) states that patients follow their postoperative instructions more closely because they have actually seen the surgical reasons for their restrictions. All in all, several important benefits have arisen from the original endoscopy studies.

Johnson, Kirchhoff, and Endress (1975) expanded their clinical work in preparing patients by teaching sensation and procedural information by studying children who were having orthopedic casts removed. Children 6–11 years of age were randomly assigned to either a control group, a group taught about the procedure, or a group taught the typical sensations that accompany cast removal. Sensations described to the children were seeing the doctor, hearing the buzzing saw, feeling the tingling and heat on the cast, and smelling the chalky dust. All children studied were told the saw would not cut or burn them. During the cast removal researchers found that the children who had had the sensation teaching showed the lowest degree of distress (facial grimaces, clenched fists, attempts to pull away, kicking or hitting and crying or screaming). This research has been the basis for other approaches for easing children's fright during procedures (Johnson, Kirchhoff, and Endress, 1976).

Another study with young women undergoing pelvic examination was conducted to determine if instructions on relaxation during the procedure would decrease distress as well as the sensation information was expected to do (Culp, 1977). Some women were taught and practiced how to relax the abdominal muscles and use abdominal breathing.

Others were given sensation and procedural instructions alone or along with the relaxation practice. The control group was told only of the importance of having pelvic exams. The results of this study indicated that sensation information alone enabled the women to remain calm and cooperative during the procedure. The women who had both sensation information and relaxation instruction reported being less frightened, had lower pulse rates, and cooperated by maintaining the appropriate position during the exam. The researchers felt confident that sensation information had assisted patients in using the relaxation techniques to cope with the threatening event.

Next Johnson (1978) and her colleagues wished to determine if teaching patients sensation information along with a coping strategy would decrease distress during postoperative recovery. To study such long-term effects elective cholecystectomy patients were taught sensation and procedural information and coping exercise strategies (deep breathing and coughing, leg exercises, and getting out of bed). The control group was given only general information about surgery and postoperative care.

There were several interesting results reported from these studies that also measured patients' levels of fear prior to surgery (Johnson, Rice, Fuller, and Endress, 1978, and Johnson, Fuller, Endress, and Rice, 1978). For patients who reported high levels of fear preoperatively, sensation information alone reduced the level of fear. The patients in the exercise group who had high levels of fear reported a greater sense of well being and less helplessness or anger following surgery. In addition, those receiving exercise instruction used significantly fewer doses of intramuscular analgesics in the first 3 days after surgery and they ambulated more frequently.

In terms of reduction of hospitalization, the patients receiving sensation and exercise instruction were discharged at least a day before the other patients. Another interesting long-term effect was that following discharge, patients taught sensation information had ventured outside their homes sooner than the others studied.

The exercise coping strategy and teaching sensory instruction significantly reduced length of postoperative hospitalization, thus saving money for both patients and hospitals. Patients obviously have one less day to be billed for and hospitals have a bed open to admit another person.

These studies also point out that sensory-instructed patients venture from their homes significantly earlier after discharge. It seems possible then to imagine these patients returning to work or home responsibilities sooner than noninstructed patients. If this is found to be the case in future studies, then productivity of the individual in economic terms could also be a benefit of patient teaching. It would be interesting to determine if money was also saved by instructed patients who took less time in completing procedures such as cast removal, endoscopy, or pelvic examination. With the current economic conditions and escalating health care costs, such savings are significant.

Overall, these surgical studies (Fuller, Endress, and Johnson, 1978) and Johnson's other clinical work support the use of sensation and procedure information along with selected psychomotor skill strategies (relaxation, deep breathing, or exercise) designed to help patients cope with the potentially threatening event. Nurses have successfully put Johnson's sensory and procedural teaching preparation recommendations into practice in a variety of settings (Skydel and Crowder, 1975). As a matter of fact, the publications of Johnson's research are listed among the most cited nursing articles of the last 20 years (Garfield, 1984). Patients do benefit from teaching they receive, both the information (sensation and procedure instruction) and the coping strategy. Other specific benefits of patient teaching have been documented extensively in the studies in surgical patients reviewed.

Preoperative Teaching Studies

There is an extensive research basis that supports the effectiveness of preoperative teaching. Investigations that use different teaching interventions and study different types of surgical patients repeatedly identify benefits from preoperative teaching. These benefits include improved coughing and deep breathing by instructed patients, reduced length of postoperative hospital stay and, in many cases, decreased need for postoperative analgesics (Healy, 1968; Horsely and Crane, 1981).

The classic preoperative research work of Lindeman (Lindeman and Van Ackman, 1971, 1972) and colleagues began with the questions and concerns of practicing surgical nurses. Nurses observed that numerous complications such as atelectasis, fever, hypoxemia, and increased bronchial secretions occur in the postoperative patient. They wanted to determine if a structured preoperative teaching routine of deep breathing, coughing, and bed exercises would make a difference. To determine if preoperative teaching made a difference in these complications, Lindeman studied 261 adult surgical patients. There was a control group that received unstructured preoperative teaching and an experimental group that received preoperative structured teaching according to a specified lesson plan. The results of this study indicated that patients undergoing the structured teaching had increased ability to cough and deep breathe as measured by postoperative vital capacity, 1-second forced expiratory volume, and maximum expiratory flow rated. In addition, the average length of hospital stay was 1.9 days shorter for patients who were taught under the structured lesson plan. No difference in the need for postoperative analgesics was found, however, between those with structured and unstructured preoperative teaching (Lindeman and Van Ackman, 1971). Lindeman's research on preoperative teaching is significant in many ways. The findings of the research certainly led credence and support for patient teaching as an effective nursing intervention. The Lindeman and Van Aernam (1971) article in *Nursing Research* is the second most cited nursing article over the past decade (Garfield, 1984). The research clearly shows that unstructured teaching approaches are not as effective as well-planned scientifically based instruction. Lindeman's study, as all research should, raised other interesting questions needing further investigation.

Lindeman addressed one of these questions by studying the differences between group and individual preoperative teaching. Lindeman (1972) found group teaching as effective and more efficient than individual teaching measuring postoperative ventilatory function, need for analgesia, length of hospitalization and also length of teaching time. The research first substantiated preoperative education as an intervention that does influence recovery from surgical procedures and then established the most cost-effective method for teaching (Lindeman, 1973; 1974).

Other nurse researchers have corroborated the beneficial effects of structured preoperative teaching (Johnson, 1975). Another study that evaluated preoperative teaching interventions found that patients instructed in expected postoperative behaviors (turning, coughing, and deep breathing, splinting the incision, foot and leg exercises, and discussion of feelings) had less anxiety and a greater sense of psychological well-being following surgery (Felton, Huss, Payne, and Sric, 1976).

In another study, Fortin and Kirouac (1976) studied the effects of a structured preoperative teaching program that was conducted prior to hospitalization. The teaching program included an orientation to the surgical experience, elementary biological facts, effects of smoking on respiratory function, importance of ambulation, routine respiratory and muscle exercises, techniques for changing position, how to cope with nausea, vomiting, dizziness or weakness and practical suggestions for self-care during the hospitalization and after discharge. The results of this study indicate that those in the structured teaching program had better postoperative physical function than patients randomly selected for the control group. In terms of costs of surgical recovery, the instructed patients used less intramuscular analgesics during the first 72 hours following surgery than the non-instructed group. On the first operative day, the instructed patients reported appreciably more comfort when walking, dressing, and using the toilet.

The benefits of the program were not only apparent in the immediate postoperative period, but also after discharge. Physical function was measured by postoperative ambulatory activity, capacity for activities of daily living on the 10th and 33rd postoperative day as well as time elapsed before returning to work. The improved physical function and earlier return to work could translate into economic returns to society.

It is also important to note there was no difference in the patients' overall satisfaction with the hospitalization experience or their beliefs that they were on their way to full recovery. The structured teaching thus did not give patients an unrealistic picture of the surgical experience or false hopes about recovery. This research project clearly demonstrated the feasibility of implementing a structured preoperative educational program on an outpatient basis. The teaching program was well received by patients and was readily integrated into the hospital's preadmission routine.

Benefits of Teaching the Chronically Ill

The benefits of teaching chronically ill patients have also been identified. Numerous education programs have been conducted with patients suffering from cardiovascular problems, respiratory disorders, renal disease, diabetes, and other long-term illnesses. The most successful programs are those in which instruction teaches patients how to integrate the treatment or therapy into their daily routine and attempts to affect the patient's home or work environment in ways to promote self-management of the illness (Hayes, Taylor, and Sackett, 1979). Use of routine self-care rituals such as daily education reminder charts (Gabriel, Gagnon, and Bryan, 1977) proved to be successful teaching interventions. In terms of learning objectives patients may need to be taught less about the pathophysiology of their disease but more about incorporating the therapy into their daily lives.

After scrutinizing the outcomes of 30 experimental evaluations of patient education programs for the chronically ill, Mazzuca (1982) concluded that teaching did improve compliance with the medical regimen especially when the programs emphasized instruction in everyday self-management. Programs that instructed patients on how to manage their therapy each day resulted in physiologic benefits such as lost weight, decreased blood pressure, or improved blood studies. Nurses and others can indeed expect to enhance compliance and even improve physical results of the chronically ill through patient education.

Benefits of Teaching the Acutely Ill

Benefits have been identified for teaching acutely ill patients. Instruction for patients treated in the emergency room have been successful as have programs in outpatient departments teaching about acute infections. Even patients and families experiencing myocardial infarctions benefit from teaching during the acute onset of the disease.

Murdaugh (1982) reviewed 11 studies of cardiac patient teaching plans using structured formats (Table 1-2). All of the studies used knowledge gain for attitude evaluation, anxiety level for affective evaluation, and compliance with medical care postdischarge as evaluation for psychomotor skills learning. The majority of patients studied did increase their knowledge, decrease their anxiety, and enhance their postdischarge compliances. Further, these studies showed that patients' anxiety is highest early in the illness, immediately after transfer from intensive care areas and just prior to discharge from the hospital. One study reported that teaching after discharge from the critical care area when anxiety was lowest, significantly increased knowledge (Guzetta, 1979). The most important aspect of the review, however, was the gathering of substantiating evidence that teaching cardiac patients during hospitalization is worthwhile. Devine and Cook (1986) found similar evidence for teaching surgical patients following their meta-analysis.

OUTCOMES OF OTHER TEACHING PROGRAMS

There are several other examples of successful patient education programs conducted with acutely ill patients. Ostomy patients can be given preoperative instruction for the surgery as well as postoperative practice sessions for caring for their stoma. Orthopedic patients with joint replacement surgeries should be instructed on physical therapy, activity restrictions, and even that their artificial joint will cause the security alarm machines in airports to ring.

Many hospitals now employ nurses specifically to provide teaching for patients and families who must manage sophisticated technical equipment after discharge. For example, artificial kidney patients are taught either home hemo- or peritoneal dialyses techniques. Patients receiving intravenous nutrition or chemotherapy are taught to manage their indwelling catheters. Victims of trauma discharged after emergency care are instructed on symptoms they should report such as inflammation of lacerations or headaches and drowsiness following blows to the head. At Children's Hospital in Boston, nurses coordinate a program to provide information for parents waiting during their child's surgery. The nurses believe that telling the parents how everything is going and estimating how much longer the surgery will last helps parents cope during the emotional crises of waiting for their child in surgery.

Community health education programs have been successful in decreasing complications of illnesses and in disease prevention (Tagliacozzo, Luskin, and Lashof, 1974). In a study where preventive diabetic care was taught to 8,000 outpatients, the number of admissions of severe diabetic ketoacidoses dropped by 30 percent, and severe hypoglycemia as well as leg amputations declined (Davidson, 1975).

Effects of another large community education program were studied by comparing three towns. In two towns, extensive mass media campaigns on reducing cholesterol, blood pressure, and cigarette smoking were conducted over a 2-year period (Farquhar,

Table 1-2
Cardiac Patient Teaching Studies

Author(s)	Design	Sample	Type teaching program	Time teaching initiated	Evaluation of success
Barbarowicz et al. (1980)	Two Groups Pretest/ Posttest: Discharge 1 Mo., 3 Mos.	Cardiac Surgery Pt., N = 232	Structured: Slide-Sound Program, Printed Material	Past Transfer From ICU	Knowledge (Written Test) Compliance (Self Report) Anxiety (STAI)
Christopherson et al. (1980)	Three Groups Pretest/ Posttest	Cardiac Surgery Pt. N = 20	Structured: Printed Material	Prior to Admis. and Immediately After Admission	Knowledge (Written Test) Anxiety (STAI) Length of Hospitalization
Miliazzo (1980)	Three Groups Pretest/ Posttest	M.I. Pt. N = 25	Structured: Individual Instruction, Slide Presentation	Past Transfer From CCU When Ambulatory	Knowledge (Written Test)
Scalzi et al. (1980)	Two Groups Pretest/ Posttest: Discharge, 3 Mos. 1 Yr, 2 Yrs.	M.I. Pt. N = 23	Structured: Printed Material, Individual Instruction, Audiotapes	Does Not State	Knowledge (Written Test) Compliance (Self Report) Denial (Denial Scale) Depression (Beck Inventory) Coronary-Prone Behavior (Written Test)
Toth	Two groups posttest only	M.I. Pt. N = 20	Structured: Individual Instruction	No Later Than 24 Hours past Admission	Anxiety (IPAT)

Study	Design	Sample	Intervention	Timing	Outcome Measures
Rahe et al. (1975)	One Group Pretest/Posttest	M.I. Pt., N = 24	Structured: Printed Material, Individual Instruction	Between 4th & 7th day post M.I.	Knowledge (Written Test)
Bille (1977)	Two Groups Posttests Only: Discharge 1 month	M.I. Pt., N = 24	Structured: Printed Material, Individual Instruction	Does Not State	Knowledge (Written Test), Compliance (Self-Report)
Pozen et al. (1977)	Two Groups Pretest/Posttests: Discharge 6 Mos.	M.I. Pt., N = 102	Structured: Printed Material, Individual Instruction, Counseling	First 24 Hours past admission	Knowledge (Written Test), Compliance (Self-Report), Anxiety (IPAT)
Owens et al. (1978)	Two Groups Pretest/Posttest: Discharge 6 Wks.	M.I. Pts., Cardiac Surgery Pt. N = 36	Structured: Group Discussions	6–10 days post M.I. or post surgery	Knowledge (Written Test)
Guzetta (1979)	Three Groups Pretest/Posttest	M.I. Pt. N = 45	Structured: Printed Material, Individual Instruction	Past CCU Transfer @ 1–3 days, 7–9 days 11–13 days	Knowledge (Written Test), Anxiety (A–D Scale, 24 Hr. Urinary Cortisol)
Linds et al. (1979)	Two Groups Pretest/Posttest: Discharge 1 Mo. 3 Mos.	Cardiac Surgery Pt., N = 55	Structured: Printed Material, Individual Instruction, Models Audiocassettes	Does Not State	Knowledge (Written Test), Compliance (Self-Report Lab Studies, Kept Appts.)

Murdaugh, C., Using Research in Practice. *Focus on Critical Care*, June/July 1982, pp. 11–15. With permission.

1977). In one of these towns, one-to-one teaching was also provided to a small subgroup of people receiving the mass media. After 2 years the cardiovascular risks had increased in the town that did not have the community education program, while the risks in the other two towns had declined. In the town where the one-to-one teaching was provided, the initial success in reducing cigarette smoking was greater than the other two towns. Health education to communities provided through various methods thus has also proven effective in enhancing positive outcomes (Breckon, 1985).

Continuing Need to Substantiate the Effectiveness of Patient, Family, and Community Education

Patient teaching was considered costly in the early 1970s. Although benefits of patient education that justify the costs have been identified, more work could be done. Nurses are told they must be equipped to provide health instruction appropriate for today's consumer. Urgently called for in prior decades, but still needed today, is evidence concerning the effectiveness of patient education in a variety of circumstances. Development and testing of a variety of instructional materials and teaching strategies for different cultural and age groups is needed. When new materials or strategies are developed the studies used to determine their effectiveness must also be instituted. Incorporation of modern technology for patient teaching is being undertaken in hospitals where closed circuit television channels and computerized health risk appraisal forms are used by patients. Evaluation of life style changes produced by such materials is needed.

In the public health arena, the American Academy of Nursing provides awards to nurses for excellence in presenting health information to the public through the mass media such as newspaper columns, television and radio features. In addition, The National Council on Patient Information and Education has begun an "Ask Your Nurse" television and radio campaign. The commercials encourage the public to use nurses as sources of information about the medications they take. Paul Rogers, the chairman of this campaign, was a former congressman and chair of the House Subcommittee on Health and Environment. Rogers states that nurses have the interpersonal skills and the education to counsel patients effectively; and he further indicated that nurses should be recognized for their role in patient education in their health care team.

Nurses can document that the process of teaching patients is worthwhile in terms of the trust and rapport developed. Indeed, instructed patients are likely to report positive perceptions of their health care (Dykes and Smith, 1976). Satisfied individuals are typically more cooperative than those who have not developed sense of trust or rapport with the staff. The educated patient who cooperates with his health care plan may benefit in terms of decreased distress, reduced length of hospital stay, and earlier return to daily activities. In addition, educated families and communities achieve greater levels of wellness and are able to prevent many illnesses. It thus behooves nurses to utilize the steps of the teaching process—assessing, planning, intervening, and evaluating so that patients can benefit. To employ these steps in a purposeful manner, the nurse must have a background in learning theories, teaching principles, instructional strategies, and evaluation. Latter sections of this text provide just such a background.

The following teaching plan utilizes the nursing process to develop a plan for the whole family. This plan illustrates the usefulness of pre- and postoperative teaching.

TEACHING CARE PLAN: INCORPORATING THE FAMILY
OF A PATIENT

Nancy R. Lackey

In recent years, the changes in our medical care system have been phenomenal. The advent of diagnostic-related groups was only the first in a number of changes in third-party payers that lead to a decrease in the length of hospital stays for patients. This has led to a decrease in actual contact time that nurses have to carry out their teaching care plans. More patients are being discharged much earlier from acute care institutions to convalesce in their homes. As a result, more of the responsibility for the patient's return to health is falling on family members. Therefore, nurses must start incorporating family members into the teaching plan as soon as the client enters the health care system.

ASSESSING LEARNING NEEDS PREOPERATIVELY

Nurses are going to have to be more innovative in the area of patient teaching. For scheduled admissions, hospitals may have to devise programs in which a nurse contacts the patient and his family before the scheduled admission date. This preadmission contact could be by letter, telephone, or a visit. The purpose of this initial contact would be to assess the knowledge base of the patient regarding the disease process and the purpose of the planned hospitalization. This initial contact could also be used to assess the strengths and weaknesses of the family members. The knowledge can be incorporated later into the patient's care plan. Some of the questions the nurse may want to ask are: How many people, including their ages, are living in the home? What is their relationship to the patient? How many hold jobs outside the home and what are the working hours? What is the overall health status of the family members? What are the roles and responsibilities of the patient in the family? Who will be taking over these roles and responsibilities while the patient is in the hospital? How much knowledge do the family members have about the condition of the patient? What types of experiences have the family had with hospitalization? What kind of questions do each of the family members have about the patient's forthcoming hospitalization?

Based on this initial assessment of the family and their knowledge base and questions, the nurse can begin family teaching by explaining the hospital admission policies and what can be expected during this time. The nurse also should encourage the patient and family members to ask questions and to express their concerns and feelings. The nurse must learn to listen to each family member's questions in order to be effective in the area of family teaching. It often is not as important to give facts as it is to listen in order to learn what facts and information family members need.

Planning: Formulating the Teaching Objectives

The nurse formulates a teaching plan that is based on the patient's diagnosis, treatment plan, knowledge base, and concerns of the patient as well as those of each family member using the data gained from the preadmission interview. The nurse needs to conceptualize, whenever possible, the period of hospitalization for the patient and plan discharge teaching. Some of the questions the nurse may ask at this time are What type of information does each of the family members need during the period of hospitalization? What kind of psychological support will they need? How can each of the family members be incorporated, to some extent, into the patient's care during hospitalization? If there are to be special treatments, dressing changes, etc., when the patient is discharged, which of the family members would be best able to carry these out? Once these questions are answered, the nurse should incorporate these family members into the patient's plan of care.

Implementing: Executing the Teaching Plan

During the actual hospitalization, it is easy for the nurse to become focused on the patient's needs and forget that the patient has a life and family outside the medical setting. Nurses are accustomed to the institutional environment and language and frequently find that it is easier to provide for the care of the patient without family involvement. While this might be true, the nurse must recall that he or she will only be caring for this patient for a limited time during the convalescent period, and that the family will be taking over this care when the patient is discharged. Nurses need to feel competent in their abilities and tasks so that they are comfortable in having family members around during specific treatment and care periods. If the nurse is administering a treatment that will be continued after the patient returns home, he or she can start the teaching procedures to the family members by explaining the treatment, its purpose, and how it might have to be adapted for the home environment. It is also best if, during this time, the nurse assesses from the family members and the patient specifics about the home environment and incorporates this knowledge into the teaching about the treatment. Gradually, the nurse can let the family members carry out the treatment with supervision.

Throughout the hospitalization period, the nurse should try to establish times to sit down and discuss the patient's progress with the family and answer questions that they might have. The nurse should actively listen to their concerns and questions and give the information they are seeking. During this period, the nurse also needs to reassess individual family members' strengths, weaknesses, and coping techniques. Nursing can no longer just care for the patient but must care for the whole family's welfare during this time.

Discharge Teaching

Discharge planning starts before the patient is admitted. The nurse should be familiar with referral sources, what types of supplies third-party payers will cover, where supplies can be obtained, and the existence of support groups. Once the nurse knows the diagnosis and the plan of treatment, he or she should be able to identify the degree of teaching needed for the patient to continue convalescence at home. Discharge teaching should be done when some of the family members can be present.

If a specific treatment is to be administered, the designated family members should be taught the treatment and have at least a couple of opportunities to perform the treatment under the supervision of the nurse. In teaching a specific treatment, the nurse must remember to demonstrate or discuss how the treatment can be adapted for the home setting. If enough supplies can not be sent home with the patient for the duration of the treatment, the nurse needs to inform the family members where these can be purchased.

Specific instructions should be written out whenever possible to lessen anxiety within the patient and family members. The family should also have written out for them the phone numbers of agencies, the physician's office, and the hospital unit itself where they can call to have their questions answered.

The following scenario demonstrates how individual family members can be incorporated into a teaching plan:

Mannee Hawke, R. N., a primary nurse on a surgical unit, has been given the list of patients who are scheduled for surgery next week and will be assigned to her caseload. One of the patients scheduled for a total abdominal hysterectomy is a 36-year-old woman, Mrs. Bruce. Mannee knows that Mrs. Bruce will be admitted the night before surgery and that the average stay in the hospital for an abdominal hysterectomy is approximately 4–5 days. Mannee decides to call Mrs. Bruce and do a preadmission assessment.

During her conversation, Mannee learns that Mrs. Bruce is a single mother with three children, Maria, 17; Lee, 15, and Nathan, 9. Mrs. Bruce's parents, both in their mid-60s and in good health, live a couple of miles from her and will be caring for her children while she is in the hospital. Mrs. Bruce is employed as a computer operator in a large industrial warehouse and has hospitalization insurance. Mannee learns that Maria is a very mature and responsible girl who helps with the cooking, cleaning, and care of the other children. Since Mrs. Bruce has not been hospitalized before except for the birth of her children, she sounded glad to hear about the preadmission procedures of the hospital. None of her family has been hospitalized either. During the conversation, Mrs. Bruce asked if all of her children would be able to visit her and was unhappy to learn that children under 12 could not visit in patient rooms. Mannee assured Mrs. Bruce that as soon as she was able, she could be taken to a visiting room where she could visit with her youngest son. During this conversation, the nurse told Mrs. Bruce how she would be prepared for surgery and that she would come from surgery to the recovery room before returning to her room. She also explained that she would have an abdominal dressing and a foley catheter. The nurse explained that since Mrs. Bruce was having a total hysterectomy, she might have periods of depression and unexplainable crying periods for approximately 6 months after she returned home. The nurse explained that these were normal for most women having this type of surgery. Mannee suggested that Mrs. Bruce discuss this with her two older children so they would understand this behavior when it occurred. The nurse asked Mrs. Bruce if she had other concerns and listened as Mrs. Bruce asked a couple of questions. Mannee encouraged Mrs. Bruce to tell her children of the discussion that they had had and stated that if Mrs. Bruce or the children had further questions to call her at the hospital.

Evaluating: Outcomes of Preoperative Teaching

Mrs. Bruce's first 2 postoperative days were uneventful. As instructed, she turned frequently by herself, coughed, and deep-breathed. She was ambulating in her room by the end of the first postoperative day and experienced no surgical or pulmonary complications. On the third postoperative day, her physician told her that her pathology report had returned and that she had a stage II cervical cancer. Cancer cells were also found in the pelvic lymph nodes, which were also removed during surgery. The surgeon referred her to an oncologist who suggested that she have radiation therapy, and Mrs. Bruce consented.

On the sixth day postoperation, Mrs. Bruce started radiation therapy, which consisted of whole pelvic irradiation as well as two intracavitary implants. Mrs. Bruce told the nurse that Maria was very upset about the diagnosis and treatment. Mannee learned that Maria was to visit her mother after school and started arranging her schedule so that she could talk with her.

Evaluating: Outcomes of Discharge Teaching

The nurse listened carefully to Maria's questions. Maria asked about the treatment, how long it would continue, and when would her mother be able to go home. During this discussion, Mannee sensed real fear in Maria's questions and asked Maria if she was afraid that her mother was going to die. Maria burst into tears and nodded her head. Mannee allowed her to cry for a period of time and then asked her if Lee and Nathan had the same fears. Maria nodded yes. Maria then told Mannee that since Nathan had been unable to see his mother and had only talked with her on the telephone, he was sure his mother was dying. Mannee told Maria that she would make arrangements the next day for Nathan to see his mother. The nurse also told Maria that she would be glad to talk with Lee about his mother's condition. Maria said that she would tell him.

Mrs. Bruce's radiation treatments were completed without side effects. However, during this period, she did develop an incisional abscess that had to be opened and drained. Because of the position of the abscess, Mrs. Bruce was unable to irrigate it by herself. After a family conference, it was decided that Maria would do the irrigation and dressing changes when Mrs. Bruce went home. The nurse also discussed with Lee and Nathan the importance of their helping with certain household tasks while Mrs. Bruce recuperated. The following teaching plan chart illustrates this family's postoperative teaching plan (Tables 1-3 through 1-5, pages 25–27).

REFERENCES

A better way to calm the patient who fears the worst. *RN.* 1977, 40, 47–53.

Beck, M. L. Preparing your patient psychologically for an esophagastroduodenoscopy. *Nursing,* 1981, *11*(1), 28–30.

Beck, M. L. Preparing your patient physically for an esophagastroduodenoscopy. *Nursing,* 1981, *11*(2), 88–96.

Breckon, D., Harvey, J., and Lancaster, R. *Community health education.* Rockville, MD: Aspen Publication, 1985.

Culp, J. K. The effect of relaxation and information on young women's responses to pelvic examination. Unpublished master's study, Detroit, MI, Wayne State University, 1977.

Davidson, J. Educating diabetic patients about diet therapy. *International Diabetes Foundation Bulletin,* May 1975, 20:1–5.

Devine, E., and Cook, T. Clinical and cost-relevant effects of psychoeducational interventions with surgical patients: A meta-analysis, *Research in Nursing and Health,* Vol 9, issue 2 June, 1986, p. 89–105.

Dykes, M. A. & Smith, C. E. Effect of a written agreement on patients' perception of their health care and adherence behaviors. Unpublished Master's Thesis, Wayne State University, Detroit, MI 1976.

Engle, V. Mental status and functional health 4 days following relocation to a nursing home. *Research in Nursing and Health,* December 1985, p. 355–361.

Farquhar, J. W. Community Education for Cardiovascular Health. *Lancet,* June 1977, 1192–1195.

Table 1-3
Teaching Plan For Postoperative Patient and Family

Assessment	Plan/Learning objectives	Interventions	Evaluation
		Affective	
•Determine how Nathan is dealing emotionally with his mother's illness and hospitalization.	•Nathan will express his feelings about his mother's illness and hospitalization. •Mrs. Bruce will talk uninterrupted with Nathan by telephone daily at a preestablished time period. •Nathan will visit his mother for at least 30 minutes at least once within the next three days.	•After establishing a rapport with Nathan, use a variety of therapeutic communication techniques (listening, reflecting, clarifying, open-ended questions) to help him ventilate his feelings. •Encourage Nathan to ask questions about his mother's disease and hospitalization. •Establish a time daily that Nathan can visit with his mother by telephone without interruption. •Arrange Mrs. Bruce's schedule so that she will have an uninterrupted time to talk with Nathan by telephone. •Obtain permission to allow Nathan to visit his mother for 30 minutes the next afternoon after school. •Arrange Mrs. Bruce's therapy and treatment schedule so that she will be as pain and stress free as possible for an uninterrupted visit with Nathan. •Give Nathan the Unit's phone number, nurse's home, and when I will be working so he knows he can call and talk to me about his feelings and about his mother.	•Nathan appears to communicate his fears and feelings about his mother's illness and hospitalization. •Nathan communicates daily with his mother by telephone at a certain time. •Nathan will be able to visit his mother for a minimum of 30 minutes in the next 3 days.

Table 1-4
Teaching Plan For Postoperative Patient and Family

Assessment	Plan/Learning objectives	Interventions	Evaluation
		Cognitive	
* Ask Mrs. Bruce what she knows about radiation therapy. —have any of her friends, coworkers, or family had radiation therapy	* Mrs. Bruce will be able to state why radiation therapy is the treatment of choice for this type of cancer. * Mrs. Bruce will be able to list verbally the side effects of radiation therapy that she should report.	* Give Mrs. Bruce information about radiation therapy. —have the nurse from radiation therapy come talk with her. —give her some pamphlets and brochures on radiation therapy. —ask the physician to describe the radiation treatment per se. * Encourage Mrs. Bruce to ask questions and ventilate her feelings regarding the radiation therapy.	* Mrs. Bruce is able to state the purpose of radiation therapy. * During the therapy, Mrs. Bruce will be able to identify the early signs of side effects she is experiencing regarding radiation therapy. * After the therapy is started Mrs. Bruce will be able to help the nurse identify the early signs of side effects by reporting.

Table 1-5
Teaching Plan For Postoperative Patient and Family

Assessment	Plan/Learning objectives	Interventions	Evaluation
		Psychomotor	
*Ask Mrs. Bruce and Maria if they have changed a dressing before.	*Maria will irrigate the incisional abcess according to the procedures demonstrated. *Maria will do a clean dressing change of the incisional abcess after the irrigation and whenever necessary.	*Explain the purpose of the irrigation and dressing change to Maria. *Let Maria practice handling the irrigation equipment and dressing materials. *Talk through the irrigation process while demonstrating it. *Talk through the dressing change while demonstrating it. *Have Maria return both the irrigation and dressing demonstration until she feels comfortable doing it and is competent and safe. *Encourage Maria to ask questions and express her feelings throughout the learning process.	*Maria will irrigate and dress the incisional abcess in a safe and competent manner.

Felton, G., Huss, K., Payne, E. A., and Sric, K. Preoperative nursing intervention with the patient for surgery: Outcomes of three alternative approaches. *International Journal of Nursing Studies.* 1976, *13,* 83–96.

Fortin, F., and Kirouac, S. A randomized controlled trial of preoperative patient education. *International Journal of Nursing Studies,* 1976, *13,* 11–24.

Fuller, S. S., Endress, M. P., and Johnson, J. E. The effects of cognitive and behavioral control on coping with an aversive health examination. *Journal of Human Stress.* December 1978, 18–25.

Gabriel, M., Gagnon, J., and Bryan, C. Improved patient compliance through use of a daily drug remainder chart. *American Journal of Public Health,* 1977, *67,* 968–969.

Garfield, E., Journal citation studies. 44 citation patterns in nursing journals, and their most-cited articles. *Current Contents.* October 22, 1984. *43,* 3–12.

Guzetta, C. E. Relationship between stress and learning. *Advances in Nursing Science,* July 1979, p. 35.

Hammer, V. B., A model relating an adult in a job, interests and needs, and continuing education. *Journal of Continuing Education in Nursing,* 1977, 8, (5), 15–23.

Hayes, R. B., Taylor, D. W., and Sackett, D. C. *Compliance in Health Care.* Baltimore, MD: Johns Hopkins University Press, 1979.

Healy, K. M. Does preoperative instruction make a difference? *American Journal of Nursing.* January 1968, 68, 62–67.

Henderson, V. *Basic Principles of Nursing Care.* London: International Council of Nurses, 1961, 42.

Horsley, J., and Crane, J. *Distress reduction through sensory preparation.* New York: Grune & Stratton, 1981.

How to include sensory information into your patient teaching. *RN.* 1977, *40,* 53–54.

Johnson, J. E. Effects of structuring patients' expectations on their reactions to threatening events. *Nursing Research.* 1972, *21,* 499–504.

Johnson, J. E. Effects of accurate expectations about sensations on the sensory and distress components of pain. *Journal of Personality and Social Psychology,* 1973, *27,* 261–275.

Johnson, J. E. Stress reduction through sensation information. In I. G. Saranson and C. D. Spielberger, (Eds.), *Stress and Anxiety* (Vol 2). Washington, D.C.: Hemisphere Publishing Corporation, 1975.

Johnson, J., Fuller, S., Endress, M. P., and Rice, V. Altering patients' responses to surgery: an extension and replication. *Research in Nursing and Health.* 1978, *1,* 111–121.

Johnson, J. E., Kirchhoff, K. T., and Endress, M. P. Altering children's distress behavior during orthopedic cast removal. *Nursing Research.* 1975, *24,* 404–410.

Johnson, J. E., Kirchhoff, K. T., and Endress, M. P. Easing children's fright during health care procedures. *The American Journal of Maternal Child Nursing.* 1976, *1,* 206–210.

Johnson, J. E., and Leventhal, H. Effects of accurate expectations and behavioral instructions on reactions during a noxious medical examination. *Journal of Personality and Social Psychology.* 1974, *29*(5), 710–718.

Johnson, J. E., Morrissey, J. F., and Leventhal, H. Psychological preparation for an endoscopic examination. *Gastrointestinal Endoscopy.* 1973, *19,* 180–182.

Johnson, J. E., and Rice, V. H. Sensory and distress components of pain: Implications for the study of clinical pain. *Nursing Research.* 1974, *23,* 203–209.

Johnson, J. E., Rice, V. H., Fuller, S. S., and Endress, M. P. Sensory information instruction in a coping strategy, and recovery from surgery. *Research in Nursing and Health.* 1978, *1,* 4–17.

Johnson, M. Outcome criteria to evaluate postoperative respiratory status. *American Journal of Nursing.* 1975, 75, 1474–1475.

Knowles, M. *Modern Practice of Adult Education.* Chicago, Follett Publishing Co., Association Press, 1980.

Lindeman, C. Influencing recovery through preoperative teaching. *Heart and Lung.* 1973, 2, 515–521.

Lindeman, C. Study evaluates effects of preoperative visits. *AORN Journal,* February 19, 1974, 427–438.

Lindeman, C. Nursing intervention with the presurgical patient: Effectiveness and efficiency of group and individual preoperative teaching-phase two. *Nursing Research.* 1972, *21,* 196–209.

Lindeman, C., and Van Aernam, B. Nursing intervention with the presurgical patient—the effects of structured and unstructured preoperative teaching. *Nursing Research.* 1971, *20,* 319–322.

Lorig, K. An overview of needs assessment tools for continuing education. *Nurse Educator,* March–April, 1977, 12–16.

Mazzuca, S. Does patient education in chronic disease have therapeutic value. *Journal of Chronic Disease.* 1982, *35,* 521–529.

McClurg, E. Developing an effective patient teaching program. *AORN Journal.* 1981, *34*(3), 474–487.

Murdaugh, C. Using research in practice. *Focus on Critical Care.* June-July, 1982, 11–14.

Nightingale, F. *Notes on Nursing.* New York, D. Appleton and Company, 1932, Preface.

Nursing A Social Policy Statement. American Nurses Association, Publication No. NP-63 35M, December, 1980.

Parker, C. B. Endoscopic movies for patient teaching. *AORN Journal.* 1981, *34*(2), 254–258.

Redman, B. K. Guidelines for quality of care in patient education. *Canadian Nurse.* 1975, *71*(2), 19–21.

Ross, H., and Mico, P. *Theory and practice in health education.* Palo Alto, CA, Mayfield Publishing Co., 1980.

Skydel, B., and Crowder, A. *Diagnostic procedures: A reference for health practitioners and a guide for patient counseling.* Boston, MA, Little, Brown and Company, 1975.

Smyth, K. Symposium on teaching patients. *Nursing Clinics of North America.* 1971, 571–690.

Tagilacozzo, D. M., Luskin, V. B. and Lashof, J. C. Nursing intervention and patient behavior: An experimental study. *American Journal of Public Health.* 1974, *64,* 596–603.

2

Ethical, Professional, and Legal Aspects of Patient Education

Carol E. Smith

With Teaching Plan by
JoAnn B. Reckling

OBJECTIVES

1. Describe ethical issues pertinent to patient education.
2. Discuss the professional mandates for patient education.
3. Analyze the legal statutes pertinent to patient education.
4. Develop a teaching plan for a renal dialysis patient that addresses ethical, professional, and legal issues to establish guidelines for teaching aseptic technique.

The ethical, professional, and legal aspects of patient education are explored in this chapter. Examples of ethical issues, professional mandates, legal statutes, and court cases will be used to illustrate the increasing responsibilities of nurses in educating their patients. Guidelines for ensuring that sensible judgments are made about what to teach are discussed. Factors with impact on patient education are discussed in terms of realistically providing quality education for patients, individuals, and groups in the community.

FACTORS AFFECTING PATIENT EDUCATION: ETHICAL ISSUES

There are numerous factors in every day practice that have contributed to increased responsibility for nurses to educate patients. One such factor is the acuity level of patients. Modern medical care enables very ill persons to survive and continue productive lives. However, this means that patients are more acutely ill during their hospitalizations. Because medical care is so very expensive, hospital length of stays is being shortened whenever the patient's condition permits. Patients thus are discharged earlier than ever before with more complicated treatment plans to follow.

The patient's ability to take care of himself after discharge depends on understanding the illness and treatment. Patients and families are better able to manage their illness or enhance their health when they are taught about their condition (Steckel and Swain, 1979). When patients are very ill, however, they may be unable to concentrate on everything the nurse is teaching them. In addition, the condition of patients at the time of discharge may still preclude their active engagement in the teaching-learning process. This presents a dilemma because the nurse's major responsibility is to educate the patient.

If the patient is not, in the nurse's judgment, adequately informed because the acuity of illness interferes with his learning, then alternatives must be developed. One would initiate teaching with the patient's family so they could be informed (Gasser, 1981). But if the family is so distraught that they are unable to learn how to manage the medications or treatments? When it is impossible to keep the patient hospitalized for teaching purposes something else must be done to ensure that the family can manage when the patient returns home. Very few patients can learn all that the health care personnel would like them to prior to discharge. This creates a difficult decision-making and often an ethical dilemma.

Making Decisions About Patient Teaching

The science of ethics can assist with decisions about patient-teaching issues. Ethical decision making can be used in solving dilemmas that involve patient teaching issues. A moral or ethical dilemma, like the one described above, occurs when there is a difficult problem with solutions that seem unsatisfactory (Davis and Aroskar, 1978) or equally undesirable (Curtin and Flaherty, 1982). Although there are various ethical frameworks or theories (Former, 1981) that can be used to solve such dilemmas, basically the nurse must compare what is "good" or helpful for the patient and family as well what is "right." Simply put it may be right or correct to teach the patient and family, but in the situation where clients are too ill and families too distraught to learn, teaching wouldn't do them any good. In such a situation, calling upon a community health nurse who would visit the client after discharge to assist with medications and treatments may be the best solution. The community health nurse would institute the teaching plan as the patient improved and the family became less distraught.

Factors such as severity of illness, short hospital stays, and significant others' level of stress must be taken into account to make an ethical decision about teaching the patient. There are unfortunately some situations where other factors influence health care personnel's teaching interactions with clients (Steel and Harmon, 1979). Factors such as the patient's race, socioeconomic level, or medical diagnosis should not bias or stop patient teaching efforts. For example, patients with herpes simplex II may be avoided by the nursing and medical staff due to prejudice against individuals with venereal disease or fear of exposure to this virus. Another ethical dilemma arose when a committee developing nutrition education programs for schools decided not to hold classes in one school because the pupils are "too poor to afford good food and would be shamed by the program." The nurse member of this committee indicated that this dilemma could be solved by engaging a dietition to speak about low-cost nutritious meals in all the schools.

Code of Ethics

As a guideline for providing ethical practice, a code was established by the American Nurses Association (ANA). The code contains several statements pertinent to patient education. The Code of Ethics for Nursing (American Nurses Association 1976) states that nursing service must be provided with respect for dignity and uniqueness of the client. Nurses should be unrestricted by considerations of patients' social or economic status, personal attributes, or the nature of health problems. When teaching a vegetarian patient, it would not be "good" to teach that meats are the best sources of protein and iron. It may be "right" or correct to teach that meats are protein and iron sources, but in terms of this patient's welfare, it ignores the uniqueness of vegetarians. The nurse in this case, should ascertain the patient's knowledge level and dietary preferences and then teach about foods that are acceptable and will meet the individual's nutritional needs.

The ANA Code of Ethics refers to other factors that may affect patient education responsibilities. For example, safeguarding patient privacy and maintaining confidentiality are underscored. Teaching appropriate hygiene measures to the patient who has repeated urinary tract infections thus should take place in a private setting to safeguard the patient against embarrassment. Persuasion of parents of a neglected child to attend educational programs on government-sponsored day care services should not be attempted in a crowded waiting room. The dilemma of the parents' refusal to obtain this education should not be compounded by breeching confidentiality.

The Code of Ethics (American Nurses Association, 1976) also states that a nurse must consider competence and qualifications prior to delegating activities to others. Registered nurses thus must consider that practical or vocational nurse training programs have little, if any, content on the teaching-learning process. Therefore, delegating the licensed practical nurse (LPN) or licensed vocational nurse (LVN) to teach patients must be limited to areas in which they have been educated, such as postoperative routine or the side effects of oral medicines. There will be times when delegation of teaching responsibilities must be done. Short length of hospitalization, emergency nature of the situation or one-time only interactions for teaching may require that less skilled personnel do the teaching. The registered nurse still carries overall responsibility, however, for evaluating the learning and designating all the necessary patient education.

For example, when delegating patient teaching for a senior citizen group's hypertensive medications, there were several considerations to be made. First, an LPN who checks blood pressures at clinic appointments may know most of these elderly clients. This LPN also routinely reviews the hypertensive medication schedule and dosages during the blood pressure check. Thus the RN could assign the LPN to instruct on oral medications at the group program. However, the RN would work with the LPN in advance of the program to prepare for any questions related to hypertension, diet therapy or the aging process. In addition, the RN would develop the learning goals and evaluation measures for this program; and the LPN would be instructed to refer questions on diet, relaxation therapy, or exercise to the appropriate health care professional. In any case, according to the Code of Ethics the nurse must use informed judgment in deciding what to teach and what not to teach or in delegating such teaching tasks.

Deciding What to Teach

Another ethical concern in patient education is deciding what to teach. The key factor in this decision is the patient himself. The public today is much more aware of the right to information and is generally well informed about health and medical services. Patients and their families are often active participants in their care and desire a great deal of information. There is always a wide range of topics that each patient and family might want to learn as part of their education. The nurse must learn to expect many detailed, well thought out questions from patients. As consumers of health care, they have the right to obtain information.

Some patient questions may be centered on a medical therapy or a controversial issue. Nurses should refer questions on medical prognosis and risks of treatment to physicians (Annas, Glantz, and Katz, 1981).

The nurse's responsibility in dealing with controversial areas of health education is to be a patient advocate. This means that the nurse will ensure that the patient obtains the information needed. Part of the nurse's responsibility for health education thus is referral. Referring the patient to the appropriate source of information is a vital part of the nurse's ethical and legal responsibility for patient education. Nurses who use appropriate referrals also gain the respect of their professional colleagues.

Another guideline for determining what to teach a patient relates to safety. The patient should be educated so that he or she will not come to harm. For example, upon hospital admission, the nurse should inform the patient where the nurse call light is and how and why the bedside rails are used; and by discharge, patients must be aware of any medication side effects that they should report.

Nurses also teach healthy people a variety of things to ensure their continued safety. Such topics as proper nutrition, immunization schedules, sound parenting practices, and the importance of using nonlead paint would help protect children. Topics such as human sexuality, drug and alcohol misuse, and developmental tasks of young adulthood would provide important information for adolescents. Topics such as early detection of disease, necessity for regular self-examinations, and ways to manage stress would also be appropriate for the adult population. Many of these health education topics are taught to community- or consumer-oriented groups.

Patients as Consumers of Health Information

When patients ask about something they have heard or read, the nurse must respond to the accuracy of that information. These situations are also opportunities to suggest sources of information that are factual, easy to read, and accessible. It is good for the nurse to acknowledge patients' information as right or correct and also to indicate other appropriate sources of health information (Benjamin and Curtis, 1981).

Some professional organizations, notably the American Dietitians Association, routinely review layman's journals and rate them on the accuracy of the nutrition information written. Other organizations also provide guidelines or suggest content deemed essential for teaching clients. For example, the La Leche League, which supports breast feeding, has several pamphlets describing appropriate topics for discussion during lactation. Also professional standards for practice, as described later in this chapter, provide specific content for teaching patients.

Through its various services, the federal government has written materials suggesting not only health-oriented content but also factors that affect patient learning. For example, through the Offices of Cancer Communications the National Institutes of Health published a packet describing the special issues of educating adult patients with cancer (U.S. Government Printing Office (1983-381-132:765). One of the issues discussed is the patient's preference for certain types and sources of information. The nurse must consider the patient's preference in determining what information sources to suggest.

Patients Who Don't Seek Health Information

Patients who do not seek information or who blindly follow recommendations also constitute an ethical dilemma for health professionals. A survey conducted by the Food and Drug Administration (FDA) determined that there is a lack of information seeking on certain topics. Of persons with new medication prescriptions 96 percent asked no questions of either their doctor or pharmacist about their drugs. Based on these findings, the National Council on Patient Information and Education has begun a campaign designed to encourage consumers to ask health professionals basic questions about prescription drugs. The campaign uses television, print, and other broadcast media, letters and posters to health care centers, and seminar packets for consumer groups. The goals of the campaign are to have patients ask about their medications and to improve the quality of health care information given to patients.

Another nationwide campaign for dissemination of patient education materials is supported by the National Cancer Institute. This institute developed a pamphlet that sets standards for public education on breast cancer. This pamphlet provides a framework for planning and implementing public education programs.

There may be times, however, when even campaigns such as these do not stimulate the patient's desire to know or learn about his or her condition. In other words, there are some patients who do not want information, who are fearful of what they will hear; who do not want the responsibility of knowing health facts. Research with cancer patients revealed that 10 percent of those studied did not want to hear information about cases where treatment had proven ineffective (Cassileth, Zufkis, Sutton-Smith, and March, 1980). There have been other studies on the assessment of patient learning needs that have uncovered areas of information that patients have found nonuseful or fear arousing (Sivarajan, 1983). Other studies have identified teaching strategies that appear detrimental to convalescence or compliance (Reddick and Reddick, 1979; Sivarajan Bruce, Almes, et al., 1981; Sivarajan, Newton, Almes, et al., 1983). And there is the common situation in which the patient gives the responsibility of learning to someone else. An example of this occurs when the nurse begins to teach a patient about his diet and he says, "Oh, just tell my wife. She watches everything I eat."

Each of these situations sets up a difficult ethical dilemma for the nurse and for other health care professionals involved with the client. It is best to document on the chart and to discuss the patient's reluctance to learn with others. Members of the health care team may be able to generate a variety of options for approaching this dilemma.

Techniques that would motivate the patient to learn are probably the right course of action. However, these techniques may result in further agitation, alienation, or confusion for the patient. Such results certainly aren't good for the patient or his family. When attempts to teach or motivate to learn are unsuccessful, nurses must document or chart their attempts at counseling, referring the patient, or other forms of intervention. It is hoped that with time and other forms of assistance the patient will engage in learning. But as in all aspects of health care, the clients do have the right to refuse treatment even if that treatment is patient teaching.

Issues in Health Education

Along with these ethical dilemmas related to direct patient teaching, all nurses are also confronted with more global issues of health education (Squyres, 1983). Many public health problems such as environmental pollution, abuse of drugs or tobacco, and alcohol-related automobile accidents have patient education implications. Nurses must be active at the national and regional levels in identifying these issues, soliciting funds for educational programming, supporting legislation to prevent such problems, and encouraging research and social policy planning for preventive health education programs.

For example, nurses in industry and education who are monitoring the impact of computer technology in the workplace, predict that social isolation, stress-related illnesses will increase as the computer becomes the mode of interaction among us (Ball and Hannah, 1984). Health issues related to eye strain, postural-skeletal problems, exposure to radiation, and computer-related psychological-social isolation will need to be explored. Today, educational programs to alert occupational nurses to these health risks are needed. Nursing organizations at a national level should encourage computer companies, as part of their social responsibility, to provide educational materials related to these health problems for the computer users.

Other social responsibility issues that nurses have been concerned with include proper product labels and instructions, misleading advertising claims for health-oriented products, and use of expensive over-the-counter materials. To address these issues, nurses have provided public education programs, testimony at congressional hearings, and examples of appropriate teaching materials.

The content or exactly what topics to teach or counsel patients on can also raise ethical concerns for the nurse. If a nurse does not believe in abortion she may have conflicting feelings when asked to do preoperative teaching for patients electing this surgery. Families or patients might feel that some content the nurse presents is not good for them. Parents of adolescents might object to nurses teaching that depression can occur during teen years, especially in the face of illness. Children whose elders are very ill might be affronted by the nurse's teaching about a living will. And significant others of the acquired immunodeficiency syndrome (AIDS) patient may reject the nurse who teaches them to help the patient prepare for death. There are any number of content or topics that will raise such ethical issues. Figure 2-1 describes some of the knowledge, skills, and values important for nurses to teach families caring for members at home. These topics were categorized into biological, personal, and social content areas that could potentially raise ethical dilemmas between patient, family, and nurse. Open discussion about such content issues must be undertaken so that a teaching plan that is termed "good" and "right" by the standards of both the patient and nurse is developed.

In addressing any of the aforementioned issues, whether individual or societal in scope, nurses must keep welfare of the clients in mind. There will be situations in everyday nursing practice as well as in a social policy context in which patient education will be tested in terms of good and right. This context is a relatively simple way of viewing ethical issues. The reader is encouraged to seek guidance from colleagues and ethicists.

	BIOLOGICAL	PERSONAL	SOCIAL
KNOWLEDGE	Pain Control Eating and Nutrition Mobility	Meaning and Purpose Depression Hope	Family Dynamics Hospice Sick role
SKILLS	Lifting, Turning Moving CPR ROM	Art of Listening Promotion of Independence Attitude to Seriously Ill	Care Giver's Function on Health Care Team Restorative Activities Resting Activities
VALUES	Need for Care *Time for Life Support Measures Community Resources	Caring Commitment Community Resource	Adjust to Changes Time Community Resource

*Relates to the *timing of the use* of life-extending treatments such as oxygen, IVs, tube feedings, etc. In Home Care experiences, family members or caretakers observe negative progression of the illness and wonder when and/or if they should institute such measures. The concern of euthanasia is often real.

Figure 2-1. Biological, personal and social content areas that might raise ethical issues. (From R.N. perspective of home health care needs of family members. Quiring, J. D. *Kansas Nurse.* April 1985, p. 11. With permission.)

FACTORS AFFECTING PATIENT EDUCATION: PROFESSIONAL ISSUES

There are several factors impacting patient education that nursing professional organizations or societies address. Professional organizations establish standards to guide practice. Standards of nursing practice are used as minimum criteria for judging quality care. The published standards, as those developed at the national level, have gone through many appraisals to ensure that they are appropriate and realistic guidelines for ensuring the safety and welfare of the patients they would affect.

Initially, the call for development of standards for a specific group of patients comes from nurses practicing in the area or from consumers or patients. This request is then turned over to a group of nurses who have education and experience in the field. After this group formulates the standards, they are reviewed by representative nurses, public, and legal experts. The review is done to ascertain each standard statement relative to scope of practice, assurance of quality care, applicability to different health care settings, and reflection of appropriate knowledge base. After the statements are revised according to these criteria, they are approved by the total organization. In this way, rigorous standards that assure the public that nursing in that area will be practiced and judged in terms of quality are established.

Standards of Professional Practice

The Standards of Nursing Practice (1973) established by the American Nurses Association (ANA) can be used to judge quality care in all settings. The standards can be obtained from ANA publications section 2420 Pershing Rd., Kansas City, MO.

Several of these ANA standards provide rationale and guidelines related to patient teaching. For example, the fourth standard was established to guide nursing actions that are planned to promote, maintain, and restore patients to well being. The following guideline for assessing achievement of this standard is listed: Teaching-learning principles are incorporated into the plan of care and objectives for learning stated in behavioral terms. Similarly, the fifth standard uses the guideline: Nursing actions employ teaching-learning opportunities for the patient.

To practice at the level of national standards, nurses should always include patient teaching. Some patients will require only informal teaching carried out while doing wound site dressing changes or even ambulation down the hallway. There are many times that patients and families can be instructed, and nurses must learn to take advantage of these situations. There will also be more formalized teaching opportunities where families are sent to classes, where educational pamphlets are discussed, or where patients are asked to demonstrate how they care for themselves (e.g., site care of amputation stumps, give insulin injections, or perform postural drainage).

Whether formal or informal, the nurse will be meeting the standard by stating the learning objectives in terms that can be measured and then describing the actions that were used. The learning opportunities for the patient must be identified and then documented in the chart. In this way, the supervisors and administrators of the agency are able to illustrate how nurses are teaching patients and practicing according to the national standards.

Standards Established by Special Interest Groups

The American Nurses Association and other organizations representing specialty areas of practice have also developed standards for critical care, oncology areas, operating room, gerontological nursing, and others. Typically, these standards are published in pamphlets, books, or journals that are available to the public and, of course, nurses. The delineations of standards by speciality groups benefit individual nurses by giving them more specific guidelines by which to practice. It is noteworthy that such detailed standards developed by a wide variety of specialty groups consistently refer to patient education. The standards of various groups are reviewed below to highlight their patient education components. Nurses working in these areas must be aware and practice according to such guidelines.

Neurological Nurse Standards

The standards for neurological and neurosurgical fields developed jointly by the ANA and the American Hospital Association of Neurosurgical Nurses (1977) emphasize the family's need for education. Several nursing goals are delineated for evaluating patient and family outcomes: (a) understand the neurological deficit and its effect on daily living; (b) demonstrate ways to maximize the use of existing abilities; (c) make use of safety measures; and (d) report changes in health status and make use of community resources.

The nursing care plan thus would list the teaching interventions used with the family and patient. These might range from providing names of community agencies to explaining the pathophysiology of the patient's head injury depending on which strategies were needed to meet the desired results identified in the standards. Teaching psychomotor skills for a patient with a head injury might simply consist of asking the patient to show you which brush to use for brushing the hair and which for the teeth. Or the parents of an epileptic patient might be asked to demonstrate how they would use a padded tongue blade during their child's seizure. Each of these teaching interventions would be based on the patient and family's needs and the goals set forth in the standards.

Cardiovascular Nurse Standards

The standards set forth for cardiovascular nursing practice (American Heart Association 1975) indicate that patients should demonstrate a knowledge level that enables them to appropriately modify their lifestyle to manage the disease. Specifically, the standards indicate that patients should be taught to maintain dietary intake, activity patterns, effective coping mechanisms, and appropriate pharmacologic regimens necessary for their therapeutic goals.

Most cardiac education programs are designed to meet these standards and address such content. Indeed, such programs draw on the skills of nurses, dietitians, pharmacists, physical therapists, and counselors who teach the patient and family. Often clients are taught new cholesterol-free recipes, rest and exercise protocols, drug purposes and side effects, as well as stress reduction strategies. Each of these topics will assist the patient and family in modifying their lifestyle and potentially reduce the recurrence of cardiac pathology in the community as a whole.

Psychiatric-Mental Health Nurse Standards

The standards for psychiatric-mental health practice include one section devoted exclusively to patient education (American Nurses Association, 1973). Basically, this section indicates that health teaching is an essential part of the nurse's role and that every interaction with clients with mental health problems can be utilized as a teaching-learning situation. Emphasis is placed on educating individuals, families, and communities to understand and cope with mental health problems.

Further, this standard follows the nursing process by stating that learning must be assessed, principles of teaching-learning used in planning and experiential learning opportunities afforded patients through nursing interventions. In addition, references to evaluation include judging the results by determining if patients, families, and communities achieve satisfying and productive patterns of living through the health teaching. Even some basic content to be taught, physical and mental health, and interpersonal and social skills, are listed in these standards.

Such specific standards certainly create a challenge, not only for those in psychiatric-mental health, but for all nurses whose patients have potentially destructive lifestyle patterns. These patterns can be found in individuals, families, or communities; examples range from communities with high rates of alcoholism to teenagers experimenting with cigarette smoking. The nurse might help the community try to combat alcohol abuse by regulating happy hours, drunk driving, and age for purchasing liquor and teen support groups might be set up to educate against smoking. Legislative, legal and ethical issues thus must be addressed to meet these psychiatric-mental health standards of practice.

Many individuals need teaching in areas of interpersonal and social skills to meet the goal of productive family and occupational lives. Individuals with these needs are seen by nurses working in all areas from pediatrics to coronary care and are not restricted to psychiatric-mental health settings. The surgical nurse who recognizes the withdrawal of the patient with amputation thus might intervene by teaching skills such as how to avail themselves of handicap accessible housing. The emergency room nurse who observes conflict between parents over how to administer their child's asthma reactions must teach them the interpersonal skills of discussion and cooperation. Nurses in all settings will still have the psychiatric standards as guides to teaching aspects of mental health.

Emergency Room Nurse Standards

There are standards established for emergency nursing practice (American Nurses Association and Emergency Department Nurses Association, 1979). These standards stipulate that the individual or responsible party demonstrate a knowledge of the problem presented, the immediate care provided, and the importance of follow-up care. Nurses in all settings would do well to make this standard a goal in all patient teaching endeavors.

Community Health Nurse Standards

The standards established for community health nursing practice (American Nurses Association, 1974) describe many aspects of patient education. The use of teaching-learning principles is delineated in terms of considering patients' readiness to learn, planning for reinforcement of learning, and developing content appropriate to the learner's level of understanding. The principles of teaching when the patient is ready, teaching what that person understands, and continually checking and reteaching are essential aspects of all nursing practice. These are especially important to Community Health nurses, however, who work over a long period of time with families in a variety of stages of learning.

Another interesting aspect of the community health nursing standards is the focus on the patient as a consumer. Also identified in the standards is the need to orient or teach groups and communities about changing roles, life styles, and patterns of health care delivery. Knowledge of these changes is thought to maximize communities' health potential. Here again, some standards delineate what is to be taught by nurses. The philosophy of consumer advocacy is essential as it underlines patients' right to be actively involved in the learning and in their care planning.

Lastly, the community health nursing standards are also oriented to clients as groups or communites. Indeed, the standards state that nursing actions are directed to influence community actions as well as the behaviors of individuals. Community health nurses thus are often involved in teaching large groups or providing educational materials for certain segments of the population.

Community health nurses can be found speaking before rotary meetings, school classrooms, and industrial groups on a variety of health issues. These same nurses may provide health education materials at shopping malls, planned parenthood centers, or housing developments for the elderly.

Operating Room Nurse Standards

Another set of standards, that of operating room practice, guides nurses in a completely different setting (Association of Operating Room Nurses, 1971, American Nurses Association, 1975). These standards guide nurses to give information and supportive preoperative teaching specifically related to the surgical experience. These standards also state that the patient and/or responsible party demonstrate knowledge of the individual's physiological and psychological responses to surgery.

In addition to these standards, the Ohio Nurses' Association has published a statement on operating room practice indicating that development of teaching aids is a measure of excellence in nursing care.

Urological Nurse Standards

Other standards specifying the requirements for preoperative teaching are those established for urologic nurse practice (American Nurses Association and American Urologic Association, 1977). Not only is preoperative teaching deemed necessary, but instruction on preservation of bladder and genital function as well as proper use of genitourinary prosthetic devices are also specified. The patient outcomes resulting from such teaching include knowledge of the urologic disorder and how this may modify the individual's life style.

According to the standards for gerontological nursing practice (American Nurses Association, 1976), the patient education is deemed to be significant in achieving a level of wellness consistent with the chronic illness or with the limitations imposed by the aging process. Furthermore, those working with the elderly are guided by the standards to orient them to new surroundings, roles, and relationships and health care resources.

Public Special Interest Groups

Several professional groups have set standards for the health education they provide. The National Task Force on Training Family Physicians in Patient Education (A Handbook for Teachers, 1979) developed manuals stipulating content essential for family practitioners. Also the Society for Public Health Education has published guidelines for preparation and practice of health educators.

In addition to the standards established by nursing and other professional organizations there are other special interest groups that have also published such guidelines. The International Work Group on Death, Dying and Bereavement consists of many health professionals and people interested in the care of dying patients.

A task force of that group published the principles and assumptions underlying the standards for terminal care. Essential to the standards for dying are the principles that the patients' wishes for information about their condition should be respected and that the family should be given the opportunity to discuss all aspects of dying and the related emotional issues. It is noteworthy that this group published its work in a leading nursing journal. Apparently it is important to this group, committed to the care of the terminally ill, that nurses are aware of the standards that ensure the dying have rights to patient education.

Another special interest group publishing standards specific to patient education is the Oncology Nurse Society. This society has published standards for cancer nursing, cancer nursing education, and cancer patient education. The standards for cancer patient education (1982) outline the knowledge needed by individuals experiencing cancer in order to maximize their ability to live with this chronic disease. These standards also provide guidelines for education strategies, criteria for quality assurance studies, and evaluation mechanisms for ascertaining teaching effectiveness. In addition the guidelines are useable in a variety of settings such as hospitals, outpatient clinics, physician offices, home, and public health agencies. The conceptual framework for cancer patient education standards draws on the nursing and research process so that guidelines for all aspects of care are presented. The usefulness of these detailed standards is apparent to all those working with cancer patients.

All standards whether developed on a national level by nursing organizations or by special interest groups provide the basis for professional practice relative to patient teaching. Other written documents provide the legal mandates for patient teaching.

FACTORS AFFECTING PATIENT EDUCATION: LEGAL ISSUES

Statutory and Common Laws Mandate Patient Education

Nurse practice acts are the legal statutes that broadly define nursing and the scope of practice. Many nurse practice acts state specifically that nurses conduct "health teaching." Health teaching is contained in either part of the definition of nursing practice or in the list of specified nursing functions. For example, wording such as this is often used: "nursing is diagnosing and treating human responses to actual (or potential) health problems through such services as case finding, health teaching, health counseling and provision of care supportive to or restorative of life and well-being." There is a model nurse practice act developed by the American Nurses' Association (1976) as an example to guide State Boards of Nursing. This model act includes the terms counsel and health teaching.

Although the wording in the licensing act of each state varies, the majority gives statutory authority for nurses to "care and counsel." Counsel has been interpreted to include teaching and thus the nurse does not need a physician's order to teach (Chaska, 1983). Most nurse practice acts prevent nurses from diagnosing disease or prescribing medications. Therefore, the nurse is restricted from teaching what medications a patient should take or about the patient's diagnosis without the physician's permission. These limitations have not proven difficult because nurses teach about medications that have already been prescribed and most physicians delegate the responsibility for teaching about the patient's diagnosis or disease. For example, orders are often written by physicians for "diabetic teaching" or "MI exercise program."

Some nurses will find little, if any, guidance in their respective state practice acts relative to patient teaching. But even when specific wording about patient teaching responsibilities is not included in the legal statute statements reflecting the nurse's obligation for promotion of health and prevention of disease imply needed areas of patient education. Indeed, common laws or case laws derived from previous court decisions also establish legal grounds for educating patients. In court cases Standards of Practice developed by professional organizations, hospital, or other employee job descriptions and statements on practice from national commissions are used as criteria for judging the registered nurses' responsibilities for patient teaching. Both statutory law and common law thus support the patient's right to have information about condition and treatment. In fact, when a patient is admitted to a hospital, he or she may be handed a patient bill of rights that clearly indicates the right to such information. The doctrine of informed consent further supports the patient's right to know.

Informed Consent and Patients' Rights

Signed consent is often required prior to surgical procedures so that patients understand the risks they are undertaking. So, too, consent is required for relatively new therapies such as the chemotherapy drugs used in treatment of cancer. Patients are also frequently asked to sign release forms that indicate that they understand and accept responsibility for the therapy or diagnostic procedures they are about to undergo.

Each of the situations requiring signed consent provides the opportunity for teaching the patients and their families. For informed consent to be considered valid under the law, the patient must understand the risks and benefits of any treatment. If the patient signs the consent form without understanding the procedure, surgery, or therapy, lawsuits against all parties involved for negligence in failing to inform patients fully can be made.

It has been established by common case law (Scakia vs. St. Paul Fire and Marine Ins. Co., 1975) that it is the physician, not the nurse or hospital, who is responsible to inform the patient about the risks and benefits of the proposed treatment or procedures (Bernzweig, 1984). The patient furthermore has the right to be informed regarding risks and consequences of *not* having diagnostic or therapeutic procedures.

The nurse's legal duty is limited to witnessing that the patient signed the form and agreed to what is stated on the form (Northrop, 1985). Rankin and Duffy (1983) state that witnessing a signature, however, indicates that the witness judged the patient to be in possession of his faculties, that the form was signed without coercion, and that the patient was able to read the consent form. Many nurses are now writing "witnessing signature only" below their name to clearly indicate the patient agreed to sign the form. Even if a nurse thinks the patient isn't sufficiently informed he or she may still legally witness the signature because the nurse is only indicating that the form was signed in his or her presence. However, concern about the patient's lack of understanding of the risks or benefits should be documented and brought to the attention of a supervisor and the physician. In these situations the nurse may certainly teach about the treatments recommended, but it is the physician's responsibility to inform the patient of the risks and the benefits.

In the case of Beck vs. Lovell (1978) a patient claimed the doctor performed a tubal ligation and the hospital nurses failed to get a validly signed consent form. The admitting nurse asked the patient to sign the consent form for a cesarean, which the patient did after striking the clause, "I am aware that sterility may result from this operation." During the cesarean section the operating room nurse was sent by the doctor to have the husband sign a tubal ligation consent form, even though state laws indicate that one spouse cannot grant authority for another (Rocereto, 1979).

There are only two instances when it is legal to have a consent form signed by someone other than the patient. That is when the patient is a minor or when the patient has been legally declared incompetent. Physicians may perform emergency life-saving procedures without signed consent if the patient or guardian is unable to do so (e.g., unconscious).

In Beck vs. Lovell the physician was found negligent but the nurses were not. The court stated that the nurses discharged their legal duties to the patient and that they were acting on the physician's order in obtaining the tubal ligation consent (inappropriately from the husband) and on hospital regulations by allowing the patient to strike the unwanted clause from the cesarean consent form.

Patient Bill of Rights

The rules and regulations for informed consent are based on the American Hospital Association stipulations that the patient has the right to obtain from the physician complete information necessary to give consent in terms that are understandable. Further, in 1972 the American Hospital Association developed a Patients' Bills of Rights. Individual states, hospitals, departments of health, and other agencies have enacted their own patient bill of rights statements. Like the American Hospital Associations' patients' bill of rights, independently developed statements stipulate the patient's right to complete information, privacy, and confidentiality (AHA, 1978). Other groups such as enterostomal therapists, mental health associations, religious groups, handicapped organizations' bills of rights issued by health-care institutions, and professional organizations are not legally binding.

Many states are following the lead of Minnesota, where in 1973 a patient's bill of rights was passed into law. A legislated bill of rights does provide the statutory authority by which courts would judge a nurse's actions should suit be brought. However, other documents developed by professional or interest groups as cited have been presented as standards for practice (Hogan, 1978). Nurses thus might find themselves judged against the National League for Nursing patients' bill of rights first published in 1959. One of the seven statements reiterated therein is the right of patients to health education by health professionals.

Whether working in a state with legislated bills of rights or not, nurses are responsible to know and understand the regulations used by their employer to fulfill the patients' rights. Furthermore, the nurse must clearly understand and follow the policies used to implement regulations that support patient rights. All personnel involved must keep the patient reasonably informed on the aspects of health care provided. The interdisciplinary team that works together thus ensures the patient's rights.

Court Cases Related to Patient Teaching

Legally the interdisciplinary approach assures that the patients' rights to information, informed consent and health education are met, and every individual on the health care team can be held responsible in court for actions related to patient education.

One case that did address the question of a nurse's liability for patient teaching was Kyslinger vs. United States (1975). In that case a hemodialysis patient was sent home after he and his wife were taught how to use and maintain the machine. Instruction on how to give hemodialysis treatments was given over a 10-month period. Two years after discharge the patient died while on the machine. His wife sued, alleging that the hospital and its staff had failed to teach either her or her late husband how to properly use and maintain a home hemodialysis unit. After examining the evidence, the court ruled there was no basis to conclude that any liability or any evidence that indicated the husband and wife were not properly informed on the use of the hemodialysis unit (Creighton, 1981).

In this case the nurses and hospital were sued for negligence. Legally, negligence is an omission of something that a reasonable person guided by ordinary consideration would do. Negligence occurs when nurses have been careless, take action that is contrary to reasonable conduct or imprudent (Cazalas, 1978). Negligence was not proven in this case because the nurses had charted the hemodialysis instructions given to the patient and his wife on a biweekly basis. Thus, this case points to the fact that providing and documenting instruction are considered reasonable, prudent, and necessary. An omission of either providing necessary instruction or documentation of teaching could provide grounds for successful suits against nurses.

In another case involving patient teaching, the court also ruled in the nurse's favor. In this case a child was injured after the mother incorrectly carried out the instructions given her by the nurse for applying a heating pad (Creighton, 1981). The charting documented that appropriate instruction had been given the mother. But, importantly, the chart also indicated the mother's response to this instruction. No grounds for malpractice thus were substantiated.

Malpractice can legally be proven if there is professional misconduct, evil, illegal and immoral conduct, or negligent conduct (Creighton, 1981). However, malpractice of a civil nature is more often cited where the practice falls below the reasonable standards or levels of competence of the profession. In this court case professional standards were upheld (instructions were provided) but furthermore the nurse's competence was substantiated in the chart that indicated the mother's documentation of the correct method for applying the heating pad.

Another classification of malpractice is ethical. Ethical malpractice includes violations of professional ethics resulting in censure by licensing boards and associations. In one case a nurse's license was suspended by the Idaho Board of Nursing for engaging in unprofessional conduct. However, this suspension was reversed by the Supreme Court of Idaho. The unprofessional conduct cited by the Board of Nursing raised the question whether nurses may suggest alternative procedures for treatment when teaching patients (Creighton, 1981). The Idaho Board of Nursing originally suspended the nurse's license on the grounds that she had interfered with the physician-patient relationship because she told the patient and family about alternative treatment. In overturning the suspension the court indicated that there was no definition in the state statute that prohibited or defined as unprofessional the discussion of alternative treatments with patients. No basis for ethical malpractice thus was found by the court.

Situations where patients and families request information about alternative treatment are best handled in collaboration with the physician. The patient's welfare is guarded by nurses who explain the patient's concern for other information to physicians. Advocating the patients' and families' right to such information exemplifies the nurse's commitment to the client's right to know. And ensuring that information about medical alternatives comes from physicians guards the nurse against charges of practicing beyond the scope of nursing.

The court faced with a question involving a nurse's responsibility for patient teaching will probably examine the question under the general category of a patient's right to know (Practices, 1984). When the right to know becomes critical to the patient's health, a court is likely to view patient teaching as a health-care provider's legal duty. This is similar to the way in which courts view the act of supplying information as essential to obtaining a patient's informed consent. Courts would also hold student nurses legally liable for their patient teaching actions as several cases have held student nurses to the standards of the competent professional (Cazalas, 1978). These decisions are based on the patient's right to expect competent nursing services.

Nurses in practice are judged liable against the highest standards that prevail. For example, if a nurse is working in the psychiatric-mental health area she may be held accountable for practice at the level specified in those standards. Likewise, if nurses represent themselves as specialists, whether they have been certified or not, they are held to the higher standards (Creighton, 1981). Nurses thus are very likely to find themselves judged against standards developed at the national level.

Local Standards Used in Court Rulings

In deliberations courts also employ local standards derived from policies, job descriptions, and expert witnesses with training and work experiences in similar employ. Nurses must be familiar with their institutions' expectations and general operating policies.

Nurses should familiarize themselves with their employer's guidelines related to patient teaching. Many agencies have a philosophy statement that clearly articulates patient education as an institutional goal.

There are also nurse job descriptions with statements that specify responsibilities for patient teaching.

Following is a list of patient teaching responsibilities found in staff nurse job description:

1. Discuss nursing care plan and interventions with patients and their significant others.
2. Identify patient's and significant others' learning needs in conjunction with them.
3. Assess learning readiness of patients and significant others.
4. Document teaching plan as component of the nursing care plan.
5. Implement and assists others in using appropriate teaching strategies.
6. Evaluate and document outcomes of patient education.

The patient teaching elements of the job description, goal, or policies for informing patients within the agency will serve as local standards for nursing practice. The locality rule of court evidence indicates that nurses can be judged against standards of practice of a particular local community. The locally accepted standards could be gleaned from expert witness testimony, agency policies, job descriptions, agency committee actions, or procedure manuals. The standards and employee expectations established by every hospital are developed to fit the local community's needs. Each nurse must, therefore, clearly understand their employing agencies' expectations related to patient teaching to ensure that their responsibilities are met according to local as well as the nationally established professional standards. One aspect of the patient teaching responsibility that is governed by these local standards relates to informal activities of teaching.

Ethical, Professional and Legal Aspects of Informal Teaching

Nurses teach informally when, for example, they answer a myocardial infarction patient's questions about a low grade (99.4°) temperature. When the nurse explains that a low-grade temperature is common for a day or two after a heart attack, the patient is reassured and taught that this sign isn't unusual. For best results, informal patient teaching should include the other health care workers involved in the patient's care.

Informal teaching usually occurs after the patient has asked a question about care, medication, diet, or other aspects of treatments. The employing agency will often have established guidelines that indicate the appropriate sources for answering patients' questions. Teaching about medical therapy even in response to patient questions may be inappropriate for nurses and better handled by physicians. Most informal teaching can be readily handled by nursing staff who should chart the patient's concern and the information provided so that documentation exists supporting the fact that local standards of providing information for the patient have been maintained.

It is important that the patient's questions be answered and that the questions be communicated to the physician, dietitian, pharmacist, or other appropriate health care worker. Many times judgments about the patients' or families' understanding of the situation, ability to manage medications or treatments, and acceptance of their illness come from the questions they pose. When such questions are asked, the nurses can explain to the patient that the appropriate health care personnel will answer it. The nurse should make sure the patient recognizes that questions are important, that it is good to ask and that an answer is forthcoming.

Another aspect of patient teaching is that the nurse must understand the local agency's policies on delegation of teaching responsibilities to other personnel. When referring the patient to the dietitian or physical therapist for teaching, the nurse must document this and the education outcomes on the chart. The personnel delegated to teach should understand what is to be accomplished. Remember LPNs and LVNs aren't taught the fundamentals of patient teaching as part of their school curriculum. And patient teaching is not included in their scope of practice. RNs may delegate to LPNs/LVNs the responsibility to reinforce what has already been taught. For example, if an RN is preparing a patient for a barium enema, she could ask an LPN or LVN to tell the patient about the x-ray room and what to expect there. (The LPN or LVN should know what to tell the patient, because they are educated in the technical aspects of patient care.) Frequently the practical nurse will have observed many of the laboratory studies that patients must undergo in her training, and have been taught the nursing care necessary to prepare the patient for these tests. This is a limited form of patient teaching that the RN would supervise and add to. The RN could add to the information as necessary and evaluate if the patient had learned.

Lack of Informal Teaching: Grounds for Litigation?

In some situations, such as the patient in postoperative pain, giving information about medication relief, instructing the patient to breathe slowly and explaining that pain is not unusual following surgery is beneficial for anxiety reduction. But the nurse must also be aware that patient-education efforts can be stress inducing. In one situation a nurse had initiated preoperative teaching when the patient stated, "I just don't want to hear about those details, it makes me too nervous." The patient repeatedly reported that he trusted everything was going to be done well and that he had anxiety when attempts at preoperative teaching were made. Thus the nurse in the situation charted the refusal, notified the physician, and informed the postoperative care nurses of the situation. In this way, the patient's choice was supported.

Another situation in which patients aren't educated occurs when they ask that you teach their spouse or significant other. Nurses hear examples of this when they begin teaching a patient about medications, only to hear him say, "Oh, just tell my wife; she gives me all my pills." Document the patient's exact words; then describe what you taught his wife, and how she responded.

Other times patients may not receive teaching are when a physician specifies that he or she does not want patients educated or to obtain certain information. This places the nurse in a difficult position because the Nurse Practice Act in most states mandates patient education. It is hoped that the dilemma will be solved by discussing the situation with the physician to ascertain concerns and with nursing administrators to review agency policy. Such discussions can lead to development of methods of imparting information to patients that are acceptable to all concerned and that allow for legal and professional nursing practice.

Courts have rarely had cases involving nurses' wrongful patient teaching acts. Yet, as health care agencies, consumer groups, and nurses become more sophisticated in this area, we are likely to see a rise of law suits related to patient education.

If nurses are sued for malpractice or wrongful acts involving patient teaching, the court will consider whether patient teaching was a legal duty to the patient. Local, national, and statutory standards of care would be used to judge if the nurse had met the legal duty. If the evidence indicates the nurse did breach his or her duty to the patient and so caused him harm, the nurse could be found liable.

Nurses must communicate routinely about patient instruction, develop in conjunction patient education plans and clearly delegate responsibilities for teaching patients.

Interdisciplinary Patient Education

As an independently licensed practitioner in a given state, the nurse's primary obligation is to the patient within the scope of practice as indicated in the nurse practice act. Within this scope the nurse executes prescribed physician orders, observes the patient's condition, reports changes, and practices independently under the statutory definition of nursing.

In this light patient education is deemed a mutual responsibility of nurses, physicians, and other health care personnel. The interdisciplinary approach is based on the notion that some aspects of patient education can be carried out by different health care professionals.

It may be difficult for nurses to determine exactly what they are independently responsible to teach. There are some general guidelines that can help with these decisions however. Nurses would most often teach patients things that they want to know or things they ask about by providing the general information and by referring the patient to others. For example, if the patient asks about the medical diagnosis, the nurse can explain the disease pathophysiology. The nurse should however, ask the physician to explain the prognosis of the disease. Or, a patient may ask about the physical therapy regimen; nurses would explain the overall goal of the exercises but then refer to the physical therapist to explain the specific techniques or schedules involved.

Judgments about what nurses should teach patients relative to the diagnosis and care they receive from other health care providers may be difficult. Physicians are often involved in teaching patients many things about surgical procedures and risks, potential complications of medical treatments, and the reasons for prescription drugs. It is important to speak with physician colleagues about their patient education plan so that nurses can reinforce their teaching and vice versa. Also, documenting teaching plans so they are communicated to other staff is important.

A unique way of documenting interdisciplinary patient teaching is presented in the Preoperative Heart Surgery Teaching Outline (Table 2-1). This table reflects the collaboration of nurses, respiratory therapists, surgeons and anesthesiologists in preparing patients for heart surgery. It is clear from the documentation required that nurses have met their obligation to carry out their independent scope of practice while also coordinating the education efforts among appropriate health professionals for the benefit of the patient. In addition, such documentation represents the institutions' expectations for patient education as a shared responsibility among disciplines.

There are many other examples of collaboration that enhance patients' educations. Dietitians and nurses often work jointly in nutrition programs. Pharmacists frequently ask nurses to evaluate the patients' medication knowledge. Physical therapists tell patients to have their nurses assist them with their crutch-walking after they have "graduated" from the physical therapy department. Because it is so important to evaulate and reinforce patient teaching the interdisciplinary approach is very worthwhile.

It is apparent that to legally, professionally and ethically meet the teaching-learning needs of patients, health care workers from all disciplines must work as a team. The

Table 2-1
Preoperative Heart Surgery Teaching Charting Sheet

I. Nursing	Teaching Presented sign and date	Teaching Reinforced sign and date (all disciplines reinforce one another's teaching)
A. Find out what patient/family understands about procedure and hospitalization.		
B. Complete the Pre-Operative Heart Surgery Information Booklet (it has photographs of intensive care unit, describes typical post-operative procedures and sensations, lists visiting hours) with the patient and family.		
C. Patient to demonstrate coughing, deep breathing and leg exercises.		
D. Family: Instruct that patient will look pale (washed out) and will be unable to talk postoperatively.		
E. Teaching tools used: Video tape: Coronary Bypass, a patient's viewpoint Pamphlets: Coronary Artery Bypass Grafts (AMA) Heart Valve Surgery		
F. Anticipatory Guidance/Discussion: a) Indicate emotional reactions to surgery reported by other patients, b) Patient and family demonstrate/verbalize they will seek seek nurse to assist them with reactions.		
II. Respiratory Therapy A. Explain blood gases laboratory purpose and technique.		
B. Demonstrate and give Maximyst; Incentive Spirometry.		
C. Demonstrate and hve patient splint chest with pillow and cough.		
D. Explain ventilator and that they cannot talk while on this machine.		
III. Anesthesiology A. Describe intravenous line insertion		
B. CVP (Central Venous Pressure) Monitoring and Position		

(continued)

Table 2-1   (*Continued*)

    C. Swan Ganz in neck for several days
    D. E. T. (Endotracheal) tube and they
        cannot talk and will have sore
        throat.
    E. Explain Foley and NG tubes started

IV. Surgeons
    A. Informed Consent Form Signed.
    B. Prognosis discussed with Patient and
        Family
    C. Description of other health care
        professionals involved in care

Signature _____ Date _____ Time _____

Modified and used with permission of Laura Gregar, R.N., M.N., Cardiac Rehabilitation Nursing Coordinator, 1985

following is a description and teaching plan for patients needing education on sterile technique. This plan is provided to illustrate the need for interdisciplinary team work in teaching such a complicated psychomotor skill to patients. Ethical, professional and legal factors are illustrated throughout the narrative.

TEACHING CARE PLAN: ASEPTIC TECHNIQUE

JoAnn B. Reckling

There will be several situations in which nurses will need to teach the patient and family aseptic technique. For example, wound dressings or instillation of eye drops may require this, as will more complicated technologic procedures such as intravenous nutrition, infused chemotherapy, and peritoneal dialysis that are routinely being managed at home by patients and their families. One set of patients who are often taught aseptic technique are those with end-stage renal disease (ESRD). This teaching plan describes the variety of procedures these individuals must learn and discusses some of the ethical, professional and legal aspects of teaching aseptic technique to these people (Reckling, 1980).

Patients with ESRD are faced with multiple life-style changes (American Nephrology Nurses Association, 1984). These changes are necessitated by the treatment required to keep them alive when their kidneys fail. Treatment options include hemodialysis at home with help or in a dialysis center; peritoneal dialysis, which can be done alone on an outpatient basis; organ transplant; or no treatment, which will result in death. Patients and families participate in selection of any one or more of the above options. Factors included in the decision-making process are the patient (state of physical and mental health), the environment (e.g., proximity to dialysis center), support systems (e.g., assistant for home hemodialysis), and/or availability of donor organ for transplant. Due to federal financing availability, monetary constraints are not a major factor except in paying for immunosuppressant medications once one leaves the hospital after a renal transplant. Thus the past ethical dilemmas of deciding who could use the limited number of machines in any given community are obsolete.

This teaching plan will deal with a patient who has selected Continuous Ambulatory Peritoneal Dialysis (CAPD) as a treatment method for ESRD, and even more specifically will deal with teaching aseptic technique to this patient (Zappacosta and Perras, 1984). Peritonitis remains a major complication of this dialysis method, and patient contamination is implicated in the majority of cases. The sequelae of peritonitis vary from discomfort and inconvenience, to loss of the peritoneal surface as a dialysis membrane because of thickening and scarring as a consequence of infection, and on some occasions systemic sepsis and even death. Patients are informed of this risk as part of the information provided by the physician when the patient and family are making the decision regarding choice of treatment for ESRD. Not only does aseptic technique have to be used when connecting and disconnecting bags, but patients also must use it when adding medications such as heparin and insulin to the dialysate bags. It usually is the nurse's responsibility to teach the patient the principles and practice of aseptic technique that apply to the peritoneal dialysis procedure, and to evaluate his learning before he assumes responsibility for self care. Meeting standards of professional practice in patient teaching is important here.

Of course, many things other than aseptic technique will have to be taught this patient to make him or her capable of safe self care. These include proper diet, medication administration and side effects, self-assessment of fluid and electrolyte balance, and "trouble-shooting" when problems arise. The whole health team, including dietitian, pharmacist, social worker, physician, and nurses are likely to be working with this patient. For purposes of this teaching plan the concepts and procedures involved in teaching aseptic technique are emphasized. But legally the nurse planning the overall educational program for such an individual must consider all the areas when setting goals and planning specific teaching interventions.

Guidelines for Development of A Teaching Plan for CAPD Patients

Assessment

Before patient teaching is begun, at least three areas need to be assessed. First, of course, is the patient's physiological and psychological readiness for learning. Second, is the level of the patient's knowledge in this area and the things he or she *wants* to know. Third, is information about the patient's environment and support systems that will have impact on the content to be taught.

Information about the patient's physiological and psychological readiness for learning can be determined by patient interview, talking with family and other care givers, and from the patient record. Return towards normal of vital signs, lab test results, etc., indicate resolution of the uremic state after dialysis is initiated.

Questions can be asked to determine if the patient has done anything in the past that uses principles of aseptic technique, such as home canning, sterilization of baby bottles, or jobs that involve working in a laboratory, or with foods. If the patient is a diabetic, specific questions about how to prepare insulin injections, and a history of past infections can provide valuable information.

The patient's home environment and support systems will affect how what is taught is carried out. The individual living in a few rooms with several children and pets will probably find it more difficult to find a clean, draft-free location to administer self-treatment than the person living alone, or with more room. Also, the work environment will need to be considered, since the CAPD patient will need to do at least one exchange at work if he or she works an eight hour day. The social worker may be able to contribute a considerable amount of information based on interviews she has with the patient and family.

On occasion it is necessary to teach another family member to do the exchanges if the patient has some temporary or permanent physical or psychological problem that interferes with the ability to perform this self care.

Plan

Cognitive goals regarding aseptic technique for the patient who plans to do CAPD include understanding the cycle of infection well enough to be able to intervene in this cycle in a variety of ways to prevent infection from occurring. The cycle of infection includes a source or reservoir of microorganisms, a mode of transmission, a portal of entry, and a hospitable host for their multiplication. In addition to knowing how to do the exchange without contamination under one set of conditions, the patient needs to be able to evaluate each environment where an exchange is performed for the absence of a reservoir of microorganisms as well as a mode of transmission.

Psychomotor goals for the person learning to do CAPD aseptically include learning to handle the equipment without contaminating anything. This includes proper cleansing of the medication port and container and sterile transfer of medication from a vial to the CAPD bag, proper cleansing of the connection of tube and bag when changing bags, proper care of the entry site of the catheter into the abdomen, and the proper method of aseptically obtaining a sample of fluid to be sent for culture. In order to achieve these goals, in addition to the cognitive knowledge, the person has to have the sensory and motor abilities to handle the equipment. There are programs available for teaching visually handicapped and blind people to successfully perform CAPD, but of course special arrangements have to be made. Assuming the person can see and read, he or she must be coordinated and strong enough to aseptically remove protective caps from dialysate bags, open sterile packages of povidone-iodine swabs and ointment, etc., insert spikes and needles into small areas, and manipulate syringes and needles and vials.

Affective (attitudinal) goals include willingness on the part of the subject to learn these procedures, patience and perseverance to carry out the procedures correctly, reduction of fear and anxiety to a level where they do not interfere with learning, and absence of immobilizing depression. The nurse initially will perform the dialysis for the patient, and can ask the patient how he or she feels about learning to do the procedure. In addition to gaining assessment information, it will enable the patient to express concerns, which is the beginning of developing coping skills. The nurse can encourage the patient to watch what is done, explaining in simple terms small amounts of information about the equipment and procedure.

Implementation

Once an initial assessment is completed and goals are developed to teach a patient the information necessary for self care while performing CAPD, the nurse can begin the task. Teaching can start as soon as the patient is coherent enough and feeling well enough for short lucid conversations. The nurse must use professional judgment to ensure that the patient's mental state has improved enough with the dialysis to comprehend the teaching.

As the patient shows improvement in physical and mental status, the nurse can move toward a more structured teaching plan. The nurse may want to develop teaching aids that can be made specifically for a family's needs, such as a list with specific do's and don'ts that apply to this patient's situation.

Also, several of the equipment companies provide excellent visual aids, such as video tapes or sound-slide programs, which detail various parts of procedures. The patient and significant others will probably want to view these items more than one time. The patient should be supplied with equipment to handle and practice with. As the patient's condition improves and comfort with handling the equipment increases, he or she can begin to assume parts of the procedure, with the nurse observing, until the patient is able to perform the whole process without prompting and assistance.

Evaluation

The nurse must keep in mind that the focus of evaluation should be on the goals she and the patient have set for the learning experience. The overall goal in this situation is that the patient be able to perform peritoneal dialysis without contaminating the system and developing peritonitis. In the process of evaluating whether the overall goal is met, the nurse and patient (and possibly involved family) will be evaluating attainment of the behavioral objectives from the three major areas (cognitive, affective, and psychomotor).

The whole area of evaluation in teaching patients aseptic technique remains a very difficult one, as no absolutely definitive measures have been developed to measure patient learning (Reckling, 1980). Overall, the nurse will want to observe to see that the patient or family member changed dialysate bags using careful sterile technique and that they described rationale for preventing touch and droplet contamination. The teaching plan described above would be completed over several sessions.

Following the principles and guidelines discussed above should assist the nurse in ensuring that ethical, professional and legal standards of practice will be met (Tables 2-2 to 2-4, pages 54–57). The following is an example of one session used to teach aseptic technique to Mrs. Peri Toneal, a 32-year-old female with a history of type I diabetes mellitus for 22 years. She graduated from high school, is married, and has one child aged 8 years. Her husband is employed in the insurance business and travels during the week. She lives 150 miles from the nearest dialysis center, and when her renal insufficiency began to develop and renal failure appeared a certainty, she and her family selected continuous ambulatory peritoneal dialysis as the preferred dialysis treatment method. When she was admitted this time with renal failure, she was irritable, confused, and vomiting. Her blood pressure was 210/120, rales were auscultated in her lung fields, and an S3 was audible during cardiovascular assessment. Her glucose was unstable (338 upon admission), and other abnormal lab values included blood, urea, nitrogen (BUN) 140, creatinine 14, potassium 5, and hemoglobin 9. She was excreting 1000 ml of urine in 24 hours.

REFERENCES

American Hospital Association. 1974 Patients' Bill of Rights. Chicago: The American Hospital Association.

Annas, G., Glantz, L., and Katz, B. *The rights of doctors, nurses and allied health professionals.* New York, Avon Books, 1981.

Table 2-2
Teaching Plan for *Principles of Aseptic Technique*

Assessment	Plan/Learning objectives	Interventions	Evaluation
		Affective	
Assess Peri's family's attitude toward her having to begin CAPD.	Peri's family will move toward a state of acceptance of this new procedure, as evidenced by verbalization and actions.	Perform similar interventions with family members as listed above individually for Peri.	Peri's family will look at her catheter and apparatus and willingly participate in her care as needed.
Assess Peri's usual coping mechanisms.	Peri will identify her usual coping mechanisms.	Ask Peri to tell you what she usually does when she's upset. Ask her how she thinks these things will help her now.	Some coping mechanisms may be impossible in this situation (e.g. going for a walk in the woods) but focusing on the possible should be helpful.
Assess Peri's strengths for dealing with this situation.	Peri will identify strengths she has which will help her cope with this situation.	Ask Peri to list what she sees as the good things about herself which will help her get through this situation.	Being able to focus on strengths can move Peri to a more positive attitude toward learning.
		Ask her to list several things she will still be able to do when she goes home from the hospital.	
Assess Peri's motivation to learn material necessary for safe self-care.	Peri will begin to show interest in learning safe care as indicated by asking questions.	See Cognitive Function Section of Care Plan.	

Table 2-3
Teaching Plan for *Principles of Aseptic Technique*

Assessment	Plan/Learning objectives	Interventions	Evaluation
		Cognitive	
Assess physical factors affecting Peri's readiness to learn (e.g., level of comfort, visual acuity, and cognitive functioning ability).	Peri will be able to concentrate for short periods of time without feeling uncomfortable.	Assess and record her vital signs and respiratory status. Note her ability to retain foods and ask her if she is comfortable.	Vital signs, respiratory status, and lab values should be within normal limits for a well-dialyzed patient with ESRD.
	Peri's recent and remote memory are functioning well enough to allow her to learn.	Assess her current lab values. Assess her orientation to person, place, and time. Ask her what her address and birthdate are. Ask her to read her menu or a newspaper paragraph out loud to you.	She should be relatively comfortable, not nauseated, and rested. She should be oriented to person, place, and time, and appear to have intact cognitive functions, as indicated by remembering her address and birthdate, (remote memory), and what she had for breakfast (recent memory), and being able to read.

(continued)

55

Table 2-3 (*Continued*)

Assessment	Plan/Learning objectives	Interventions	Evaluation
Assess Peri's knowledge base regarding aseptic technique and cycle of infection.	Peri will recall and discuss instances in her life when she has willfully concentrated on preventing spread or growth of microorganisms.	Discuss definitions such as microorganism and arrive at terminology comfortable for Peri ("germs" or "microorganisms").	Ask her to tell you what terms mean to her and evaluate her understanding.
		Ask Peri if she can think of any way she has controlled microorganism growth or spread in the past.	Determine if she is aware of microorganism spread in everyday life (e.g., food preparation, prevention of disease and spread in a household); her answers should enable you to make this judgment. Determine if she is applying her previous knowledge to the cycle of infection.
		Explain Cycle of Infection (Reservoir, Mode of Transmission, Portal of Entry, Host) and ask Peri to tell you how she might have interrupted this cycle when someone in her household was ill with a cold or the flu.	

Table 2-4
Teaching Plan for *Principles of Aseptic Technique*

Assessment	Plan/Learning objectives	Interventions	Evaluation
		Psychomotor	
Assess Peri's visual acuity (diabetes affects vision as well as renal function).	Peri must be able to see well enough to make aseptic connections and to read material in the training manual.	Ask Peri to read her menu or a newpaper paragraph to you.	Observe and listen to determine if she is capable of these motions. If she is not, options might be a special training program for the visually impaired, or teaching an available family member.
Assess Peri's ability to make fine coordinated movements (uremia causes peripheral neuropathies which interfere with this).	Peri must have enough strength and steady, fine motor coordination to be able to connect tubing spike to dialysate bag.	Ask Peri to place a needle on a syringe. Ask Peri to spike a bag of dialysate.	
Assess Peri's ability to perform a CAPD exchange using aseptic technique.	Peri will be able to perform a CAPD exchange using aseptic technique.	Along with the Cognitive Teaching Plan, encourage Peri to begin participating in her own dialysis, one step at a time, with close observation by the nurse.	Observe the steps as she begins doing them, encouraging and praising her, and correcting errors as they occur.
		Encourage her to increase her involvement until she can do the whole procedure without help.	A specific procedural checklist could be helpful in evaluating this step.

Aroskar, M. A. Ethics of nurse-patient relationships. *Nurse-Educator.* March-April, 1980, pp. 18–20.

Benjamin, M., and Curtis, J. *Ethics in nursing,* New York, Oxford University Press, 1981.

Bernzweig, E. Don't cut corners on informed consent. *RN.* December 1984. pp. 15–16.

Boll, M. J., and Hannah, K. *Using Computers in Nursing.* Reston, VA: Reston Publishing, 1984.

Cassileth, B. R., Zufkis, R. V., Sutton-Smith, K., and March, V. Information and participation preferences among cancer patients. *Annals of Internal Medicine.* 1980, 92, 832–836.

Chaska, N. L., (Ed.) *The nursing profession view through the mist.* New York, McGraw-Hill, 1978.

Cazalas, M. W. *Nurses and the Law.* Germantown, MD: Aspen System Corporation, 1978.

Creighton, H. *Law every nurse should know.* Philadelphia, W. B. Saunders Co., 1981, pp. 25, 134.

Curtin, L., and Flaherty, J. Nursing Ethics: Theories and Pragmatics. Bowle, MD: Robert J. Brody Co.-Prentice-Hall Publications, 1982.

Davis, A. and Aroskar, M. *Ethical dilemmas and nursing practice.* New York, Appleton-Century-Crofts, 1978.

Fromer, J. J. *Ethical Issues in Health Care.* St. Louis, C. V. Mosby, 1981.

Gasser, L. All nurses can be involved in teaching the patient and family. AORN. *Journal.* February 1981, 39, 217–218.

Henderson, V. *Basic principals of nursing care.* London, International Council of Nurses. 1961, p. 42.

Nightingale, F. *Notes on Nursing: what it is, and what it is not.* New York, D. Appleton and Company, 1932.

Northrop, C. E. The ins and outs of informed consent. *Nursing 85.* January 1985, p. 9.

Outcome Standards for Cancer Patient Education. Oncology Nursing Society, 1982.

Professional Accreditation and Legal Statements Supporting Patient Education, *American Hospital Association,* 1978.

Rankin, S. and Duffy, K. *Patient Education: Issues, Principles and Guidelines.* Philadelphia: Lippincott, 1983.

Reckling, J. B. Assessment of peritoneal dialysis patients' understanding and performance of sterile technique. Unpublished master's thesis, University of Kansas, 1980.

Reddick, J. M., and Reddick, P. J. Intellectual changes following closed heart surgery. *New Zealand Nursing Forum.* 7:10, 1979.

Rocereto, L., and Maleski, C. *The legal dimensions of nursing practice.* New York, Springer Publishing Co., 1982.

Sivarajan, E. S., Bruce, R. A., Almes, M. J., et al. In-hospital exercises after myocardial infarction does not improve treadmill performance. *New England Journal of Medicine.* 1981, 305, 357–362.

Sivarajan, E. S., Newton, K. M., Almes, M. J., et al. "Limited Effects of Outpatient teaching and counseling after myocardial infarction: a controlled study. *Heart and Lung.* Vol. 12, 1 January, 1983, pp. 65–73.

Standards of cardiovascular nursing practice. American Heart Association Council on Cardiovascular Nursing and American Nurses Association, 1975.

Standards of Clinical Practice. Pittman, NJ; American Nephrology Nurses' Association, 1984.

Standards of community health nursing practice. American Nurses Association, 1974.

Standards of emergency nursing practice. American Nurses Association and Emergency Department Nurses Association, 1979.

Standards of Medical-Surgical nursing practice. American Nurses Association, 1974.

Standards of neurological and neurosurgical nursing practice. American Nurses Association and American Association of Neurosurgical Nurses. AM5-8. 1977.

Standards of nursing practice, American Nurses Association, 1973.

Nursing's role in patients' rights. NLN Publication No. 11-1671. New York; National League for Nursing, 1976, p. 37.

Practices. Springhouse, PA, Springhouse Corp., 1984. pp. 152–156.

ANA Model Practice Act. Kansas City, KS, American Nurses Association, 1976. Publication number NP-52M5/76.

Patient education: a handbook for teachers. Kansas City; Society of Teachers of Family Medicine, 1979.

American Nurses Association Model Practice Act, Kansas City, ANA. *Code of Ethics for Nurses.* 1976.

Code for nurses with interpretive statements. American Nurses Association, Kansas City, 1976, 6–56.

Adult patient education in cancer. U.S. Department of Health and Human Services. Public Health Service National Institutes of Health, U.S. Government Printing Office. 1983, *381–132; 765.*

Standards of Nursing Practice: Operating Room. Association of Operating Room Nurses and American Nurses Association, Pub. No. MS-220M, February, 1975.

Standards of psychiatric-mental health nursing practice. American Nurses Association, 1973. PMH-1.

Standards of urologic nursing practice. American Nurses Association and American Urologic Association, Allied, 1977.

Squyers, W. Challenges in Health Education Practice. *Journal of Biocommunication,* 1983, 10(3), 74–9.

Steckel, N., and Swain, M. Contracting with patients to improve compliance. *Hospitals.* 1979, *51;*81–843.

Steel, S. M., and Harmon, V. N. Values clarification in nursing. New York, Appleton-Century-Crofts, 1979.

Zappacosta, A. R., and Perras, S. T. CAPD: Continuous ambulatory peritoneal dialysis. Philadelphia, PA, J. B. Lippincott Co., 1984.

3

Using the Teaching Process to Determine What to Teach and How to Evaluate Learning

Carol E. Smith

With Teaching Plan by
Sister Ann Schorfheide

OBJECTIVES

1. Explore methods of assessing learning needs.
2. Discuss the activities associated with planning for the teaching interaction.
3. Describe successful strategy, techniques, methods, and aims for implementing a teaching plan.
4. Develop basic approaches for evaluating teaching and learning.
5. Develop a community-oriented networking education plan that illustrates the use of each step of the teaching process.

This chapter follows the steps of the teaching process from assessment, planning and implementing through evaluation. The details necessary to carry out each step of the process are presented. Examples of individual, family, and community-based patient education are used to illustrate the content.

ASSESSMENT, THE FIRST STEP OF THE TEACHING PROCESS

Assessment of the learning needs of individuals, families or communities basically encompasses three areas of data gathering. First, the nurse must determine what the patients already know. Next, the nurse must decide what is important for the individuals or groups to learn. Finally, a judgment must be made to determine what the patients are ready to learn.

PATIENT EDUCATION: NURSES IN PARTNERSHIP
WITH OTHER HEALTH PROFESSIONALS

Assessing What is Already Known

It is important to assess what is already known by an individual or a group so that teaching builds on present levels of knowledge. The use of a quick review to ascertain what is already known and then building on that knowledge base is important. Assessment of past health information or what people already know is essential as nurses should not assume that patients don't need teaching just because they have had their illness for a while or managed their medical regimen for several months. For example, patients who have taken diuretics in the past must be informed when they are changed to the potassium-sparing types, so they realize less potassium intake is necessary.

Assessment of what is already known is also important because there may have been a misinterpretation by the patient or even misinformation conveyed in the past. The postoperative patient who is straining to keep his fractured leg as still as possible because he was instructed "not to dislodge his leg pin with active exercise" is one such example. This misunderstanding from previous teaching was corrected by clarifying for the patient the differences between excessive and potentially harmful movements and the need for quadracept exercises that promote circulation. In addition, there may well have been a change in the patient's status or the family's ability to cope with the progression of the illness since their past patient education took place. The knowledge or attitude changes gained from the previous teaching thus may need reinforcement and additional development.

Sample Interview to Use in Assessing What Patients Already Know About Their Health Care

1. Can you tell me what you have learned about your illness?
2. You have had surgery before. Can you tell me what you remember from that experience?
3. When you spoke with your doctor or pharmacist, what did they tell you was important to know about your medications?
4. Have you heard about your therapy from anyone else who has had your health problem?
5. Have you read or heard reports about the treatments your doctor wants you to undergo?

Assessing what the learners already know can assist in determining what has changed and correcting any misinformation they may have (The Educated Patient, 1974).

Health Care Professionals' Perspective of What Should be Taught

Assessment also includes determination of what the health professionals believe the individual or group should be taught (Kratzer, 1977). Nurses, physicians, pharmacists, and others may have difficulty in deciding what the patient should be taught. There is a fine line between teaching too much and too little. There are difficult distinctions to make in what is essential for the patient to know and what is excessive and potentially confusing detail for them. Patients and community groups, no matter their espoused level of interest in the health topic at hand, should not be taught as though they were medical or nursing students.

Health care personnel often err on the side of teaching too much detail in terms of anatomy, pathophysiology, and medical terminology. These same teachers err on the side of teaching too little detail in terms of expected side-effects of therapy, self-care management, coping strategies, or anticipation of the psychosocial impact of the health problem. The latter topics are as essential for patients to know as are the risks and consequences of that therapy.

It is important for nurses to make conscious decisions about what individuals, families, and community groups need to be taught. Consensus from all health care personnel involved in caring for the patient is ideal in determining what is to be taught.

Important Information to Consider For All Teaching

Cognitive information about the health risk or illness and demonstration of manual or psychomotor skills necessary to manage at home are certainly essential areas of content of all patient teaching plans. In addition, attention must be paid to the affective areas of learning. Affective areas of learning emphasize the attitudes, emotions, and methods of adjustment that the person must be taught. The importance of affective teaching cannot be overlooked when learning is defined as change in behavior. The person or community must be aided in adjustment to the new health behaviors by learning positive attitudes or by experiencing positive feelings and emotions.

Nurses must assess factors that have an impact on the affective domain and then provide learning experiences that allow for adoption of positive attitudes. When affective learning is ignored, neither knowledge nor skill is put into practice. The most pervasive evidence of this type of failure is the poor results reported for teaching hypertensive patients. Hypertension underlies most of the cardiovascular illnesses that account for the greatest morbidity and mortality statistics in the United States. Public health officials teach numerous hypertension programs aimed at large segments of our population as well as programs taught for individuals. Yet the rates of compliance with the medication regimen necessary to combat hypertension and ensure the therapeutic health benefits of lowered blood pressure are low. Hypertension teaching programs have significant impact only when the health education assists people to integrate the demands of the medical regimen into their daily routine (Mazzuca, 1982).

Gerard and Peterson (1984) studied the congruence between nurse and myocardial infarction patients' perceived learning needs. The patients agreed they needed the information nurses thought important. However, the patients did request a greater emphasis on risk factors of the disease and the medications prescribed.

There are several texts and articles that provide content outlines for teaching individuals with particular illnesses or health risks. When using such references, it is important to critique them to ensure that affective learning content and strategies are among their recommendations. Published guidelines for patient education can also suffer from suggesting that too much or too little detail be taught. Suggested content must be individualized to meet the needs of each patient, family, and community.

Judging When People Are Ready to Learn

Possibly the most challenging aspect of the assessment step of patient teaching is judging when people are ready to learn. Readiness to learn is optimum when both motivation and ability to take in new information, develop new skills, and acquire new attitudes are present. In other words, the individual or group must be willing and able to learn.

Willingness or motivation to learn determines the amount of effort the individual or group will put into the activities for learning. At the very basic level willingness to listen to what the nurse is saying reflects motivation to learn. So too, does the family's or significant others' willingness to be involved in the psychomotor aspects of the patient's care. For example, if the parents of a child with cystic fibrosis are fearful that chest percussion is painful for their daughter they may be unwilling to learn it. On a different scale, community groups may be unwilling to set aside time at their regularly scheduled meetings for discussing health topics. Each of these situations indicates a lack of motivation that will impede learning.

Assessing Ability to Learn

The nurse must also assess for abilities to learn when considering a patient's readiness to learn. There are certain perceptual abilities such as hearing, sight, reading level, that are necessary for learning. Individuals with limitations in perceptual abilities, however, can still learn. The blind person has many options for learning, as does the hearing-impaired individual. Nurses must assess for such limitations and then select teaching methods appropriate for the individual's or group's perceptual abilities. If, during the assessment for learning readiness, a person's perceptual skills are found deficient, then the nurse must take steps to improve these. If there is a hearing or sight impairment then the appropriate learning materials (e.g., large print pamphlets or audiotapes of health information) should be obtained. If there are other perceptual problems such as receptive aphasia as from a stroke or inability to speak while on a respirator then referral to occupational therapy can be helpful in setting up picture boards or other useful communication techniques.

The ability to read and the level of difficulty at which patients can read is another aspect of perceptual ability that should be assessed. Techniques for judging reading level of materials are presented in Chapter 7. The school nurse must judge the reading level of the fourth graders before selecting written materials used to present health topics such as bicycle safety, drug abuse prevention, and sexual development. Medical/surgical nurses must also judge the reading level of their patients before using dietary instruction sheets, activity limitation pamphlets, or drug information fliers. It is suggested that health education materials be written at the sixth to eighth grade level for ease of comprehending the content.

Besides judging the person's readiness to learn, the nurse must determine if the situation supports learning. Remember that reading ability as well as perceptual skills can be hampered by a noisy, disruptive environmental situation, or by the anxiety of the family and the patient or a community's fear of the health problem. Nurses thus may need to alleviate disruptive situational factors or environmental distractions so that the patients can use their perceptual abilities to the fullest.

Assessing Past Learning Experiences

Another aspect of learning readiness depends upon the person's or group's experience. Individuals who have experienced illness in the past may have confidence that they can learn what is necessary to manage in their current situation. Families who have partaken in health care services that emphasized teaching may be very motivated to learn based on that past experience. Community groups that have benefited from past programs may readily accept responsibility for conducting a health fair.

Other experiences that may have contributed or detracted from a person's readiness to learn include mass media campaigns, peer or cultural pressures, satisfaction with health care and the availability of health information.

The nurse should assess the learners to determine if any of these factors has influenced their readiness to learn or, on the other hand, decreased their desire to learn. For example, individuals seeking nutritional instruction to control obesity often state how discouraging national advertising is because the unrealistically thin people are often portrayed as the ideal. This may decrease their motivation to change their eating behavior because they fear they can't live up to this ideal. Community groups may become so dissatisfied when health care personnel can't provide them with the culturally oriented information that they give up including health topics speakers at their meetings. Nurses must be alert for these barriers so that past learning experiences won't interfere with current teaching (Bille, 1981).

Past experiences, perceptual skills, and motivation to learn thus are important factors to ascertain in determining learning readiness.

Questions to Answer When Assessing Readiness to Learn

1. Does the person or group display willingness or motivation to learn, e.g., do they listen attentively, ask appropriate questions, or participate in the discussion?
2. Are there barriers such as reading or hearing disabilities that must be addressed?
3. Has the patient or group come to accept the condition?
4. Is the environment conducive to learning?
5. Have past teaching experiences provided information or confidence in learning?
6. Is there congruence between the patients and the professional perceptions of what should be taught?

Enhancing Readiness to Learn

Steps may be needed to enhance readiness or desire to learn prior to the education program itself. Individuals may need to discuss past experiences so that any negative attitudes or misinformation they received from health care workers can be altered. For example, the patient might say, "Well, they ordered me to be on this diet, but they just didn't listen to how hard it is to cook for the whole family that way." This discussion should clue the nurse into inquiring about ways that the new diet can be fitted into this person's lifestyle so the attitude that health care workers don't listen can be altered. If patients feel the health care teacher is not listening, they may not listen to their teachings.

It is also important to assess past experiences that the person feels resulted in failure to learn. A family caring for a frail, elderly parent in the home may lament that they did not remember side-effects of a medication that they should have reported. This family needs reassurance that the symptoms that should be reported will be written on a list for them to take home and refer to. It is also helpful to point out to this family the many things they did learn about caring for their elderly loved one.

Negative attitudes toward taking on new health care responsibilities can also detract from an individual's or group's readiness to learn. For example, people in a community who now have to partake in a public health education program on well water testing may resent having to learn this procedure, as the county health officer had always done this in the past. In this case, the public health worker responsible for the educational program would first want to explain the reason for the change in service in positive terms (e.g., saving the taxpayers' money) to defuse the group's displeasure over the change. Once any negative feelings are dealt with, the group will be more attentive to the informational program.

If, during assessment for learning readiness, there appear to be negative attitudes or a lack of motivation to partake in the teaching process, then other measures must be used (Wise, 1979). Counseling may be initiated to reduce the patient's anxiety, behavior modification to reward difficult changes, social service referral to ease financial difficulties, or values clarification to highlight the necessity for learning.

Enhancing Readiness to Learn Through Counseling

It must be remembered that a person's readiness to learn is greatly influenced by interpretation of the illness and the treatment. It may be necessary to counsel the patient regarding these concerns before teaching takes place. To assess for counseling needs, nurses listen to any fears the patient or family may have about the prognosis, severity of limitations, cost of the therapy, body image changes, or other disruptions that the patient might feel concerned about. *help solve problems*

Learning readiness will be enhanced if the patient's concerns are attended to before teaching. The nurse thus should ask if the patient has anything to talk about or any concerns about the situation.

Another way of enhancing readiness to learn is to identify and utilize the patient's support systems. Support systems are persons, groups, or activities that assist the individual to cope with the situation. Find out who are the most important people to the patient. Determine if family or friends share the patient's concerns for or faith in the therapy. Ask if family or friends can help with any treatments or procedures to be performed. Are there activities, hobbies, or social groups from which the patient must withdraw because of the illness? If so, can alternative activities be used?

The nurse can encourage family and friends of the patient to enhance learning readiness. Ask the family to talk with the patient about particular worries, encourage the patient to learn; emphasize that he or she can manage the illness, and to praise the patient for compliance with prescribed therapy. Most techniques the nurse employs to reinforce the patient's learning or to counsel for enhancing readiness to learn can be used by family, friends, and others in the patient's support system.

Enhancing Willingness or Motivation to Learn

1. Explore past teaching experiences that created negative attitudes toward learning.
2. Compliment individuals and groups on information already learned.
3. Determine what the person wants to learn and teach this first.
4. Take steps to overcome in deficiences in perceptual skills, e.g., vision limitations, memory loss.
5. Provide counseling to reduce patient or family anxieties.

6. Refer for discharge planning so that financial, housing or other needed assistance can be found to decrease patients' worries.
7. Include the person's significant others in the teaching process.

Several of these techniques will be discussed in later chapters so that nurses can use them to increase patients' readiness to learn. Succeeding chapters will also expand on the important issue of motivation to learn. Assessment for learning needs will also be discussed in greater detail in remaining chapters.

PLANNING: THE SECOND STEP OF THE TEACHING PROCESS

Planning for teaching patients, families, or communities is a comprehensive endeavor. Plans must be made about the actual information to be taught. Learning objectives must be determined. The techniques or strategies of teaching must be selected. The learning evaluation mechanisms must be established. Several chapters in this book are devoted to specific aspects of planning such as developing objectives based on learning domains, selecting teaching strategies based on learning theory, and establishing mechanisms for evaluating the effectiveness of the teaching process.

This section provides general discussion of the types of information that should be taught to patients, families, and communities. Guidelines for systematic planning will also be offered. Later chapters and each of the teaching plans will discuss specific content and information that would be used with individuals or groups having certain health care needs or problems.

Planning the General Content to be Taught

The content or actual information the patient, family, or community will be taught is specified in measurable learning objectives. These objectives are written to specifically reflect the learners' needs based on the assessment that was conducted. However, there are general areas of content related to preventive health education that can be planned into almost any patient teaching situation.

Preventive Health Education - Content Topics to Plan

Preventive health education is the process of teaching people to maintain their highest level of wellness. Highest level of wellness is a popular phrase used to emphasize that there are several levels of being well. Preventive health teaching occurs in conjunction with preventive health medicine and other types of prevention. The goals of all such endeavors are to enhance levels of wellness.

Preventive health teaching is very broad in scope and not limited to "healthy" or disease-free individuals. For example, the postmyocardial infarct patient continuing an appropriate exercise program is maintaining his or her highest level of wellness. So is the teenager who is healthy but undergoing a developmental crisis. The myocardial infarct patient's highest level of wellness will be enhanced by preventive teaching about strenuous exercise to avoid. The teenager will require preventive teaching about bodily changes, self-concept, and adulthood responsibilities appropriate to the developmental level. In general practice there are thought to be three types of prevention: primary, secondary, and tertiary (Leavell and Clark, 1965). The example of the teenager reflects secondary prevention because the teaching is aimed at stopping the progress of the problem, in this case the developmental crisis. The example of the myocardial infarction patient is considered tertiary prevention because the teaching is aimed at preventing further impairment of a person already suffering from disease limitations. Primary preventive teaching would incorporate endeavors aimed at averting a disease, injury, accident, or other health problems.

It is important to understand the distinctions between the types of preventive teaching so that every opportunity is used. It must be emphasized that a patient, family, or community will often have needs for all three types of prevention teaching at the same time. Nurses must learn to predict the types of preventive teaching needs that their patients, whether individual or group, will need. In this way the nurse will plan the appropriate content or topics for teaching according to the level of wellness of those involved.

Primary Preventive Teaching - Examples of Content to Plan

The nurse who recognizes the need for primary prevention (averting a disease, ailment, or accident) can teach individuals how to avoid problems that commonly occur in their age or cultural group. For example, the mother who is taught how to provide a safe home for a toddler can avoid accidents that too often occur at this age. Nurses who are working with newly arrived immigrants such as the Asian Boat People or migrant workers can provide primary teaching about illnesses such as tuberculosis or malnutrition common to the refugee camps. In this way, it is hoped, the newly enculturated groups will avoid these preventable ailments.

Primary preventive teaching can be used with families in various levels of wellness. For example, teaching a family communication skills is important for the adjustment of a youngster being hospitalized. Parents will need to know that regression in behavior is not uncommon during hospitalization. The family needs to know how to talk to the child about the hospitalization and that children do return to their normal behavior patterns after the crisis is over. Families can also be taught games that help the child cope with treatments. Teaching the family ways in which they can assist their loved one enhances all members' ability to adapt with the situation. (Smith, Garvis, and Martinson, 1983).

Families that have concerns about their older adult members can also benefit from a variety of preventive health teaching topics. Discussing the developmental tasks of aging, normal physiologic changes, and importance of constant communication can help family members accept their aging members. Teaching is essential for the whole family to prepare for the oldster being admitted to a retirement center or nursing home. It is hoped that open family communication in these cases would assist the patient in accepting the need for a supportive, loving environment and avoid the fear of institutionalization.

Normal growth and development is another primary preventive teaching topic that is helpful to families as well as individuals. The middle-aged men and women who are about to become grandparents need teaching to help anticipate their new roles, just as the new mother needs instruction to adapt to parenthood. Families who are entering the retirement stages of life need teaching in many areas. Information to prepare for disengaging from work and becoming involved in leisure, hobbies, or volunteer work can enhance this life style adjustment. Nurses can see that retirees obtain needed instruction from social service workers on financial planning and budgeting. Families who are taught about normal developmental tasks and stages can anticipate and adjust to these changes with a minimum of stress.

Another primary prevention area in great need of teaching programs is stress management. People of all age groups, levels of wellness, and socioeconomic backgrounds face stress in everyday life. When taught to avoid and/or deal with stress, individuals at any stage will attain higher levels of health. These general areas of preventive teaching can be linked together under the topic of anticipatory guidance, which will be discussed in detail later in this chapter.

There are, however, examples of more specific preventive teaching topics that would be considered primary because their purpose is to avoid or avert occurrence of illnesses, ailments, or accidents. These include teaching families the importance of such health care practices as immunization, vision and hearing screening, and even pre-operative instructions for coughing and deep breathing. Teen groups can be involved by their school nurse in nutrition programs. Cafeteria workers can be instructed on hand-washing to decrease spread of infection, and plant workers can be taught safety measures to decrease chemical exposure or industrial accidents. With more specific preventive teaching individuals will maintain high levels of wellness by avoiding many common health problems.

Secondary Preventive Teaching - Examples of Content to Plan

There are numerous incidents when persons need teaching about secondary prevention. Secondary prevention is when problems resulting from ailments or accidents are treated very early so that normal or near normal function can be maintained and complications avoided. Secondary preventive teaching programs are valuable for many different age and ethnic groups. The occupational nurse who is working with young Black employees would be wise to provide hypertension screening and secondary preventive teaching programs describing the warning signs of stroke, need for salt-reduced diets, and the necessity of maintaining drug therapies. There are many general topics that serve as secondary prevention teaching for groups of people who experience the same health problems. Diabetics need diet and foot care instruction to prevent complications. The families of head injury patients need instruction about activities that may be confusing due to the patient's mental state. Families of anorexic youngsters need instruction on strategies that build positive body image.

Any teaching program that is aimed at stopping the progress of disease or injury would be considered secondary in nature. The programs designed for the patients and families struggling with oncologic, cardiovascular, respiratory, and renal diseases thus are fine examples of secondary prevention teaching.

A nurse typically will coordinate the early recovery programs that include teaching about basic pathophysiology of the illness or injury, need for changes in diet, activity, or occupation; explanations of medical or surgical regimen; descriptions of necessary pharmaceuticals or equipment; required physical or respiratory therapy; and a clear understanding of expectations and responsibilities of patient, family, and health care workers. In addition, the emotional reactions and impact of the health problem on sexuality, daily activities, spouse-family communication, and role changes of daily life should be explored in these teaching programs.

The general content of these programs is very informative. Specific content of these programs is based on the assessment of individual patients and their family's experience with the disease. Examples of results from such teaching programs include diabetic patients who control their ketoacidosis, renal transplant patients who maintain their immunosuppressive medications and thus their donor kidneys, athletes who avoid further injury by using joint stabilizers, arthritics who retain range of motion by following their exercise instructions, and chronic pain victims who continue their respective social lives by using visualization techniques versus sedating medications to manage their problem.

These specific outcomes indicate that the goal of secondary preventive teaching programs are being realized. Secondary prevention utilizes patient and family education programs to support adaptation to the health problem, ensure early detection of any untoward side effects, and instill a sense of mastery or control over the potential complications of the illness. In essence, the secondary prevention education programs are used to teach individuals and families coping abilities.

Tertiary Preventive Teaching - Examples of Content to Plan

The third type of preventive teaching is also used to increase the individual, family, or community's coping abilities. The aim of tertiary prevention is to rehabilitate the person who has suffered from illness or injury. Permanent damage or dysfunction has already been sustained and tertiary prevention is employed to stop potential sequelae from occurring and restore function. For example, the person with paralysis, whether from cardiovascular accident (CVA) or spinal fracture, would have bladder retraining to avoid the sequelae of urinary infection so common in these individuals.

As with the other types of prevention, individuals of all age groups, families from all ethnic backgrounds and communities of all socioeconomic strata will have needs for tertiary prevention teaching at some point or other. The leukemic child will need teaching about chemotherapy if he or she is to withstand the tauntings of schoolmates about the loss of hair. The nurse would teach the child ways to sustain a positive body image so he or she does not become depressed or anorexic. Similarly, a family who has lost a baby to sudden infant death syndrome will need the preventive teaching of the local support group to work through the guilt and grief that follow this tragedy and to avoid divorce and/or depression that follow. It would be unfortunate for this family to elect to not have other children because their guilt and fear were not eased by reliable information provided by the health care personnel sponsoring the support group. In another situation, the diet-controlled 40-year-old diabetic will need information on physiologic changes of aging if he or she is to contend with the changing caloric needs, decline in energy, and weight gain of middle age. Each of these sequelae has the potential for causing severe problems and multiple social, emotional, or physical limitations.

With tertiary preventive teaching, patients already experiencing problems can arrest the sequelae, maintain their highest level of wellness, and actively contribute to their family and community. The themes of high level wellness, enhancing coping strategies, and rehabilitation thus are all components of preventive teaching, especially the tertiary type. Anticipatory guidance, another type of preventive teaching can be used for patient education also.

Anticipatory Guidance—A Must in All Health Education

Predicting and teaching about expected life events, states of health, or potential problems is called anticipatory guidance. In working with the healthy patient, family, and community, or with those who already have experienced illness, the nurse must anticipate the potential problems that may occur and develop teaching programs on these topics. If individuals can be educated to anticipate stressful and even normal events, they will learn what to expect and how to manage such changes or problems.

— Anticipatory guidance often centers around the following topics: normal growth and development, health risk identification and management, control of community and environmental factors influencing health and, of course, primary, secondary, and tertiary preventive teaching relative to illness or injury.

Anticipatory Guidance for Growth and Development

To provide anticipatory guidance related to normal growth and development, the nurse would describe the stages of growth, developmental tasks, and the concomitant emotional hurdles that might be experienced at various ages. Also the psychophysiologic changes and cultural or societal expectations of various age groups would be explained.

Such preventive teaching programs titled "parenting the preschooler," "surviving those teen years," "middle aging and liking it," or "financial planning for retirement" all include components of anticipatory guidance and primary prevention. The parents of the preschooler who learn the techniques of limit-setting discipline will better prepare the child for what is expected of him in first grade. The teenagers who are taught the normal physiologic changes of puberty will feel less stress about menarche or voice changes. The middle-aged couple who is guided to manage the emotional reactions of being in between and responsible both for their youthful children and their older parents will be better prepared for the stresses of this life stage. The individual who has learned to plan for finances as well as new hobbies or activities certainly will better adjust to retirement.

Nurses will also find themselves needing to give anticipatory guidance about growth and development issues in situations complicated by a health problem or risk. The teenager who must adjust to a leg amputation needs to anticipate and prepare for difficult situations such as being asked to dance or to go swimming after the surgery. The oldster who must stop night driving needs to consider other options for transportation in advance. In each of these cases the normal growth and development changes have been complicated by a health risk or problem.

Health Risks

Anticipatory guidance can also be used to develop teaching programs about common ailments or injuries. The significant predictable health risks of Americans today include cardiovascular and oncologic diseases, motor vehicle and other accidents, as well as emotional or mental stress resulting in depression, suicide, or mental breakdown. These ailments are by no means the only possible health risks in the United States, but they are the most common.

Anticipatory guidance can be used to decrease these problems. Individuals can be taught the risk factors that contribute to cardiovascular disease. In addition, people can be guided to healthier lifestyles through diet, exercise, stress management instruction, and smoking cessation programs. Americans can also be taught the early warning signs of cancer, informed of the success of current treatments and dissuaded from the myth that cancer is a death sentence. Anticipatory guidance for accident prevention in sports and use of car safety belts could prevent senseless losses and wasteful crippling that occur yearly. So too, could anticipatory guidance enlighten us to the risks of mental strain that result in drug and alcohol abuse, withdrawal and isolation and a variety of mental disorders. It is hoped that such anticipatory guidance would change people's behavior so that they would maintain a healthy lifestyle, monitor early signs of illness, and seek health care services routinely.

Environmental Factors

Providing anticipatory guidance and preventive teaching about community and environmental factors that have impact on health can also improve levels of wellness. Nurses often deal with the results of communicable disease, air or chemical pollution, lack of environmental safety or sanitary precautions and the health consequences of natural and man-made disasters. Communities that have taught their residents what to do in case of weather emergencies or how to report suspect health and safety risks will be able to avert many health-related illnesses. Nurses are providing their communities with anticipatory guidance in terms of disaster preparedness, sanitation standards, and various types of preventive health teaching programs. These topics and those suggested under the preventive teaching sections can provide much of the content that nurses will plan to teach. Planning also includes preparing for the actual teaching interaction also.

Plan for the Teaching Interaction

The learning environment is the physical space where the teaching interaction will take place. This may vary from the patient's living room or hospital room, auditorium, or a learning booth. The learning climate is the atmosphere created between the health care personnel doing the teaching and the individuals or groups learning. The learning environment and the learning climate both affect the outcomes of the teaching interaction.

Arrange for an Environment Conducive to Learning

To plan for a positive learning environment several factors must be taken into account. Certainly, it's best to decrease extraneous noises such as the television of the patient in the next bed or traffic sounds outside a classroom window. Such distractions decrease concentration and detract from the teaching. Nurses have reported that couples coming to prenatal sessions are unable to concentrate when their classroom is near the labor room and women's sounds of discomfort can be heard. Nurses have also noticed that patients who are being taught to change their colostomy bags learn best when the curtain is pulled or the patient in the next bed has left the room.

Ideally, the nurse would seek out an environment that is quiet, where interruptions can be avoided, and where normal speaking voices can be used in the teaching interaction. Health care workers must be cognizant that routine noises in the hospital may be very distracting to patients who are trying to learn (Grosser, 1981). For larger audiences attending public health–oriented sessions the noise level in the environment can also be a deterrent to learning. Other aspects of the environment such as lighting and temperature should also be considered in the planning. An individual patient can be very motivated to learn and the community group can be very enthusiastic about the topic, but if they are unable to concentrate on the materials used or if they are distracted by room temperature, noise, or activity, learning will be disrupted.

It is also important to consider seating arrangements. In the hospital room it may be difficult to adjust the bed and chairs used by the family during the teaching session. But the few moments it will take to arrange seating is worth the effort because the individuals who are comfortable can listen longer and people who can see all the instructional tools will comprehend more. The fact that the nurse has taken time to ensure seating that allows all those present to participate is motivating in itself. It's best to plan to ask about comfort at the beginning of any teaching session. Something as simple as raising the head of the patient's bed or turning down the room thermostat in an auditorium may make all the difference in the learning outcomes.

Creating a Positive Climate for Learning

Creating a positive learning climate is another planning challenge. An atmosphere that positively influences the person's learning is essential. Nurses teaching patients or groups can create a positive atmosphere by conveying respect for them, giving them a sense of control, and by enhancing their self confidence. Respect can be conveyed by introducing one's self, stating appreciation for the person's interest in learning and by asking if they are comfortable. Giving learners a sense of control is conveyed by asking if there are specific topics or questions they would like to discuss prior to the teaching session. Also teachers can focus on the patient and family self-management responsibilities in efforts to illustrate they do indeed have much control in their situation. Self confidence can be enhanced by encouraging active participation. The teacher should plan in advance several questions that could be posed during the learning sessons to draw the learners into the discussion. Plans can also be made to have learners demonstrate what they are learning throughout the teaching sessions. For example, when giving diet instructions to cardiac patients, at appropriate intervals during the teaching session the nurse might plan to ask the family to name foods high in sodium or select the meat lowest in cholesterol from a list.

Provide Time for Learning

Time is another factor that affects the atmosphere or learning climate and should also be considered in planning. If it is possible, the patient should be allowed to select the time to set aside for learning. In this way the patient gains a sense of control. The nurse can ask patients to select a time when they are the most alert and comfortable (e.g., following heat therapy to the arthritic patient's joints or after the new mother breast feeds her infant).

Do encourage the patient to select a time when the family member or significant other can be available for the learning session. Remember also to consider the timing of medications when scheduling teaching sessions. Some medications may interfere with understanding or attentiveness. And remember to be flexible and reschedule any teaching sessions if you find the patient is in pain, restless, or anxious.

Another aspect of timing that must be considered is the length of the teaching sessions. Patients in acute care settings may tire quickly or families may be overwhelmed if too much material is presented at one time. It is hoped that the learning sessons will be instigated early in the hospitalization so that several information sessions can be planned. Time is often better spent in short sessions with plans for review and questions in between.

In planning the schedule for group sessions or large meetings the audience for that health education program must be considered. It would be best to offer programs at the times the target group is most likely to have available. Offering health education programs for teens on weekends is probably unwise, although this might be a good time to

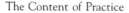

The Content of Practice

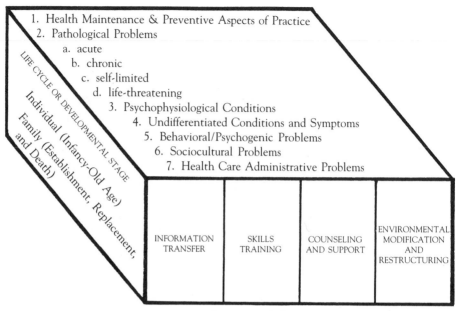

Figure 3-1. Content areas and techniques of patient education. (Reprinted from Society of Teachers in Family Medicine, *Patient Education Handbook,* Kansas City, KS 1979. With permission.)

schedule meetings for working adults. The timing of a program as well as the location and availability of parking all affect the attendance. These factors may seem mundane compared to the importance of planning for the topic or content but health education programs are most successful if the environment and climate have been prepared and any barriers to learning eliminated.

The importance of planning for preventive teaching, considering the life cycle stage, counseling and support, as well as environmental modifications is depicted in Figure 3-1. This figure was developed by a national task force to guide family practice physicians in planning for their patient teaching. The figure calls attention to several other significant variables essential to comprehensive planning. This figure points out how interpersonal communication strategies underline transfer of information and skill training. Communication strategies are the essence of any teaching methods that are implemented. Several methods for teaching are discussed in the following sections on implementation.

IMPLEMENTATION: THE THIRD STEP OF THE TEACHING PROCESS

Implementing the teaching plan involves several steps. First, any counseling interventions the patient or family may need to decrease anxiety and enhance self confidence about managing the situation should be undertaken. Next, strategies that will enhance readiness or motivation to learn should be used. Several of these strategies were described in the section on assessing learning readiness. Then the environment must be prepared so it is conducive for learning. Finally, the nurse can implement the chosen teaching method or strategy with some assurance that emotional, motivational, and environmental barriers to learning have been dealt with.

There is a great variety of teaching methods used in health education. These range from simple information statements delivered at the bedside to sophisticated computer-assisted instruction delivered to a home terminal. Whatever teaching strategy is used the nurse must be aware of the importance of establishing a relationship with the learners, communicating clearly, enhancing transfer of learning, and establishing realistic measures of evaluation.

Develop a Respectful and Caring Relationship

An individual, family, or large group can readily discern the amount of respect or caring the nurse teacher has for them. A simple but often forgotten tenet for starting a teaching interaction off on a positive note thus is to introduce yourself and other teachers. When handshakes, good eye contact, and a pleasant demeanor are part of the introduction, respect and caring are demonstrated. Even the characters on film strips and the narrative responses on computer screens can be made "user friendly."

This is not to suggest that overly cheerful attitudes should be employed. This would be inappropriate, for many health-related topics such as ostomy site care, care of a handicapped child, or community care of the mentally disabled are not easily managed. However, a caring attitude of accepting not only the health problem of the patient, family, or group, but also their feelings about it, will help establish a mutually respectful relationship. This respectful atmosphere encourages individuals to ask questions, pay attention, and participate in the learning activities. When individuals participate they more readily learn the information being discussed, whether it is imparted by a nurse, physician, audiovisual presentation, or a computer program.

Implement Summary and Overview Statements

Another technique that has proven successful with all types of teaching methods is the use of overviews and summaries of the information to be learned. Good teachers have a way of clearly stating at the onset what is going to be taught. In other words, the person or group is given a picture of what they will be able to accomplish by the end of the learning sessions. For example, the dietitian speaking to mothers of diabetics might start off by saying "at the end of our sessions you will be able to plan menus for picnics, birthday parties, and eating out that will fit into the whole family's routine. We will start by learning about food groups and specific quantities that you'll be selecting during your weekly grocery shopping." These types of statements give an overview of what will be learned and also convey the notion that the necessary changes can be transferred into the family's current routine or lifestyle. It is important that the dietician in this example indicated that "food groups and specific quantities" are essential content. The more difficult information to be learned thus was identified at the onset. And when this challenging material is associated with everyday behavior such as menu planning for the children's birthday parties, motivation to learn is enhanced and a sense of confidence that the new food selection skills can be mastered is projected.

Throughout the instructional sessions this same dietitian would also use summary statements to motivate learning, enhance participation and provide constructive feedback. Summary statements such as "now that you can select appropriate choices within the starch, vegetable, and fat groups we'll move on to learn the allowable meat and dairy product foods on a diabetic exchange diet." Or, "you have all planned good meals and snacks, now let's decide what to exchange for these if your child comes down with a cold, eats at a friend's house, or just doesn't want what you've planned." Each of these statements summarizes what has been learned, praises the mothers for what they have already accomplished, and then directs them to the next step of learning. In this way, summary and overview statements become reinforcements to learning.

It is essential that these statements be planned for because many summaries or overviews will be lengthy. To give an overview of preoperative teaching including everything from skin preparation to postoperative pain management may take several minutes. And, of course, summaries of the teaching used to prepare a family to care for the patient on oxygen at home, for example, should be written down. The safety, comfort, mechanical and even purchasing information taught can be written down for review at home. Because overviews and summaries may be lengthy and because they are essential to learning, it is important to plan time for their inclusion in the teaching interaction.

Even written and audiovisual materials should have overviews and summaries included. It may well be that printed materials and illustrations can be used to orient and summarize.

Stimulate Participation in the Learning Activities

Participation in the teaching process will enhance learning. Participation by the patient can be as simple as asking questions and reading pamphlets or as complex as giving a lecture to other patients and demonstrating their skill at managing their home dialysis equipment. There are many other methods of implementing patient participation in their learning. Nurses teaching cancer patients about infection prevention following chemotherapy can use graphs to summarize the information they have given on typical white blood cell level reductions after treatment. Further, the patient can be asked to write his own blood cell counts down on the graph as a way of illustrating the material and enhancing participation in the learning. The active participation leads to a clearer understanding of the need for the procedures and enhances self responsibility. In this case when the patient recognizes his white blood cell counts are low on the graph, he will know to take precautions against exposure to infections.

Participation can also be enhanced by using examples, analogies, and stories that are similar to the patient's, family's, or community's experiences. In planning to use such techniques be sure the examples you select are brief, clear, and do not convey any negative attitudes. It's essential to plan enough time to use the stories and to be sure analogies are understandable, do not generate fear, or offend any of the audience. For example, a story used in teaching adults about body image changes resulting from arthritis and steroid therapy might be experienced very negatively by teenagers with the same illness. An example selected by an occupational health nurse to illustrate an on-the-job safety program may be very effective in one industrial plant but insulting to workers in another. It's always wise to have a colleague familiar with the audience to review your examples, analogies, or stories prior to your use of them.

One person or a whole group also can misinterpret any part of the teaching program from the basic information to the examples. The nurse thus should plan to observe the audience's reaction throughout, ask questions about the material being presented, and reflect back to the patient any quizzical looks observed. When these communication techniques are used any concerns or misinterpretations can be identified and corrected before the remainder of the teaching session.

Obtain Feedback Throughout the Teaching Interaction

Communication that is personal and encourages participation will add to the respect, clarity, and mutual feedback necessary for successful implementation of any teaching strategy. Good communication involves using language appropriate for the audience, conscious awareness of nonverbal cues the patient gives and careful listening to the questions asked, issues raised, or concerns expressed.

Good communication also involves observing and listening to those being taught (Patient Education Handbook, 1979). For situations where media such as pamphlets or films are used, listening and observing for learner reactions is still vital. In large lecture groups, on radio, or with telephone teaching interactions the communication may appear to be virtually one-way. Setting up time for questions and answers, however, instructing families to write down their concerns, and referring individuals to other health information resources will communicate concern for patient's continued learning.

Indeed, in this day and age technology can be used to elicit feedback. For example, some health educators are asking individuals to describe to a telephone answering machine their reactions or questions following a television education program they have viewed. The educator later listens to the person's comments so that clarification can be provided to individual patients and so that group evaluation of the programs can be done.

Similar techniques can be used with individuals or families who are engaged in teaching techniques such as self-instruction diet guides, baby care films, or practicing insulin injections on a model. When it is clearly stated that the nurse will return to address questions or problems, patients recognize that their participation and feedback are important even when the teaching strategy used is largely self directed.

Types of Teaching Strategies

A teaching strategy encompasses the total interaction that takes place during the implementation phase of the process. The term or concept of strategy implies that the teaching aids, techniques and methods employed were preplanned, well thought out, appropriate for the learner and the information to be conveyed. Teaching aids include the materials used in teaching such as handouts, audiovisuals, pamphlets and the like (Woldum, 1985). The techniques of teaching as previously discussed are based on good communication skills, development of a respectful relationship, and reinforcing learning throughout the interaction. The methods of teaching range from lecture and use of simulation games to role playing. These will be discussed below and throughout the remainder of the text.

Teaching Methods

Teaching methods can be categorized in a general way into individual, group, and mass type formats (Knowles, 1980; Houle, 1976). The individual methods include teaching activities that are based on interpersonal one-on-one interactions. Some examples of these types of methods are giving explanations, demonstrating a manual skill, exploring concerns or answering questions, role modeling appropriate behavior or discussing pamphlets, films, or other exhibits. The teaching aids that might be used with individual type formats include self-study materials, computer simulations or pamphlets. Other techniques that might be beneficial in individual interactions are contracting for learning, scheduling for self-monitoring, and discussion conducted by other patients with the same problem.

The group methods include teaching activities that are based on group dynamics and interactions. Some examples of group type methods include lecture discussion, role-play or drama, practice sessions, seminar conferences, and review of past experiences. The teaching aids that are helpful in group situations include audiovisuals such as films, overhead projectors, poster and flannel boards. Other techniques that might be employed are problem-solving or task completion exercises, and exhibits or models that can be used for practice.

The mass type formats include teaching methods that are oriented toward mass media and large audience programs. Some examples of these types of methods are local and national television campaigns or closed circuit television available in hospital rooms, lecture series or presentations for large groups, radio talk shows that provide health information, billboards or signs posted in highly visible areas, and tape recordings available from libraries.

If the teaching is conducted through a technologic learning method such as television or computer programs, then summarizing techniques should be built in at the end of each session. The television narrator can summarize what the individuals should have learned, and the computer program can pose questions or guidelines for patients to evaluate their own learning. Questions that can be used to evaluate learning after some of these self-study teaching materials have been used are listed here.

Questions to Use After Self-Study Teaching Materials Have Been Used

1. What have you learned from the materials you have read?
2. Were the questions posed at the end of the pamphlet useful?
3. Was it difficult to use the computer program?
4. Has the film raised any questions or worries in your mind?
5. Were the examples or illustrations in the materials clear to you?

When using methods from any of these three categories it is important to remember the communication techniques that help listeners to focus their attention on important content, to use overview and summary statements and planned repetition of essentials. These techniques can be built into mass media or audiovisual materials as well as the individual and group methods. A variety of teaching aids can also be employed with either individual, group, or mass teaching methods. These teaching aids are discussed in detail in Chapter 7. It is to be hoped that the nurse considers the communication techniques, instructional methods, and teaching aids in a cohesive, well-thought-out manner hopefully, during the implementation phase. When a strategy for implementing the teaching plan is used, evaluation becomes a rewarding review of good teaching and patient learning.

EVALUATION: THE LAST STEP OF THE TEACHING PROCESS

Evaluation is the last phase of the teaching process. Evaluation is used to judge several aspects of teaching such as cost-effectiveness of the program, appropriateness of the teaching materials, and quality of the teacher. Each of these areas of evaluation will be discussed in chapter 8 of the text.

Emphasis will be placed here on the essence of evaluation however: to determine whether the patients have learned or changed their behavior. Evaluation of learning involves comparing the expected behavioral outcomes to the patient's actual behavior following the teaching.

Evaluating the Assessment and Planning of the Teaching Plan

The expected outcomes or behavioral changes are determined by the assessment obtained in the first step of the teaching process. For example, many learning needs were found following the assessment of the family of a patient undergoing extensive surgery for cancer. The family revealed knowledge deficits about the disease, lack of resources for managing this long-term illness, and fears that the patient would suffer chronic debilitating pain. From this family's assessment data, specific plans and behavioral objectives were written to guide both the teaching interventions and the evaluation of learning. Sample objectives for this family are presented.

Objectives to Evaluate After Teaching the Family With a Member Diagnosed With Cancer

1. *Knowledge.* Family members state that cancer is a long-term illness that is treatable.
2. *Psychomotor.* Family members demonstrate use of comfort measures with a patient.
3. *Affective.* Family members state they no longer fear the patient will have great pain because they are aware of comfort measures and medication.

Evaluating if these objectives are realistic, measurable, and appropriate for the family will determine if the planning phase was adequate in this case.

Evaluation of the Implementation and Teaching Methods Used

Teaching methods were implemented to increase the family's knowledge about cancer, provide experiences with the necessary psychomotor skills, and reduce their fears by enhancing their confidence that pain can be relieved. A variety of teaching techniques, materials and teaching aids were implemented. To increase the family's knowledge, the nurse conducted discussions at the bedside and left pamphlets from the American Cancer Society. The nurse had the family assist with bedside care of the wound dressings and showed a film on how to transfer a patient from bed to chair to provide experiences and psychomotor skills. To reduce the family's fears the nurse described the medications that are being used and explained how they relieved the patient's pain. Also, the nurse would describe to the family several pain control interventions such as distraction, visual imagery, application of heat or positioning and back rubs. It might also be useful to have the patient and family discuss pain control with another person who has successfully managed after similar surgery.

Many other techniques certainly could be employed to meet the patient's and family members' needs. No matter what methods are used to implement the teaching plan, the objectives are used to evaluate if learning has taken place.

In this example, if the family continues to express a fearful attitude towards pain control management and cannot employ comfort measures with the patient, then learning has not taken place. The family has not changed behavior in either the psychomotor skills or affective learning areas. Upon discussing this with the family, it may well be that describing the comfort measures to the family did not give them confidence to actually carry these out.

In evaluating the appropriateness of the behavioral objectives, both family and patient agreed they did want to manage the pain by using comfort measures, thus no change was made in these. However, evaluation identified a need for readjustment of the teaching methods. In the changed teaching plan, the nurse used the teaching technique of demonstration and involved the family in providing the comfort measures they deemed most beneficial to the patient. In this way, the evaluation has enabled the nurse to revise the teaching plan and employ a method more successful with this family.

Evaluating the Evaluation Used

It is even necessary to evaluate the evaluation step of the teaching process! If ineffective measures of evaluation are used, it may appear learning has taken place when in reality it has not, or that learning hasn't taken place when in reality it has. For example, a patient may be asked, "Do you understand how to do your physical therapy exercises?" and respond, "Yes." However, this should not be misconstrued to mean that the patient has the psychomotor skills to perform the exercises, the positive attitude to do them religiously, or even the knowledge to schedule them at the appropriate times. The original question and answer were too general to be a valid evaluation measure. It is important that the techniques or measures used for evaluation be valid criteria that precisely measure the expected outcomes. Otherwise, general information could falsely be used to determine that the patient had learned.

Evaluation techniques or measures must also be instituted at the appropriate time for them to be valid. If evaluation is conducted too early, it may falsely appear that the patient has not learned, or if the evaluation is conducted a long while after the teaching has taken place, many of the details of the information may have been forgotten even though the behavioral change still is intact.

Poor timing interfered when public health officials were evaluating the effectiveness of a community lecture/demonstration of self breast examination six months after the program. The evaluation questionnaires revealed that the women were unable to re-member some of the facts about cancer described in the pamphlet used to illustrate the technique. Unfortunately, this was taken to mean that the practice of self breast exam was not being done correctly and therefore the program was unsuccessful. Yet, the expected behavior of conducting monthly mid-menstrual cycle breast examinations using the appropriate technique was reported by a majority of the women attending the lecture and demonstration. This example shows that timing of the evaluation should be consid-ered when judging if the technique is an appropriate one for eliciting accurate evaluation data.

Evaluation is best conducted throughout the teaching process. Evaluation of bedside teaching should be done to judge the short term effectiveness of the teaching plan. It is important that the evaluation of learning take place soon after the teaching so that other teaching needs can be assessed, new objectives developed, different teaching interven-tions tried, and reevaluation conducted. It is not unusual to revise a teaching plan after the first evaluation is completed. In the short span of a hospital stay or in the week between home visits, learning needs may have altered, teaching aids may have been misplaced, inaccurate information obtained elsewhere, or possibly the family had learned the necessary procedure but the patient refused to have the treatment. The desired outcomes, therefore, may have not been achieved. The evaluation techniques or mea-sures used must be comprehensive enough to uncover all factors that affect learning.

Evaluation Techniques or Measures

Factors that either hamper or enhance learning, must be identified by the evaluation techniques used. It is important to identify factors that enhance learning so these can be reinforced. Factors that deter learning certainly must be extinguished whenever possible. Because such factors are very diverse and individual to the learning situation, no one evaluation technique or measure is favored.

Any evaluation technique or measure should use skilled observation by one who can adequately judge if the desired behavioral change has occurred. To guide skilled observa-tion the evaluation technique should ideally obtain both objective and subjective data. Objective data is information that can be observed or measured. Some examples of objective evaluation measures are observing for signs of anxiety such as rapid speech, tachycardia, and lack of cooperation with procedures. Laboratory data such as blood tests, respiratory measures, or medication levels are also used to gather objective data. Evaluation of observable information such as compliance with return appointments and return to work after hospitalization are also measurable data. Such objective data can reflect the expected outcome of a variety of teaching plans.

Subjective data should also be gathered in the evaluation step. Subjective data is information expressed by the patients about their learning. This may include their descriptions of their ability to manage the new behaviors, their perceptions that they have learned, and their commitment to following the prescribed health care program.

The evaluation techniques used for collecting either subjective or objective data vary. Some informal methods of evaluation include asking questions, observing facial expressions, or using group conversations to elicit information. Even though these techniques of evaluation are informal the questions asked should be specific to the expected behavior. Asking "How many pills do you take each day?" is much more specific than asking, "Are you taking your medicine?" The information obtained from the more specific questioning is more accurate data than that obtained from the general question.

A respectful relationship allows for constructive informal evaluation of the learning. The family or group who feels respect from the teacher will not be affronted at the end of the session when they are asked to demonstrate what they have learned. Instead of reacting to this type of evaluation by thinking, "Oh, the nurse thinks I didn't understand," the family will think, "Oh, the nurse wants to let me practice." The nurse, of course, sets the stage for these positive perceptions throughout the teaching interaction by using good communication skills and conveying a nonjudgmental attitude when using informal techniques for evaluation.

There are also many techniques of formal evaluation and research that can be conducted to judge if persons have learned. A research study evaluating patients' understanding of a teaching manual on cardiac catheterization was conducted by Lamb (1984). This nurse researcher found that regardless of age, education, or time under a physician's care, the cardiac patients learned from the teaching manual. Other formal evaluation procedures such as paper and pencil testing, telephone and survey follow-up questionnaires and research techniques that can be employed to evaluate the results of patient education (De Joseph, 1980).

Informal or formal research evaluation of any educational program should provide data on the changes in knowledge, attitudes, or psychomotor behavior that can be used to judge if learning has taken place. If learning has not occurred then further evaluation must be undertaken to identify the interfering factors or barriers.

Barriers to Learning Must be Identified

Once it has been established that the expected change in behavior was not forthcoming, then further evaluation must take place. There are several barriers that can disrupt learning and interfere with behavior change.

Time Can be a Barrier

Possibly there was insufficient time to complete the teaching. Perhaps the rushed nature of the short time session gave the patient and family the impression that the information wasn't important. Or maybe one of the teaching aids, such as a film, was too lengthy for the fatigued patient to attend to.

On the other hand, the family and patient may simply not have had time to practice the expected psychomotor skills, read the pamphlets, or not had time to praise one another for their positive attitudes.

Lastly, time may have been a negative factor even before the teaching was instituted. The patient, family, or community may not have had time to come to grips with the health problem before the teaching was begun. A patient may still be in denial over a diagnosis of Parkinson's disease. Parents of a depressed child may still be in shock from a suicide attempt. Even a group of people in a community needs time following tragedies to develop readiness to learn.

One community that had experienced a severe flood used Red Cross Volunteers to teach about boiling drinking water. Unfortunately, there were still many cases of contamination because the teaching was conducted in the town hall within a day or two after the flood. The evaluation revealed that the teaching was ineffective because it was instituted too soon for the people to be able to come to a community meeting. As a result of the evaluation, mass media (radio alerts) were used for a week after the flood. The reported cases of contamination decreased after this adjustment in the teaching plan.

Other Priorities May Deter Learning

The previous example also points out another barrier to learning; the communities or patients may have priorities that must be taken care of before they can attend to new information. Possibly there are financial arrangements that must be made, work schedules that must be altered, loved ones that must be contacted, or even living situations that must be changed. It may be necessary before teaching for the family to set up a first floor room with enough electrical outlets for the suction, intravenous pump, and electric bed that will be necessary in caring for their loved one after discharge from the hospital. On a different scale it might be a priority for a community to establish drug rehabilitation centers before the public education programs on this topic are underway. The environment of the hospital or convalescent center may be so abhorrent to the patient that until the patient has adjusted to the surroundings, he or she may not be able to attend to teaching. Such priorities as these should be identified in the assessment step of the teaching process. It is not uncommon, however, for evaluation to reveal that other priorities created the barriers that precluded learning.

Difficulty of the Learning Material May be a Barrier

There are several other barriers to learning that might be identified by a thorough evaluation. One very common but often overlooked barrier is how difficult and challenging the information patients are expected to learn is. The medical regimen for the patient with cardiovascular disorders often includes three to ten medications per day. The parents of a cystic fibrosis child must gain positive attitudes towards the respiratory therapy treatments they must learn to give for their daughter's well being. Families of patients with a cancer involved in the Make Each Day Count program must learn to share complicated and often personal ways of coping with depression, uncertainty, and the all too frequent withdrawal of friends. The teaching plans used by the cardiac, pediatric, and oncology nurses working in these situations would necessarily be lengthy and comprehensive. It is not a surprise then that the difficulty of the content or the many changes required in everyday life account for lack of learning in some situations. The evaluation step of the teaching process should uncover these problems and distinguish them from other more elusive barriers to learning.

Psychological Deterrents to Learning

There are some subtle but very powerful psychological barriers to learning such as patients' learning disabilities or health beliefs. Learning disabilities such as restricted vision or receptive aphasia can be managed if they are identified in the assessment step of the teaching process. If these problems are not identified or the measures taken to correct them, then the patient may be unable to learn. The evaluation phase should reveal that the physical aspects of the disabilities were attended to by such methods as using large-size print materials or picture sign board for printing art objectives. It is important to remember that even when the physical aspects of these disabilities are addressed the patients' frustration and notion that they can't learn may still prevail. In this situation, working on some mutually determined objectives for enhancing a positive attitude toward learning may be the only revision necessary in the teaching plan.

In other situations, however, the patients' beliefs about their health may overpower any learning that took place. One patient stated she didn't take the prescribed medications because no one in her family ever had that disease and it was unlikely that she had it either since she felt so well.

Even groups or communities have health beliefs that can deter learning. Some city councils have turned down offers for preventive education programs about battered women believing their community couldn't have such a problem. The lack of belief that they will be affected by the problem or the fact that the disease is asymptomatic (as hypertension) may lead to such reactions. If the evaluation indicates the patient or community has a health belief that interferes with their desire to change the necessary behavior, then counseling techniques might be used to explore this issue and motivate readiness to learn.

Another subtle psychological barrier to learning is called secondary gain. Secondary gain is the term coined to describe the benefits a person receives from being ill. These secondary benefits may include increased attention from family and friends or decreased pressures to work or perform up to par. Unconsciously the patient may not be motivated to learn how to manage the illness because the secondary gains would be lost. If the evaluation uncovers a situation involving secondary gain, this should be discussed with clinical nurse specialists, medical colleagues, or psychologists so further assessment can be undertaken.

Barriers Created by the Teaching

The evaluation might also uncover problems pertaining to the instruction that interfered with learning. Possibly the teaching was unclear or confusing. If self-study teaching materials were used, they may have been unclear or sometimes conflicting instructions are given to patients and their significant others from various health team members. Often asking about puzzled expressions on the patient's face reveals conflicting values are being presented. Some information that is imparted for legal reasons such as risks of therapy may be so frightening that the patient shuts out other instruction.

Another unfortunate problem that negatively affects learning is an audience's or patient's perceived lack of respect or regard from the health care personnel teaching them. Lack of eye contact and restlessness in an audience may reveal a sense of embarrassment or discomfort stemming from the feelings they're being patronized or spoken down to.

Typically problems such as these can be identified by short-term evaluation that is conducted during the teaching interaction. Observation of the patient's facial expression or an audience's attention span throughout a presentation can uncover such problems. It would benefit future learning a great deal if such problems could be evaluated and corrected at the time they occurred.

When the nurse uses good communication techniques such as praising the individual or family for all they have learned, stating exactly what is expected to be learned and responding to questions in a thoughtful manner, the learners will feel respected. This type of communication also sets the stage for meaningful evaluation.

When barriers and deterrents to learning are eliminated by a meaningful evaluation and when objectives and techniques for teaching have been correctly employed, preventive health teaching is achieved.

The discussion that follows illustrates the use of each step of the process with a community group.

USING THE TEACHING PROCESS
FOR COMMUNITY EDUCATION

Community education is the process of providing teaching programs to groups and communities. The nurse's role in providing community education and numerous examples of such programs are discussed below. Community education programs may center around the individual's concerns about the environment, a group's common health problem or even regional and national issues. Some of the topics covered in these health education programs will raise ethical issues within the community. Issues such as use of controversial speakers, availability of sex education and discussion of health problems associated with emotion-laden topics (e.g., acquired immunodeficiency syndrome [AIDS], child abuse, environmental pollution, etc.). Even legalities such as how funds should be appropriated for health-oriented programs should be addressed. The nurses involved in community education wll need to develop skills in dealing with these issues as well as the ability to use the steps of the teaching process with communities.

Because the scope of community education is very broad, nurses teaching in such programs may find themselves working along side political, religious, and health care or consumer advocates. For example, a community education program on "safety in day care" may include presentations by local city council members, a sunday school teacher, a pediatric nurse and a lawyer who all contribute their particular expertise on the topic.

The groups most frequently seen by public health nurses are mothers and children, workers in industry and the elderly. The groups most frequently seen by hospital nurses are families who have a member with an acute or chronic illness. All these people are members of the community who share some common concerns about health, personal safety, environmental protection, and disease prevention. Nurses working in different spheres thus can be involved in community education.

Involvement in the education of community leaders and governing bodies so that goals for community health are clearly stated should be given priority by nurses.

Community education goals include health promotion, disease prevention, and personal and environmental protection and safety. There are many community education programs aimed at these goals. They include all the prenatal courses for mothers during pregnancy and courses for fathers taking an active role in childbirth and parenting. Another example of a health promotion education topic, "good nutrition on a shoestring" can be used with newlyweds, college students, single parents, retired couples or others on a limited budget.

Disease prevention is another goal of community education. Each person's ability to be emotionally or mentally and physically healthy is enhanced when he or she is disease free. Nurses thus must be aware of the typical illnesses or ailments that occur in different age groups within the community so they can provide education on prevention of these problems. Programs for safety such as use of seat belts and child restraints can go a long way to save lives. So too, can programs informing the public of health hazards in the environment. The process of asking what persons learned and how they feel the educational program affected their lives is the essence of evaluation.

Certainly, observing the statistics on the health and accident cases in the community following educational programs is also indicative of the outcomes depending on the topic. Overall there are several outcomes expected in any health education program whether for individuals, families, or communities. The teaching plan at the end of this chapter illustrates the teaching process used in community education.

Nurses often find themselves in the role of coordinator of these programs. Coordinators are expected to assess the community for its health education needs and develop learning objectives. Another aspect of the nurse's role in community education is that she or he must be ready to plan teaching programs for groups rather than for individual patients and/or families. Community health education nurses may stage large health fairs at shopping malls, provide industrial groups with CPR (cardio-pulmonary resuscitation) training through the Red Cross or conduct programs at regional senior citizens centers.

Reaching large numbers and groups of people is an essential part of community education. The nurse must expand his or her teaching role to utilize broadcast media such as radio and television to deliver and advertise programs. Nurses currently produce health columns in newspapers and on local TV news programs. Yet even with use of mass media, teaching groups is similar in many ways to preparing programs for individuals.

The steps of the process of teaching individuals, families, or communities (assessing, planning, implementing, and evaluating) are the same. There are particular points, however, that must be considered when teaching large groups of people.

Using the Teaching Process in Community Education

Assessing the learning needs of communities or large subgroups is a challenge. Some members of a community will volunteer topics they are interested in learning; some will point out what they think others need to be taught and finally there will be evidence of health problems in the population that will dictate the content of the education programs. Assessment from these three sources should be undertaken so that the most appropriate and beneficial topics can be developed into educational programs that will be well received by the community or the target groups.

Assessment

Target groups are made up of persons expected to be interested in the program. A general interest checklist of topics can be sent to people expected to be interested in attending a community education program on the topic. For example, in preparing for a series of programs on middle age, the nurse might send out checklists ascertaining interest in topics such as maintaining health, parenting teen-agers and providing for elderly parents. These surveys could be sent randomly to a sample of the community members in the 40- to 60-year age brackets. The target group of middle aged persons thus was assessed about topics of interest to them. Assessment of people's interests in topics is referred to as determining their perceived learning needs.

The community or target group should also be assessed for "ascribed learning needs". Ascribed needs are gathered by speaking to persons who could identify learning needs of the group to be taught. For instance, the community health nurse who is interested in conducting educational programs for battered women could interview or survey counselors at women's shelters or support groups. These counselors would be able to describe these women's needs for assertiveness techniques, self-image enhancement, and self-defense training. To obtain ascribed learning needs, physicians serving the community should be asked to suggest topics for teaching persons about their medical problems, pharmacists can be asked what to teach elderly people about over-the-counter drugs and dieticians could be asked what nutrition topics to discuss in local schools. It is important that the individuals selected for obtaining ascribed needs be unbiased in their view of what the learners need to know. All too often "authority figures" such as parents of teenagers, managers of employees, or religious clerics of denominations are asked to determine their "charges" or groups' learning needs. Biased self-serving programs such as "Responsibility in the Teen Years", "Maintaining Health to Decrease Absenteeism" or "Morality of Giving" might result from these needs assessments. Unfortunately programs based on biased needs assessment, or even on ascribed needs that come from nonbiased sources, are not always seen by the target group as worthwhile.

Even in the previous example of the battered women, where needs were actually ascribed by their counselors, might result in the perception of the educational topics as not interesting by the target group. It is, therefore, always best to compare the perceived and ascribed needs assessment data and develop topics in conjunction. If perceived needs had been collected along with the aforementioned authority figure ascribed needs the following topics might have resulted: "Sexual Responsibility in Teen Years," "Healthy Employees are Happy Employees" or "Volunteering is Giving but also Receiving." These topics represent a match between the learners' perceived needs and the authority figures' ascribed needs. The educational programs would most likely be better attended by the target groups than the previously mentioned biased topics.

The third technique of learning assessment often used in the community health context is referred to as determining "demonstrated needs." Demonstrated needs are those needs revealed by facts, figures, or other forms of statistical data. For example, the prediction that one in four families will have a member who has cancer certainly demonstrates the need for teaching community groups the early warning signs of oncologic disease. The fact that local industry workers have had an increased incidence of preventable eye injuries over the last year points out that programs on use of protective goggles must be repeated. The population figures of a community that indicate there are many retirees, few teens, and an increasing number of newborns. Thus programs with topics for elders and for new mothers would take precedence over those for adolescents.

Demonstrated needs can be gathered from a variety of sources. Health care workers and agencies such as the American Red Cross, Salvation Army, or Family Planning clinics provide statistical data that reveal incidence of illnesses, repeating community health problems, and target groups in need of educational programs; as well as political, financial, and public works information that indicate policy, legislative, or expenditure changes related to health or sanitation. For example, many states can no longer afford the free preschool screening and immunization programs previously required. Community education about these changes thus is needed. Day care centers and pediatricians' offices would be an ideal place to set out educational brochures explaining these changes and describing where these services can be obtained.

Other sources of demonstrated needs such as community health statistics, environmental studies, school or industry reports and hospital admissions data can be used also. For example, if frostbite cases in the emergency room during the first month of winter are above normal the community health nurse would promptly put out a media bulletin on this dangerous health hazard. Then the nurse would further determine if a particular cross-section of the population had been affected. The emergency room records would reveal if the frostbite victims were youngsters walking to school, overzealous outdoor sportsmen and hunters, or the elderly who didn't know of the free transportation service available to them. The nurse can be assisted in developing a specific worthwhile educational program by finding the exact target group affected by the health problem. When-ever demonstrated learning needs are gathered the most specific data thus should be obtained (Green, Lewis, and Levine, 1980).

There are several needs assessment techniques that can be used with large groups or communities. First, the assessment used to determine the learning needs for large groups must look at a cross-section of the general population in the community. To determine learning needs, survey types of assessment techniques are often used with the "target group." Other techniques include the matrix assessment, pyramid assessment, delphi approach and models for diagnosing educational, epidemiological and socially oriented health education needs (Bell, 1978, Knowles, 1980, Skiff, 1981). These techniques are often used in research procedures so that the nurse may work with statisticians, sampling experts, or epidemologists when using these needs assessment approaches.

Planning for Community Education

Even after sophisticated assessment techniques have been used to elicit perceived, ascribed and demonstrated needs, it's best to plan for an on-the-spot assessment with the audience at the beginning of any community education program. Because the groups attending programs will vary in their knowledge of subject matter, they may have differ-ent questions or learning needs they can articulate at the teaching session (Klimecki, 1982).

Another important part of the planning for community education is the writing of the behavioral objectives. The learning objectives should reflect introductory, as well as in-depth information on the topic. A community program on drug abuse in teenagers thus might begin with simple definitions and symptoms of abuse and move to the more complicated issues of rehabilitation. In this way, information that is informative to the person with little knowledge can be presented and important attitudes towards the necessary treatment explored. Always plan in advance to have ethical or legal issues related to the topic discussed.

Implementing Community Education

Implementation must take into account the size and composition of the group, as well as where, when, and how long the program will be planned for. Teaching bicycle safety to the local third graders is probably best done during playground recess where the children are spread out and actually try signaling stops or turns appropriately, and teach-ing CPR to local adults might best be arranged in repeated short sessions at a variety of sites with large numbers of employees.

Some community health educators present their community education topics by the "season". The community is often ready for fitness and exercise topics in the spring, skin care and itch treatment in summer, household safety procedures in the fall, and cabin fever or antidepression programs in the winter. Unfortunately, many communities be-come "ready" for programs only after problems or issues have surfaced. For example, programs on toxic shock syndrome or protection against child abduction may be called for after these problems have occurred. The nurse must be ready to implement asked for programs quickly.

Implementing urgently needed programs is made much easier if materials necessary for presenting programs to large numbers of people are readily available. This means that audiovisual equipment, microphones, mass media or other needed teaching resources should be on hand and the nurse skilled in using each.

Evaluating Community Education

Evaluating educational programs for all the diverse groups in the community is a challenge. First, the nurse must recognize that several groups are at risk for a variety of illnesses, environmental hazards, or other problems. Second, the nurse must realistically determine which groups the educational programs can reach. Then the nurse must judge where implementation is most needed and where it will be most effective. Nurses should not conclude that their program has been unsuccessful just because the evaluation reveals only a small number have attended. It may well be that the program reached the most appropriate segment of the community. The process of asking what persons learned and how they feel the educational program affected their lives is the essence of evaluation.

Observing the statistics on the health and accident cases in the community following your programs certainly is also indicative of the outcomes depending on the topic (Fletcher, 1974). Overall, there are several outcomes expected in any health education program whether it be for individuals, families, or communities. The teaching plan at the end of this chapter illustrates the teaching process to be used in community education.

TEACHING CARE PLAN FOR THE AGING COMMUNITY: A NETWORKING PLAN

Sister Ann M. Schorfheide

The graying of America is one of the most significant demographic trends of contemporary twentieth century and beyond. The number and proportion of older persons has grown dramatically and will continue to grow more rapidly than the general population. A larger population surviving into their 70s, 80s, and beyond will create some important shifts in the structure of families and communities.

The nursing implications of these figures are extensive. There will be increasing numbers of elderly who will need assistance with activities of daily living together with a host of other dependency needs. Informal and formal support network services for the elderly and their families will be used to address these needs. A network is an informal or formalized mechanism for connecting or communicating that ensures that all available resources will be utilized. People must be taught to network.

By far the largest groups of caregivers to the elderly and those with dependency needs of all ages are their families, friends, and neighbors. This is the unorganized informal natural support system of the community. These systems need to be nurtured, cultivated, maintained, and praised.

Where these natural networks fall short, however, formal organized services are increasingly needed. People need to be aware of what services exist.

Family; friends; neighbors; co-workers; clergy; and religious institutions; neighborhood, ethnic, fraternal, or social organizations, mutual aid groups, and health and human service professionals and institutions can provide meaningful assistance in times of need and are all part of the network system for the aging. To facilitate this awareness, community education is an important and viable methodology.

The aging network system can serve individuals, families, and communities at primary, secondary and/or tertiary levels of prevention if the elderly and their caregivers are educated to use their network services. Primary preventive network activities might include exercise and nutrition classes, accident prevention, stress reduction, and crime prevention awareness and/or programs.

The network might include a variety of secondary preventive measures such as screening programs, health fairs, and professional care programs. The caregivers should also take advantage of resources in the community network designed to give them time away from the elderly they care for. Respite care, day care, and support groups should be utilized.

For the elderly, disability has been defined as the inability to live at home without help. Important conditions leading to disability in the elderly include neurological, cardio-pulmonary, arthritis, obesity, and visual impairment. Tertiary preventive measures to deal with disability might include in-home services, informal support groups, various types of respite care and choosing a long-term care facility. However, if the elderly or their families are not aware of these preventive services, these services will be unused along with their benefits. This is where educating about the community networking becomes essential.

Teaching Plan

Assessment

Several techniques can be used to assess what a community needs and wants to know about the aging network. Interviews, surveys, polls, forums, and town meetings can all be part of the assessment process. Key service agencies, individual citizens, and epidemiologic data can all feed into the data base. In processing the data received, priorities are set and availability of resources are determined. If there seems to be general interest in broad services available, then an overview program might be planned. Perhaps then follow-up programs could be determined from participant indication. For example, an overview program describing services in the network for shut-ins might include information on meals on wheels, private duty nursing care, or at home physical therapy. A follow-up program providing all the details about day care and respite for the elderly could be given for those interested. The objectives written during the planning step would guide the detail of each program's topics.

Plan

Any plan involving a network program should take into account the multitude of detailed information necessary to convey about the services. Written handouts that list resource names, telephone numbers and short descriptions of services thus might be given for later reference.

Planning should also encompass locating an appropriate site for the program. Care should be taken to find a location that is convenient, adequate in size and comfort, and easily accessible.

Using appropriate experts as program presenters is usually very effective. However, it is important to have the expert address the planned objectives and use appropriate teaching strategies. The expert must be able to speak respectfully to the elderly participants at each program.

Table 3-1
Teaching Plan for *Caring for the Caregiver*

Assessment	Plan/Learning objectives	Interventions	Evaluation
		Affective	
Recognize potential stressors of caregiving.	*Minimize stressful situations experienced by the caregiver. *Participants will ventilate feelings about caregiving.	*Illicit and identify caregiving affect on the caregiver. Fear of the unknown Loss of freedom Isolation Guilt Grief	*Caregivers will recognize and use new coping strategies.
Assess for areas of secondary preventive teaching that might be needed for the caregiver.	*Caregivers state the need for rest, relaxation, time to themselves. *Caregivers will practice filling out the necessary forms (paperwork) required for obtaining assistance from a network agency.	*Informal resources Mutual support groups Family coordination and coalition *Formal resources: Agency outreach meals on wheels homemakerservice skilled nursing Respite care: home helps adult daycare temporary admission	*Caregivers will utilize resources available in the community network that provide them with support.

Table 3-2
Teaching Plan for *Caring for the Caregiver*

Assessment	Plan/Learning objectives	Interventions	Evaluation
		Cognitive	
Needs assessment indicates an increasing number of dependent elderly being cared for at home.	*Preplanning includes: Presentor potentials could be a nurse, social worker, psychologist, physician, or any combination.	*Presentor should be creditable, sensitive and dynamic.	*Ask participants to rate effectiveness of the presentors.
	Location of program should be convenient, comfortable, and safe.	*Environment should be conducive to learning.	*Ask participants to rate environment and location.
	Varied marketing techniques could use fliers, radio, TV, posters, word of mouth.	*Material should be clear, simple, eye catching and placed in church and club newsletters that the elderly and caregivers read.	*Ask participants to identify where they heard about the program.
Recognize alterations in aging.	*Learning objective is: Maximize independence of the dependent elderly.	*Primary preventive teaching of an overview of the aging process: Body Mind Emotions (Use audiovisual augmentation.)	*Ask participants to rate the helpfulness of the information.

Table 3-3
Teaching Plan for *Caring for the Caregiver*

Assessment	Plan/Learning objectives	Interventions	Evaluation
		Psychomotor	
Observe for concerns of sensory diminishment, particularly vision difficulties.	*Recognize sensory losses as tertiary problems.	*Simulate sensory loses.	*Participants will state usefulness of information and apply suggestions.
	*Demonstrate examples of vision alterations:	*Tertiary preventive teaching for intervening with visual deficits:	
	Coordination Squinting Positioning Depth perception Nonrecognition of familiar people and objects.	Simplify visual fields Place objects within visual fields Label with large print Consistent placement of objects Prewarning	
Gather information about services in the network available to assist the caregiver in working with the frail elderly with limited site	*Caregiver names local services for site impaired individuals	*Give handout with names and telephone numbers of resources in the network.	*Caregivers share handout with others working with the frail elderly.

Implementation

In implementing the teaching/learning strategies relevant spoken and written information and audiovisual materials can be used. It is important also to provide opportunities for the participants to talk about the topic, problem, or issue with the speaker and other participants. Sessions are enhanced when participants have the opportunity to question, explore, clarify, discuss, and digest information. Question and answer formats and small group break-out sessions with a facilitator have proved to be effective and safe for participants. Opportunities for practice sessions or simulations, when appropriate, are also enriching. Practice could include giving an example of how to fill out forms to apply for one of the services in the network, as this is always a frustrating problem that might stop people from using a service.

Evaluation

Community education evaluation is as vital as in any mode of patient education. Evaluation starts at the beginning with assessment and culminates in the progress (process) and outcome (product) evaluation. Summative evaluation should include written and/or verbal feedback after the education process and then later observed behavioral changes, which include lifestyle alterations and demonstrated problem solving and survival techniques. With the networking programs, one essential evaluation is to determine if there has been an increased use of services by the elderly and their caregivers in the community.

In the teaching plan on pages 91–93 the community teaching plan targets a population of caregivers for the frail, dependent elderly. The focus is caring for the caregiver. Those providing care for the frail elderly must be more aware of network services available to assist them.

REFERENCES

Bell, D. F. Assessing educational needs: Advantages of eighteen techniques, *Nurse Educator*, September-October, 1978, 15–21.

Bille, D. Barriers to the teaching-learning process, in *Practical Approaches to Patient Teaching*, Little, Brown and Company, 1981.

DeJoseph, J. F. Writing and evaluating educational protocols. In W. P. Squyers, (Ed.), *Patient Education: An Inquiry into State of the Art*. New York: Springer-Verlag, 1980.

Fletcher, S. W., and others. Improving emergency-room patient follow-up in a metropolitan teachng hospital. *New England Journal of Medicine*, 1974, *291*, 385–38.

Gerard, P. S., and Peterson, L. M. Learning needs of cardiac patients. *Cardio-Vascular Nursing*, 1984, *20*, 7–11.

Green, L. W., and Figa-Talamanca, I. Suggested designs for evaluation of patient education programs. *Health Education Monographs*, 1974, *2*, 54–71.

Green, L., Lewis, F., and Levine, D. Balancing statistical data and clinician judgement in the diagnosis of patient education needs, *Journal of Community Health*, Vol. 6, No. 2, Winter, 1980, pp. 79–91.

Gress, L. D., and Bahr, R. T. *The aging person: a holistic approach*. St. Louis: C. V. Mosby, 1984.

Grosser, L. All nurses can be involved in teaching the family. *AORN Journal*, February 1981, 217–218.

Houle, C. O. *The Design of Education*. Washington, Jossey-Bass Publishers, 1976, 131–220.

Klimecki, C. Patient education center benefits hospitalized patients community. *Hospital Progress,*
  August, 1982, 54–55, 68.

Knowles, M. *The Modern Practice of Adult Education From Pedagogy to Andragogy.* Chicago, Associated Press, 1980, 222–247.

Kratzer, J. What does your patient need to know?, *Nursing,* December, 1977, 82–84.

Lamb, L. Patient understanding of a teaching manual on cardiac catheterization. *Heart and Lung,*
  May 1984, 267–271.

Leavell, H., and Clark, E. *Preventive Medicine for the doctor in his community. An epidemiological
  approach* (3rd ed.) New York: McGraw-Hill, 1965. p. 21.

Mazzuca, S. Does patient education in chronic disease have therapeutic value? *Journal of Chronic
  Disease,* 1982, 35, 521–529.

Phillips, H. T., and Gaylord, S. A. (Eds.), *Aging and public health.* New York: Springer Publishing,
  1985.

Skiff, Ann, et al. A practical approach to assessing patient learning needs, *Journal of the National
  Medical Association,* 1981, 73, 6, 533–537.

Smith, C., Garvis, M., and Martinson, I. Content analysis of Interviews using a nursing model: A
  look at parents adapting to the impact of childhood cancer. *Cancer Nursing,* Aug. 1983, 269–
  275.

Society of Teachers in Family Medicine, *Patient Education Handbook,* Kansas City, KS: 1979.

Springer, D. and Brubaker, T. H. *Family caregivers and dependent elderly.* Beverly Hills: Sage
  Publications, 1984.

Wise, P. Barriers (or enhancers) to adult patient education, *Journal of Continuing Education,* 1979,
  10, 6, 11–16.

Woldum, K. M. (ed.). *Patient education tools for practice.* Rockville, MD, Aspen Systems Corp.,
  1985.

The Educated Patient: A new health care resource. *Hospital,* September 1, 1974, 48, 88–90.

4

Distinguishing Counseling and Discharge Planning from Patient Teaching for the Chronically Ill

Bonnie L. Westra

OBJECTIVES

1. Distinguish between counseling, patient teaching and discharge planning.
2. Assess the needs of the chronically ill.
3. Use a model for selecting appropriate interventions in caring for the chronically ill.
4. Develop a teaching plan for a neurologically impaired patient and his or her family that distinguishes among patient counseling, teaching, and discharge planning.

The previous chapter explored the nursing process in relationship to patient teaching in chronic and acute care settings. In this chapter, the nursing process will be used to explore the counseling and discharge planning needs of the chronically ill. The nurse must be able to distinguish counseling techniques and discharge planning from patient teaching strategies. The appropriate use of each of these nursing care strategies is essential to providing quality care.

Chronic illnesses, such as high blood pressure, heart and lung diseases, and cancer affect more Americans than ever before. Cure is not possible for most chronic illnesses, rather the goal is to control disability over a long period of time. Nurses are in a key role to affect the lives of chronically ill persons and their families through the appropriate selection of counseling, teaching, and discharge planning. When used appropriately, these strategies can facilitate attitude and behavioral changes such that patients and families will be able to manage their chronic illnesses and achieve their highest level of functioning (Ardell, 1977).

Many chronic illnesses have a downward progression or intermittent declines with remissions or stable periods in between. The patient's condition does not necessarily proceed in an orderly manner, and is influenced by the stage of the illness, response to treatment, other related health problems, and complications that may occur (Anderson and Bauwers, 1981). The nurse must know when to focus on the patient's and family's emotional needs versus their learning needs. Furthermore, the nurse must be aware of

PATIENT EDUCATION: NURSES IN PARTNERSHIP
WITH OTHER HEALTH PROFESSIONALS

what support the patient and family will need as they move from one health care setting to another. Through awareness and flexibility in the use of patient counseling, teaching, and discharge planning, the nurse can help patients and families to achieve their highest level of functioning (Hockbawn, 1980).

ASSESSING THE NEEDS OF THE CHRONICALLY ILL

Chronic illness is the number one health care problem in the United States today. As used here, chronic illness, is synonymous with chronic disease, disability, or limitation. Chronic illness encompasses any dysfunction of a person's bio-psycho-socio-cultural-spiritual dimensions. The dysfunction has a lasting effect, requiring the individual to change some aspect(s) of lifestyle to accommodate the limitations. These illnesses are not one-time episodes, like an appendectomy. Rather, the illnesses involve a series of intermittent or continuous health care problems. These problems strike persons of any age, sex, or nationality. They include those born with congenital diseases or anomalies such as cystic fibrosis or cardiac defects and those who develop illnesses or disabilities such as myasthenia gravis, coronary artery disease, paraplegia resulting from a motor vehicle accident, or mental illnesses such as schizophrenia. Chronic illness/disability is not discriminating, in that it can occur to anyone at any point in the life cycle.

Incidence and Impact of Chronic Illness

The incidence of chronic illness has continued to escalate with the increase in technology and advances in medicine, resulting in people living longer. The leading causes of death today are related to chronic diseases. Table 4-1 presents causes of death and morality rates for 1983. Greater than 80 percent of deaths in Table 4-I are related to chronic health problems. This figure does not, however, provide a complete picture of the impact of chronic illness.

The majority of a health care dollar is spent on chronic illnesses compared to acute illness or health promotion. A study conducted by Smyth-Staruch Breslau, Weitzman, and Gortmaker, 1984 compared 360 pediatric patients afflicted with cystic fibrosis, with 456 randomly selected children from a large urban clinic. The comparison demonstrated that the chronically ill children had a ten times greater use of health care services as well as ten times greater health care expenses. The Social Services Administration estimates that chronic obstructive pulmonary disease disability payments have been known to exceed $150 million per year (Kass, 1978). Cardiovascular disease alone was estimated to cost $64.4 billion in 1984 (AHA, 1984).

The expense of chronic illness is also seen in older population groups. It is estimated that 85 percent of all persons over the age of 65 have at least one chronic illness and many have multiple illnesses, according to the National Center for Health Statistics in 1976. The increasing aging of our population will create even more chronically ill elderly persons. Palley and Oktay (1983) found that 11 percent of the elderly used 29.4 percent of the health care dollar in 1978. Chronic illnesses, which require intermittent care over a long period of time, use the majority of health care monies.

Chronic illness affects more than use of the health care dollar. Chronic illnesses result in many changes for the individual such as ability to carry out activities of daily living, ability to work, and perform usual roles within the family. Limitations occur as a

Table 4-1
Causes of Death and Mortality Rates for 1983

Rank	Cause of death	Death rate	Percentage of total deaths
...	All causes	858.9	100.0
1	Diseases of heart	327.6	38.1
2	Malignant neoplasms	188.3	21.9
3	Cerebrovascular diseases	66.8	7.8
4	Accidents and adverse effects	18.7	4.5
5	Chronic obstructive and pulmonary diseases	28.4	3.3
6	Pneumonia and influenza	22.9	2.7
7	Diabetes mellitus	15.2	1.8
8	Suicide	12.4	1.4
9	Chronic liver disease and cirrhosis	11.9	1.4
10	Atherosclerosis	11.1	1.3
11	Homocide and legal intervention	8.2	1.0
12	Conditions originating in perinatal period	8.1	0.9
13	Nephrotic conditions	7.9	0.9
14	Septicemia	5.5	0.6
15	Congenital anomalies	5.5	0.6
...	All other causes	100.0	11.6

Data from Monthly Vital Statistics Report, 1983 Annual Summary Report, p5

result of illness and the person's whole lifestyle may be changed. This results in potential losses for the family and significant others.

Nurses must learn to assess for the individual, family, and community response to losses resulting from chronic illnesses and provide the appropriate interventions.

DISTINGUISHING AMONG COUNSELING, PATIENT TEACHING, AND DISCHARGE PLANNING

Nurses must select appropriate interventions to meet the needs of patients and families. Three effective strategies used to help patients and families experiencing chronic illness are described:

1. Counseling, which is the process of helping patients and families cope with changes, that is, deal with situations that are threatening in a manner that resolves uncomfortable feelings such as anxiety, anger, fear, grief, and guilt;
2. Patient teaching, which is the process of assisting patients and families to make a change in their behavior as a result of learning and
3. Discharge planning, which is the process of obtaining resources, such as financial, support groups, equipment, direct care, etc. for patients/families' ongoing needs after dismissal from a health care setting.

Counseling involves many diverse skills, from confrontation to reflective listening, or group therapy aimed at resolving feelings to exploring feelings on a one-to-one basis. Patient teaching can be accomplished in many ways, including providing written information about a disease, demonstrating how to give an injection, or having the patient and family discuss changes in performing activities of daily living. Discharge planning, which should always begin on the day of admission, incorporates planning for environmental changes at home, referral to community resources, and preparing the patient and family for necessary adaptations at home. Selection of appropriate strategies to meet the needs of patients and families experiencing chronic illnesses is a challenge.

Differences in Interventions

The differences among counseling, patient teaching, and discharge planning stem from the goal to be accomplished. The goal of counseling, ideally, is that the patient and family will gain an acceptance of their feelings and cope with their experiences. The goal of patient teaching is for the patient and family to learn about the illness, its treatment, and how to change their respective lifestyles. This assures that the patient and family have the resources enabling them to adapt after dismissal.

Selection of interventions is dependent upon the goals. Take for example, the case of Sally Watson, who is a 28-year-old woman with multiple sclerosis (MS). Short- and long-range goals related to patient counseling were established. The initial short-range goal was for Sally to express her feelings. Prior to discharge, the goal was to have Sally and her sister, who she lives with, state how they will manage at home. Patient counseling strategies included helping them recognize their feelings and assuring them that those feelings are normal.

When Sally first heard her diagnosis, two goals related to patient teaching were established. The first was to have her discuss bodily changes caused by multiple sclerosis, and the second manage her medication regimen. Specific patient teaching strategies included having Sally read and discuss two pamphlets from the National Multiple Sclerosis Society, "What everyone should know about multiple sclerosis" and "Grounds for hope." The nurse shared written information about each of Sally's medications and discussed them with her.

A discharge planning goal was that her sister would utilize available resources to administer prescribed treatments at home. A referral to the local MS Foundation was made for the Watson's to obtain the assistance they needed to manage at home. Counseling, teaching, and discharge planning thus were all strategies appropriately used with this patient and her significant other.

Similarities in Interventions

Many aspects of counseling, patient teaching, and discharge planning interventions overlap. The ultimate goal for the patient and family is the same: the patient and family will be able to function at the highest level possible.

Another overlap occurs when one intervention accomplishes goals related to counseling, patient teaching, and discharge planning. For instance, Sam Genoi is a 66-year-old man with Parkinson's disease. His ability to perform a skill, such as walking with a walker, affects his ability to cope with angry feelings from immobility. It also demonstrates learning from psychomotor teaching. In addition, by walking with a walker, Sam is better able to function after discharge. One nursing activity thus helps meet the patient's counseling, teaching, and discharge planning needs.

Even though one intervention may accomplish three things, the nurse must always be mindful that the patient's needs for counseling, teaching, and discharge planning are separate and distinct. Each area of need must be individually assessed. Then, in the planning step of the nursing process, one or several interventions are selected to meet the needs. It is often possible to use one intervention to meet aspects of the patient's counseling, teaching, and discharge planning needs.

Selecting the Appropriate Strategy

The process of selecting the appropriate strategies to help patients and families requires awareness and flexibility of the nurse. The chronically ill patient's condition does not necessarily proceed in an orderly manner, and is influenced by the stage of the illness, response to treatment, other related health problems, and complications that may occur. The nurse must know when to focus on the emotional needs of the patient and family versus their learning needs. Furthermore, the nurse must be aware of what outside support the patient and family will need to incorporate changes in behavior resulting from the patient's illness, as they move from one health care setting to another. Through awareness and flexibility in the use of patient teaching, counseling, and discharge planning, the nurse can help patients and families to achieve their highest level of functioning.

Typically the order of priority of interventions is counseling, then patient teaching, then discharge planning. Psychological needs, are met by counseling to relieve anxiety and help the patient and family cope with the chronic illness. The type of coping tasks chronically ill adults often face are listed below (Miller, 1983).

Types of Coping Tasks of Chronically Ill Adults

1. Maintaining a sense of normality
2. Modifying daily routine, adjusting life-style
3. Obtaining knowledge and skill for continuing self-care
4. Maintaining a positive concept of self
5. Adjusting to altered social relationships
6. Grieving over losses concomitant with chronic illness
7. Dealing with role change
8. Handling physical discomfort
9. Complying with prescribed regimen
10. Confronting the inevitability of one's own death
11. Dealing with social stigma of illness or disability
12. Maintaining a feeling of being in control
13. Maintaining hope despite uncertain or downward course of health

Unfortunately some health care workers may not recognize the patient's needs for counseling, or they may not completely attend to the patient's basic concerns, but instead use teaching or discharge planning. The effects of selecting inappropriate strategies (eg teaching when patients aren't ready or referring to outside resources that families will not use) in patient care result in increased health care costs. These increased costs are related to wasted time of the nurse when results are not achieved, potential complications from noncompliance when patients and families do not understand, potentially repeated hospitalizations when complications occur and lost time for the patient and family when problems arise. It is therefore critical for nurses to be able to select the right intervention counseling, patient teaching, or discharge planning—at the right time, if they wish to achieve success and provide cost-effective care. To avoid inappropriate use of counseling, patient teaching, discharge planning, or wasting time and money, a thorough assessment of the family must be conducted.

The family or significant others have a great impact on the health of the individual. A patient's acceptance of counseling, teaching, and discharge planning is influenced by their families' attitude. Families act as a support system, either prescribing various reme- dies and/or referring for medical treatment. The family provides norms for determining if an illness exists and when to seek medical care. The family may be responsible for the patient's perception of and response to the illness and hospitalization. Studies have even shown that negative or upsetting interactions among family members may have astoun- dingly negative effects on cardiac physiology of patients (Lynch, 1974).

Families play a crucial role in the patient's rehabilitation. For instance, if the family members see the patient's illness as overwhelming or unmanageable, and the treatment program as threatening and confusing, they may be likely to withdraw from the treatment programs and support the patient to withdraw as well. Families are an integral part of the patient's life and must be considered in his or her care.

Strauss (1984) states that divorce or separation is the most common solution to the multiple stressors that occur with chronic illness. Finances are another major concern. Twenty percent of families with a chronically ill member must seek additional revenue sources according to a study by Sultz, Schlesinger, Mosher, and Feldman (1972). This figure would likely be much higher today with increasing costs resulting from inflation. Additionally, social activities for families with a chronically ill member are limited. Respite care is difficult to obtain. Furthermore, if the chronically ill person requires care that involves technology, finding someone who is willing or able to provide care is difficult.

Hill and Hansen have delineated factors influencing the family's ability to cope with illness (1964, p. 803). These are listed below and provide guidelines for the nurse's counseling of families experiencing a chronic illness.

Factors That Influence the Family's Ability to Cope with Chronic Illness

1. Characteristics of the event
   Type of disease, disability, prognosis, potential for rehabilitation and family's perception of illness
2. Perceived threat to family relationships status and goals
   Positions and roles—changes required as a result of the illness
   Stage of development—stable versus transition
   Family goals—the more congruent goals of treatment are with family goals, the more likely the family is to be supportive
3. Past experience with the same or similar situations
   Chronic illness leads to a sense of lack of control—need to identify coping styles and determine their effectiveness
4. Resources available to the family
   Family strengths
   Finances

> Cost of illness
> Potential loss of family income
> Support systems
> > Extra family support systems—often are available for acute illnesses, but
> > decrease with length of illness
> Access to health care services

Selection of appropriate interventions is based on the assessment and goals related to each area of concern. During the acute phase of illness, the nurse, along with other health care members, provides direct care until the situation becomes manageable for the patient and family to resume care. Whenever possible, the patient and family should be incorporated in decisions about the patient's care, even during the acute phase. Patient counseling, teaching, and discharge planning should begin at the time the nurse has contact with the patient and family. While the patient is in the acute phase of care, where basic needs must be met, the nurse will focus on the "here and now" and use counseling techniques with the patient and family. As the patient progresses, the nurse will be able to focus on future needs and start teaching and discharge planning. Those needs that are not entirely met during acute care of the patient, should be communicated to health care providers in whatever setting the patient next experiences, whether the home, supervised living, or long-term care facilities. By incorporating the family in the patient's care, the nurse builds support systems to help the patient comply with treatment, adapting it to his or her lifestyle.

Assessing Counseling Needs of the Chronically Ill

Table 4-2 is a list of questions used to assess the emotional needs of the chronically ill. These questions are listed according to the common problems of grief, powerlessness and crisis.

The chronically ill experience many feelings and reactions that often need to be sorted out. The most common reaction is grieving. This is a result of the many losses

Table 4-2
Assessment Questions for Counseling the Chronically Ill

Grieving	What losses have the patient and family previously encountered as a result of the chronic illness?
	How have they coped with these losses?
	Will these coping mechanisms work for them now?
	Who are their support systems?
	Are they available now?
	What stage of the grieving process is each member of the family experiencing?
Powerlessness	What factors contribute to the patient's and family's sense of powerlessness?
	Lack of energy?
	Lack of information?
	What factors are contributing to their sense of control?
Crisis	Do they have realistic perceptions?
	Do they have adequate coping skills?
	Do they have an adequate support system?

experienced with chronic illness including loss of a normal physical body, self-esteem, self-satisfaction, recognition, and normalcy (Miller, 1983). Unlike grief related to the death of someone or loss of things outside of a person, the constant personal reminder of decreased abilities experienced by a person with a chronic illness may lead to chronic grief. This is experienced not only by the ill person, but also by significant others due to the loss of normal role interactions.

Kubler-Ross (1969) has defined five stages of the grieving process. These are: denial and isolation, anger, bargaining, depression, and acceptance. These stages do not necessarily proceed in an orderly sequence, especially for persons experiencing a chronic illness. By definition, chronic illness is not a one-time episode of an illness. It is a series of intermittent or continuous health care problems. Patients and families are continuously having to adapt to losses as a result of illness and/or treatment. Consequently, each person affected by the illness experiences a recycling of the stages of the grieving process. Assessment of patients and families during these cycles may reveal the common problem of powerlessness.

Powerlessness is the perception of the individual that one's own actions will not significantly affect an outcome (Miller, 1983). It is a feeling of loss of control. Lack of control leads to depression, and a belief that one can't do anything about the situation. A vicious cycle develops, where the patient and/or family is actually incapacitated. They are unable to take action based on their beliefs that they have no control.

Studies have confirmed that a sense of powerlessness or lack of control leads to inability to take action and/or depression. For instance, Ferrari (1962) found that elderly patients who were admitted to a nursing home were assessed to determine how well they would do based on their choice to live there. Of the 17 who stated that they had no alternative, 8 died after 4 weeks and all but 1 were dead at the end of 10 weeks. Of the 38 who felt they had alternatives, only 1 had died at the end of 10 weeks. None of the deaths were expected. Patients who feel hopeless (powerless) after being diagnosed with a terminal illness compared with those who decide to "take the bull by the horns," have a shorter life expectancy (Kastenbaum and Kastenbaum, 1971). Unfortunately, many people feel powerless when diagnosed with a chronic disease.

Counseling Based on Crisis Theory

Each time a person with a chronic illness again becomes ill or deteriorates in abilities, a state of crisis occurs. That is, a sense of disequilibrium exists wherein a perceived threat is felt that disrupts function. If the patient and family have a realistic perception of events, adequate coping skills, and adequate support systems, they will be able to resolve the crisis and may even grow from being able to manage the experience. However, if one of these three factors is not present, they will continue to experience a sense of disequilibrium and a crisis results. When the patient and family are experiencing a crisis, it is difficult for them to make decisions, retain information, or function in their usual manner. Crises are self limiting in that they will either be resolved, or deteriorate to more complex problems, such as more illness, injury, or potentially destructive behavior.

Crisis theory provides an overall framework for assessing the counseling needs of the patient and family, as the patient experiences exacerbations in his chronic illness. The patient and family experiencing a chronic illness continuously face loss as the patient moves in and out of the health care setting. Each new episode of health care problems represent a loss for the patient and family. This may be a loss of function, permanent health status, or temporary disruptions of the usual roles and functions within the family and community. Resolution of these losses must occur before teaching can be effective. Furthermore, when the patient once again experiences disruptions, due to health problems, both he and his family are likely to feel powerless. In spite of everything they may have been doing to alleviate the patient's symptoms, problems may occur. Crisis theory, along with the concepts of loss (grieving) and powerlessness provide quidelines for the nurse counseling the chronically ill patient and family.

Crisis theory states that an upset in a steady state (a crisis) provides an individual with both opportunity for growth or potential for deterioration in functioning (Aguilera and Messick, 1982). An individual who encounters a crisis can perceive the event as a challenge, threat, or a loss. The perspective taken is dependent upon the individual's unique makeup and resources available to handle the situation. Growth occurs when there are sufficient resources or problem-solving skills available. This theory indicates that resolution of the upset in the steady state (disequilibrium) results in ability to deal effectively with similar problems in the future and increased ability to deal with other problems.

Crisis theory also applies to groups. When an individual experiences a crisis, such as an exacerbation of a chronic illness, it also affects the groups to which the individual belongs. Likewise, the equilibrium of group members reciprocally affects each individual. Social groups and families can therefore hinder an individual through their own stage of crisis or can be a source of support for an individual. For instance, Evan Wilmer was chairperson for his district Republican party. Just prior to elections in the fall, Evan was rehospitalized for psoriasis. He was unable to provide guidance for the chairpersons in charge of the State Senate and House campaigns. His family received many phone calls requesting information about the best time to do door-to-door campaigns, telephone calling, and fundraising activities. They were unable to provide this information, which raised their level of anxiety in addition to Evan's hospitalization. As their tension increased, Evan's psoriasis became worse, despite treatment. When planning care for chronically ill individuals, normal feelings and reactions of both the individual and family must be considered. Crisis theory provides a framework for anticipating the counseling needs of both.

Planning and Intervening to Meet Counseling Needs

Based on the assessment a plan should then be developed with the patient and family and implemented to meet counseling needs and support their coping skills. When patients and families are coping, they will be in a better position or "state of readiness" to learn to manage their lives. However, readiness to learn is often dependent on meeting the patient's counseling goals. These goals are listed in Table 4-3. It is not intended that the nurse will be everything to everyone, but rather that these goals be considered in meeting counseling needs.

One method of meeting the emotional needs of chronically ill patients and their families, is to help them work through any grief they may experience as a result of changes brought on by the illness. The first is to accept the stage of the grieving process that they are experiencing. Statements such as "You seem angry that this is happening to you," lets them know that the nurse understands how they feel. Assuring them that angry feelings are normal and that most people experience these feelings prevents guilt and helps to resolve feelings more easily. The nurse should encourage people to share feelings

Table 4-3
Goals for Meeting Counseling Needs

Grieving	Patient and family able to verbalize losses anticipated or experienced
	Patient and family able to identify previous successful coping strategies and employ with existing problems
	Patient and family able to identify and secure support from existing support systems
Powerlessness	Patient and family able to identify factors that contribute to sense of powerlessness
	Patient and family able to mobilize power resources, e.g., physical strength, psychological stamina, hope, etc.
	Patient and family actively participate in planning and management of chronic illness
Crisis	Patient and family have a realistic perception
	Patient and family have adequate coping skills
	Patient and family have adequate support systems

even though it is uncomfortable to do so. By showing feelings, patients and families can let go of them and move on to acceptance of what is occurring.

Anticipatory guidance is a useful technique to help chronically ill patients and their families predict the grief they are likely to experience. Anticipatory guidance is the process of informing patients and families what reactions might occur, and that these feelings are normal. By teaching what to expect patients and families are able to accept their feelings without experiencing alienation. They will thus more readily be able to share their feelings, and resolve them.

Counseling for Powerlessness

Nurses are able to intervene in feelings of powerlessness by the use of three interventions: providing behavioral, cognitive, or decisional control (Averill, 1973). Behavioral control is control over the environment, e.g., the ability to reach objects such as a glass of water, or controlling of personnel entering the room by having people knock before entering. Cognitive control is control over information and its interpretation or evaluation, e.g., knowing the results of tests and procedures. Decisional control is control over selection from various alternatives affecting the individual; for example a patient with chronic low back pain should be informed about the use of medications, bed rest and traction versus surgery, with their resulting consequences. These interventions can easily be incorporated into daily routines to meet the counseling needs of patients and families, with little or no extra effort on the part of the nurse.

There are other interventions that help patients to gain a sense of power (control) while experiencing an acute episode of a chronic illness. Nurses can use stress management techniques to help keep distress within personally acceptable limits. Generating encouragement and hope provide motivation for recovery. Nurses should not provide false hope by informing patients that "everything will be alright," since often this may not be the case, especially with chronic illnesses. However, patients can hope that they will regain some sense of functioning above their present condition, or at least hope for a peaceful death if it is imminent.

Valuing opinions of the ill individual helps them to maintain a sense of personal worth. For instance, asking a person with a colostomy to demonstrate how they prefer to have it changed, acknowledges their capabilities and experiences in previously managing their illness. By encouraging visiting, and not restricting visiting hours, support from significant others can alleviate powerlessness. Furthermore, when nurses provide for basic needs, e.g., oxygen, food, etc., physical power is regained by the ill individual. Many interventions can be employed to help chronically ill individuals meet their emotional needs and prepare them to learn skills needed to adjust to limitations and treatments.

Planning and implementing counseling strategies to meet the emotional needs of the chronically ill and their families provides a creative opportunity for the nurse. For example, Mary Spooner is a 78-year–old widow being cared for in her home by the public health nurse. She has had repeated hospitalizations for "small strokes," and is supposed to be on a low-sodium diet and taking medication for her blood pressure. Mary verbalized concerns that she couldn't do the things she used to; she felt old and a bother. She also stated she didn't think her low-salt diet made any difference. The nurse, after assessing Mary, established that she had feelings of worthlessness related to chronic illness and aging and that she was noncompliant with diet because of feelings of powerlessness.

The public health nurse knew that Mary would be more successful with her diet if she felt better about herself. A program including senior citizens and adolescents provided an opportunity for Mary to feel worthwhile. Senior citizens could receive food from cooperative community shelter in exchange for teaching adolsecents who worked there some type of skill. Mary loved to knit and crochet, a skill that was valued by the adolescents at the co-op. Through sharing her talents, Mary achieved a sense of being needed, and could verbalize this to the nurse.

The nurse developed a plan, after discussion with Mary, whereby she could make choices. These choices included how Mary would realistically modify her lifestyle to incorporate the changes necessitated by the low-sodium diet. For example, on Sundays Mary visited her daughter. She didn't want to be restricted from eating the family meal, or having her daughter change how she cooked, so Mary and the public health nurse agreed to Mary following her diet 6 days a week. Allowing the patient control over this one important meal will decrease her sense of powerlessness.

Mary's situation shows nurses can empower patients by giving them a sense of control. The nurse can provide control by encouraging Mary to determine when the nutrition aid would come. The nurse can help Mary gain control by providing information and involvement in decision making in the plan of care, supporting Mary's choices. There are several other techniques that can be used to counsel patients and provide them with choices. Interventions are related to problems frequently experienced by chronically ill patients. Most chronically ill persons have a decline in psychological stamina and support. When relapses in illness occur, even when following medical regimes, a sense of futility can develop. Nurses need to provide opportunities for patients to express their feelings, so they can regain the stamina to face the work of recovery once again. Reinforcement that the patient and family has been able to cope successfully in the past and therefore is likely to do so now, also helps support their psychological stamina. Illness creates barriers between the chronically ill person and his or her support network. Liberalizing visiting hours is another method of enhancing support and was previously discussed.

Counseling for Positive Self Concept

Another common problem frequently experienced by chronically ill patients is a negative self concept. A positive self concept can be developed by emphasizing abilities rather than disabilities. This was demonstrated in the example with Mary. The use of persuasion to influence beliefs and values consistent with the goals of therapy is another method of increasing motivation. Nurses need to provide the patient with a sense of hope. If a patient is active in a religion, involvement of church members can support a sense of hope. Minimally nurses can support the patient in hoping to be as comfortable as possible.

Counseling to Conserve Energy

Chronically ill patients frequently experience a decline in physical strength or reserve at some point, due to their disease. When this occurs, the nurse can help them plan activities to conserve their strength by combining such things as going to the bathroom, getting up to sit in the chair and ambulating in the hall, all at the same time, instead of three separate activities. Family members frequently neglect their own basic needs when concerned with the illness of their family members. They need to be encouraged to get adequate nutrition and rest while the patient is in the hospital.

Counseling to Keep Informed

Obtaining knowledge to understand the illness and its treatment is a constant consideration. This is essential to empower patients and their families. The nurse should provide information about the results of tests and procedures, as well as help them interpret the meaning of this information. Interventions that help meet the needs related to frequently encountered problems in chronic illness, provide the patient and family with the power necessary to cope.

Counseling to Manage Crisis

In addition to the aforementioned interventions, assessing the chronically ill patient and family in terms of crisis theory, lends itself to some new ideas. There are three goals for helping families resolve a crisis. These include assuring that the patient and family will (a) have a realistic perception of the situation, (b) employ adequate coping mechanisms, and (c) utilize adequate support systems.

Providing knowledge and clarifying misunderstandings helps patients and families have a realistic perception. For instance, many families panic when first hearing the diagnosis of a chronic disease such as amytrophic lateral sclerosis (ALS). They are certain that the patient is going to die. Providing them with accurate knowledge of the disease, treatments, and prognosis, helps them to develop a realistic perception, decreasing their crisis.

Counseling to Support Coping

Miller (1983) assessed coping strategies used by chronically ill patients. Two general categories were noted: approach methods and avoidance. Approach coping strategies are those behaviors that use active engagement in "tackling" the task of getting well and regaining a sense of normality. These include: seeking information, choosing diversional activities, expressing emotions, using relaxation exercises, verbalizing concerns, using positive thinking techniques, setting goals and striving to achieve them, using humor, and utilizing problem-solving approaches.

Avoidance methods of coping are intellectual strategies used to minimize the seriousness of the threat to the individual. Avoidance strategies include: use of denial; minimize problems, signs and symptoms of illness; social isolation, sleeping; delay decision-making on personal health matters; blaming others; refusing to participate in treatment; excessive dependence on significant others; and setting unrealistic goals. Neither method of coping is considered good or bad. They are two different approaches and either is appropriate to use as long as it helps the individual and family to successfully cope. The nurse's responsibility is to assess whether they are working. If not, the nurse should help the patient develop coping strategies that will decrease anxiety and help the patient and family to cope.

Counseling to Maintain Support Systems

Another strategy to resolve a crisis is to be sure that there is an adequate support system present for the patient and family. The simplest step, is to enhance the natural support system. One way of doing this is to not restrict visitors and visiting hours whenever possible. Some limits may need to be set so the patient gets adequate rest and staff are able to provide care. Allowing visits at the convenience of visitors, easily enhances the natural support system. The second method of increasing support is to encourage involvement in existing support systems such as patient support groups, e.g., multiple sclerosis club, church, or community groups. Not only must they be instructed in what support systems are available, but involvement in them must be reinforced by the registered nurse. During routine activities, the nurse also functions as a support. For example, by smiling and stating "I'm pleased that you are attending the 'head injury rehabilitation group'", the nurse easily provides support. However, when the nurse does not have extensive time to spend with patients and families, a referral to others for further support, such as the chaplain, psychiatric clinical specialist, social worker, or psychologist is essential.

Evaluation of Counseling Strategies

Evaluation of counseling goals with patients most often is done by listening for verbalization of feelings, such as acceptance of the illness, or a sense of control through decision making. Resolution of crisis also results in ability to make decisions, so observation of decision-making ability is another method of evaluation. Observation of involvement in support groups further provides another method of evaluating meeting of emotional needs.

Because teaching in the affective domain may encompass various counseling strategies the nurse will also want to evaluate these learning outcomes. Acceptance of outside resources suggested in discharge planning is another indication of the success of the nurses counseling strategies.

DISCHARGE PLANNING

Discharge planning is the process of planning for the patient and family's ongoing health care needs as they move from one health care setting to another. It encompasses determination of direct care needs, as well as teaching and counseling needs that are unmet, or require ongoing assistance after discharge. Discharge planning also includes identification of resources available to meet these needs. After such a determination, the nurse organizes a plan with the patient, family, and health care team that most effectively and efficiently meets these needs.

Discharge planning includes strategies of teaching and counseling in preparing the patient and family for dismissal. It also includes an assessment of community resources and referring patients to provide for continuity in meeting their needs. Discharge planning should occur in every health care setting, e.g., hospital, nursing, home, and public health agency. The ultimate goal is to facilitate continuity of care, as the patient moves from one setting to the next during the course of the illness (Bristow and Stickney, 1982).

There are many benefits from discharge planning. Money is saved when the most appropriate resources are used that provide effective care. For instance, Noel Johnson was receiving Amphotericin B intravenously for cryptococcal pneumonia. His therapy was daily for six weeks. Since he was basically able to care for himself with the aid of his wife, it was determined that he could come into the emergency department for intravenous therapy once a day while remaining at home. This prevented six weeks of hospitalization.

Another benefit of discharge planning is assuring that the patient has easy access to diagnostic and treatment services. When Noel was discharged, the nurse arranged with the emergency department to provide his intravenous therapy, preventing time-consuming waiting that would have occurred if he was not expected in the emergency department. Relapses and needless hospital stays, as well as unnecessary emergency visits to the hospital can be prevented with good discharge planning.

Other benefits of discharge planning include: increased patient coping, prevention of premature discharge and coordination of services. Discharge planning helps patients to develop a sense of responsibility for their own care. By developing schedules for treatments after hospitalization, and having patients demonstrate their treatments, confidence is developed in their ability to cope. Planning for needs to be met after discharge can also prevent premature discharge. For example, arranging for a nursing home placement often requires time. If this were not identified early in the hospital stay, patients may be discharged back to the home before a nursing home bed could be arranged. When discharge planning is started early in the hospitalization, many services can be coordinated together to maximize utilization of health man power. Often the public health nurse involved prior to discharge, can facilitate transportation, housekeeping services, personal care services, and specialized treatment. Discharge planning thus has many benefits for all involved.

Discharge planning starts when the patient first seeks health care and requires continuous assessment throughout the care of the patient. During the initial interview, the nurse begins to collect data that will help to plan for discharge. As the patient progresses, the nurse collects additional data or modifies preexisting data, reflecting the change in the patient's health status and ability to function. Discharge planning that occurs only at the beginning of the patient's care, will not take into consideration changes that may have occurred. On the other hand, discharge planning undertaken immediately before dismissal does not allow time for a total assessment and plan by interdisciplinary health team members, patient, and family.

Discharge planning must include the patient and family along with all health care providers involved in the patient's care. The patient and family are the key members of the team. By involving all health team members who have provided care for the patient and family, such as the physician, dietitian, social worker, etc., a more comprehensive assessment and planning are developed. The nurse is, however, in the best position to coordinate discharge planning with the patient and family, because of his/her broad range of knowledge and constant interaction with the patient and family.

The nurse accomplishes discharge planning by determining the patient and family's needs and what community resources are available to them and discusses these with the patient and family. Effective discharge planning provides for use of the least costly services. Some hospitals have a discharge planning nurse who helps with this function.

Another method of assessing community resources can be done by documenting information about agencies, services provided, contact person, phone number, address and fee structure in a loose-leaf notebook for all the nursing staff to use. An example of this format is provided.

Table of Contents for a Community Resources Book

1. Policies and procedures related to discharge planning
2. Resources for direct patient care
   Home health services
   Nursing facilities
   Other community services
3. Transportation and equipment
4. Brochures from agencies and community services

The advantage of a loose-leaf notebook, is that it can easily be modified when changes occur, keeping it up-to-date.

Assessment for Discharge of the Chronically Ill

Discharge planning follows the same steps of the nursing/teaching process, beginning with assessment. The initial step begins at the time of admission and it should include a holistic assessment of the patient's bio-psycho-social-cultural-spiritual needs. The nurse will want to assess the home situation by asking several questions. Who does the patient live with? What is the living arrangement? Does the patient live in a house, or apartment? Are there stairs to get into it, or stairs within the premises? Are all essential rooms on the same floor, such as the bathroom, bedroom, and kitchen? Is it adequate to meet the patient's needs at the time of discharge? Adequacy can include basics such as heat, cleanliness, indoor plumbing, etc.

The nurse will also want to assess the patient's support systems. Who will be available to the patient when discharged? This includes immediate family living with the patient, but also other support systems. What groups has the patient previously engaged in to meet his social needs? Will the patient be able to interact with the groups upon discharge?

Other areas of assessment are similar to assessment for patient counseling and teaching. Do the patient and family have adequate coping mechanisms? Will previous coping strategies work for them now, or will they require assistance in developing new ones because of a change in the patient's condition and its subsequent impact on the family? What learning needs will the patient and family have? Can these be adequately met in the hospital, or will they require ongoing support?

Lastly, during the initial assessment, the nurse will want to determine if the family is currently using any community resources to meet their needs. If so, how many, and how frequently? Are these satisfactory to the patient and family? If the patient and family are using community resources that are satisfactory, the nurse will want to consider these at the time of discharge when making a referral, of one is necessary (Rasmussen, 1984). Any patient who is at high risk requires a referral.

Planning for Discharge of the Chronically Ill

Discharge planning may or may not include a referral to another agency. If the patient and family are able to meet their own needs after discharge, they may not require any further assistance at home. The chronically ill have many complex needs and even if they are able at present to meet their own needs, however, a public health nurse visit can help to prevent problems from arising by early detection. A referral, therefore, to a public health agency would be helpful, if acceptable to the patient and family. Criteria identifying patients at high risk for relaspe are listed below.

High Risk Patients Who Require a Referral*

1. Activities of daily living dependent (those who cannot manage self care safely on their own)
2. Comatose, semicomatose
3. Disoriented, confused, forgetful
4. Dressings and wound care (patients with complicated dressings; patients who cannot do the dressing themselves; patients who will probably not do the dressing unless supervised)
5. Equipment and transportation (this function is shared with social service)
6. Medication schedules (patients with complex schedules, injections, patients who are noncompliant)
7. Ostomies (colostomy, ileostomy)
8. Social problems (patients who live alone and could manage with some assistance; those who do not live alone but the person at home cannot care for patients adequately; those who have no home to go to, or those whose present home is no longer adequate)
9. Special teaching needs (e.g., new diabetic, complex diet, injections)
10. Terminal, preterminal
11. Therapies (occupational, physical, speech)
12. Tubes (foley, gastrostomy, suprapubic, nasogastric, tracheostomy)
13. Transfers (transferred here from another hospital or nursing home; patients who will be transferred to another hospital, nursing home, Veterans Hospital, etc.)

Most commonly seen diagnoses of patients who need referrals are those with chronic illnesses, e.g., arthritis, cancer, cva, chronic renal failure, congestive heart failure, diabetes mellitus, emphysema, hypertension, myocardial infarction, respirator patients

---

*Adapted from Rasmussen, L. A screening tool promotes early discharge planning, *Nursing Management*, May 1984, pp. 39–40.

Discharge planning can be either a formal process or informal process. The formal process should include regularly scheduled team conferences, where members of various disciplines involved in the patient's care can share their unique perspectives of how the patient is progressing. These do not always include the patient and family directly, but at times should. This formal process, although worthwhile, is costly when you consider the expense of the physician, chaplain, etc. for an hour's time. Many institutions therefore use the more informal process.

The informal process also requires sharing of information, but all team members may not meet altogether or on a regularly scheduled basis. When an informal process is used, all team members must have access to written data, so they can keep apprised of the patient's progress. Regardless of which method of planning is used, written plans are essential.

Documentation should include: both short- and long-range planning goals. For instance, Ho Chung who is a 57-year–old Chinese male, hospitalized for Lyme's disease (an infection from a tick bite that causes neurological dysfunction). The short-range goals for him included being able to eat and bathe with assistance as his neurological function improved. His long-range goal for discharge included his performing his activities of daily living (ADL) with assistance from a home health aid three times a week after discharge. The written plan should include how the goal will be accomplished. What the patient is doing in physical therapy and occupational therapy should be documented with nursing reinforcing these activities on the unit. Who is responsible for a goal or specific activity related to that goal should also be documented. The date of evaluation should be written, so the nursing staff reassesses progress toward the goal. A standard format incorporating this criteria helps to assure that the process is accomplished.

Evaluation of Discharge Planning

Discharge planning, like any other nursing interventions, should be evaluated to determine if it was effective. There are several methods of evaluation that can be used. One is feedback from those caring for the patient after discharge. This can be accomplished by telephone, using a guide sheet. Table 4-4 provides a format for an evaluation sheet that can be sent out with each referral to obtain feedback from agencies.

Another method of evaluting the effectiveness of discharge planning is a follow-up phone call to the patient and family to determine if planning was adequate. This is most effectively done by the nurse planning discharge with the patient. Not only will this phone call evaluate effectiveness of discharge planning but can also be used to evaluate effectiveness of patient teaching and counseling.

Romano, McCormick, and McNally (1982) have identified criteria for evaluation. The patient and/or family should be able to state in simple terms the patient's medical diagnosis and how it has affected the patient's physical and psychosocial functioning. Furthermore, they should be able to state what was done (during the care of the patient in that particular health care setting) in relation to the problem. They should be able to identify what type of adjustments were necessary as a result of the illness and/or its treatment. The patient and family should be able to state under which circumstances the patient needs to contact a health professional and who or where to call for questions regrading treatments or changes in health status. The patient and or family should also be able to explain the reason for any special diet, medications, special equipment or procedures necessary for maximal functioning. They should be able to state that they have

Table 4-4
Evaluation of Discharge Planning

Name of patient: _____
Diagnosis: _____
Reason for referral: _____

_____
_____

Please respond to the following questions:
1. Was the referral complete? _____ yes _____ no
   If not, what further information would have been helpful? _____
   _____
   _____

2. Were all the necessary forms included? _____ yes _____ no
   If not, what other forms were needed? _____
   _____

3. Were you notified about the patient prior to discharge?
   _____ yes _____ no

4. Was the patient/family informed about your visit? _____ yes _____ no
5. Were there needs you identified that were not identified?
   _____ yes _____ no   If yes, please list _____
   _____

6. What information on the referral was most helpful to you? _____
   _____
   _____

7. How is the patient/family doing since discharge? _____
   _____
   _____

the necessary equipment to carry out treatments or ability to function. Lastly, they should be able to list the date, time, and place of follow-up appointment(s).

Patient counseling, teaching, and discharge planning are all interventions the nurse can use in care of chronically ill patients. Selection of the most appropriate strategy can increase its benefit to the patient and family, while providing cost effective care that meets standards for quality nursing care. These strategies overlap in specific methods used to help patients and families. The nurse must be cognizant of the current needs and goals, as the patient's course of illness and treatment change and the family's ability to cope with these changes. Furthermore, the nurse must identify unmet needs, to facilitate the continuity of care when the patient moves from one health care setting to another. Patients and families experiencing chronic illnesses must be actively involved in the process, since they are the day-to-day managers. This assures a more successful outcome.

TEACHING CARE PLAN FOR PATIENTS
WITH A CEREBRAL VASCULAR ACCIDENT (CVA)

Patients and their families that experience a CVA require counseling, patient teaching, and discharge planning to effectively manage their illness after the acute phase (Smith-Brady, 1982). This teaching plan is not intended to comprehensively address all the needs of the CVA patient, but rather to demonstrate how the nurse should first consider counseling, then patient teaching, and lastly discharge planning.

Mr. Mura Yoko is a 72-year-old Southeast Asian male, married with three children. His children are also married and have children of their own. Mr. Yoko had a left CVA 2 years ago with residual moderate right weakness, intermittent confusion, expressive aphagia, and occasional incontinence. After rehabilitation, he was able to walk with the use of a leg brace and three-pronged cane. He could perform most of his ADLs with minimal assistance. Mr. Yoko had learned to use his left hand for most activities.

Since his hospitalization 2 years ago, Mr. Yoko was able to be at home with the help of a home health aid three times a week and a neighbor two times per week. Mrs. Yoko has a history of cardiac illness and was unable to help Mr. Yoko with physical care. As Mr. Yoko became more independent, he required the home health aid only once a week to help with his bath. The public health nurse continued to visit him once a month to monitor his blood pressure, and regulation of his medications. His blood pressure ranged from 150/90 to 180/110.

Mr. Yoko had recently been rehospitalized for another left CVA. After Mr. Yoko's condition stabilized, the nurse caring for him formulated the following problem list, with Mr. Yoko and his wife, in anticipation of his dismissal. Patients experiencing a CVA have certain common problems similar to Mr. Yoko, including:

1. Grieving/loss of normal physical functioning secondary to CVA
2. Powerlessness/ chronic illness and hospitalization
3. Self-care deficit/weakness and loss of motor function Right side
4. Limited mobility/need for wheelchair

The following care plan developed for Mr. Yoko is not all inclusive of his needs, but illustrates how to distinguish and prioritize patient counseling, teaching, and discharge planning needs (Tables 4-5, 4-6, and 4-7, pages 116–118).

REFERENCES

Aguilera, D.C., and Messick, J.M. *Crisis intervention: theory and methodology.* St. Louis: The C.V. Mosby Co., 1982.

American Heart Association, *1984 heart facts,* Dallas, TX: National Center, 1984.

Anderson, S.V., and Bauwers, E.E. *Chronic health problems, concepts and applications.* St. Louis: The C.V. Mosby Co., 1981.

Ardell, Donald B. *High level wellness: an alternative to doctors, drugs and diseases.* Emmaus, PA: Rodale Press, 1977.

Averill, J. Personal control over aversive stimuli and its relationship to stress. *Pyschological Bulletin,* 1973, 80,286.

Bristow, O., and Stickney, C. *Discharge planning for continuity of care,* 10 Columbus Circle, New York, N.Y. 10019 (Catalog #21-1604). 1982.

Ferrari, N.A. Institutionalization and attitude change in aged population: A field study on dissidence theory. Unpublished doctoral dissertation, Cleveland: Case Western Reserve University, 1962.

Hill, R., and Hansen, D.A. Families under stress. In H.T. Christensen, (Ed.). *Handbook of Marriage and Family,* Chicago: Rand McNally and Co., 1964.

Hockbawm, G.M. Patient Counseling Vs. Patient Teaching, *Topics in Clinical Nursing,* July 1980, 1–7.

Kass, I. *Disability benefits for chronic lung disease.* New York, American Lung Association, 1978.

Table 4-5
Teaching Plan for *Mura Yoko*

Assessment	Plan/Learning objectives	Interventions	Evaluation
		Affective	
Grieving/loss of normal physical functioning secnodary to CVA	Patient/family will verbalize feelings about the illness, the patient's prognosis and its impact on their lives. (*Counseling Strageties*)	Promote a trusting relationship by:	Ask the patient/family to explain how the patient's impaired functioning is related to the CVA, expected outcome and adjustments that will be necessary.
ʿAssess the patient/family's perception of the illness and feelings about relapse		Taking time for patient/family	
Asking them what losses changes they anticipate or are experiencing as a result of the patient's illness.		Displaying a caring attitude Using sincerity	Listen for patient/family to verbalize ability to cope with necessary adjustments
Asking them how they have coped with losses in the past.		Encourage patient/family to verbalize feelings by Utilizing silence and therapeutic leads for discussion in regards to condition	Observe absense or presence of support systems
Determining if these coping mechanisms are being used now, and if they are effective.		Providing information about grief stages Allowing for established time to meet and discuss feelings	Family realistically describes future level of function
Observing and questioning about adequacy of support system	Patient/family display hope that patients function will resume to level prior to hospitalization (*Counseling Strageties*)	Encouraging family to share positive statements about patients future Offering support and assurance	

116

Table 4-6
Teaching Plan for *Mura Yoko*

Assessment	Plan/Learning objectives	Interventions	Evaluation
		Cognitive	
Limited mobility/wheelchair	• Patient will use wheelchair in home environment after discharge in order to obtain mobility in a safe manner (*discharge planning*)	• Refer to Public Health Nurse (PHN) for assistance with home environment planning and follow-up to assure that patient is able to be mobile	PHN will report back on evaluation of discharge plan if all home modifications had been anticipated
• Assess home environment for safety and need for modifications			
Assess for environmental factors that could inhibit mobility		• Have family talk with other families who have made modifications for wheelchair dependent person	In follow-up phone call one month after discharge, patient and family will verbalize that patient has remained mobile
Ask family about barriers to mobility, e.g., width of doorways and rooms for use of wheelchair, rugs that could hinder use of wheelchair	Family accepts need for assistance from public health agency (*discharge planning*)	• Give family a check list of criteria for use of wheelchair in home evironment	Family reports acceptance of environmental modifications suggested by public health officials
		• Ask family to report back to nurse of any environmental modifications that will be needed	

Table 4-7
Teaching Plan for *Mura Yoko*

Assessment	Plan/Learning objectives	Interventions	Evaluation
		Psychomotor	
Self-care deficit/weakness and loss of motor function right side	The patient will demonstrate ability to feed self with assistance (*patient teaching*)	Ascertain what foods Mr. Yoko likes consistent with his prescribed diet	Mr. Yoko will be able to feed himself with the use of assistive deviced by the time he is discharged
Assess ability to feed self by		Reinforce the use of any assistive devices obtained from Occupational Therapy, e.g., padded spoon, plate guard, etc.	
Observing if patient is able to perceive food on tray			
Observing if patient is interested in eating		Provide for eating environment that is not embarrassing to Mr. Yoko	
Observing if patient is able to feed self with or without adaptive devices.		Pull curtain around bed	
		Minimize personnel in room during meals	
	Patient/family responds to questions evaluating poststroke education (*patient teaching*)	Provide only the amount of supervision and assistance necessary for relearning to eat	Patient/family demonstrate activities of self care listed in poststroke education pamphlet

118

Kastenbaum, R. and Kastenbaum, B. Hope, survival and the caring environment. In E. Palmore, and F. Jerrers, (Eds.), *Prediction of Life Span,* Lexington, MA: Lexington Books, Division of D.C. health, 1971, pp. 249–271.

Kubler-Ross, E. *On death and dying.* New York: The Macmillan Co., 1969.

Lynch, W. *Images of hope.* Notre Dame, IN: University of Notre Dame Press, 1974.

Miller, J. *Coping with chronic illness: overcoming powerlessness,* Philadelphia: F.A. Davis Co., 1983.

Palley, H.A., and Oktay, J.S. *The chronically limited elderly: the case for a national policy for in-home and supportive community-based services.* New York: The Haworth Press, 1983.

Rasmussen, L. A screening tool promotes early discharge planning. *Nursing Management,* May 1984, pp. 39–40.

Romano, C., McCormick, K., and McNelly, L., Nursing Documentation - a model for a computerized data base. *Advances in Nursing Science.* January 1982, pp. 43–56.

Smith-Brady, R. Assessing adherence in stroke victims. *Nursing Clinics of North America,* 1982, *17* (3), 499–512.

Smyth-Staruch, K., Breslau, N., Weitzman, R., and Gortmaker, S. Use of health services by chronically ill and disabled children. *Medical Care,* 1984, 22:310–328.

Strategies to Promote Self-Management of Chronic Disease, Chicago: American Hospital Association, 1982.

Strauss, A., Glaser, B., Fagerhaugh, S., Suczek, B., Weiner, C., Corbin, J., and Maines, D. *Chronic illness and the quality of life.* St. Louis: C.V. Mosby Co., 1984.

Sultz, H.A., Schlesinger, E.R., Mosher, W.E., and Feldman, J.G. *Long-term childhood illness,* Pittsburgh: University of Pittsburgh Press, 1972.

Only the Educated are Free.

Epictetus (50 A.D.), Greek Philosopher

5

Assessing Knowledge Deficit and Establishing Behavioral Objectives

Judith A. Kopper

OBJECTIVES

1. Analyze multiple factors that predispose an individual to have knowledge deficit.
2. Apply defining characteristics to writing nursing diagnoses related to learning needs.
3. Identify essential and optional components of measurable learner objectives.
4. Differentiate four domains of learning: cognitive, affective, psychomotor and perceptual.
5. Utilize action verbs from various taxonomy levels in writing behavioral objectives.
6. Develop a teaching plan for the diabetic patient that illustrates objective writing in the learning domains.

We are reminded by Epictetus of the first century that education is the forerunner of freedom, the freedom of choice, the freedom to influence one's outcomes. This basic maxim, "only the educated are free," provides the rationale for educating health care consumers. As participants in determining their own health goals, the consumer must be educated in order to make a free choice, an intelligent decision of whether or not to follow the health professionals' guidelines and treatment modalities. Only as we educate the consumers can they become full partners in their health care.

This chapter describes assessment of a patient's knowledge deficit and how to analyze various factors that contribute to the learning needs so that a nursing diagnosis can be established. A variety of factors that might affect an individual's knowledge deficit are discussed.

The major focus of the chapter is how to write measurable learner objectives that represent different domains of learning. Tips on how to avoid common errors when writing objectives are included.

The content of the chapter is applied in a sample teaching plan. Patients with different types of diabetes mellitus are referred to throughout the chapter to illustrate the content.

PATIENT EDUCATION: NURSES IN PARTNERSHIP
WITH OTHER HEALTH PROFESSIONALS

© 1987 by Grune & Stratton, Inc.
ISBN 0-8089-1833-8 All rights reserved.

ASSESSING LEARNING NEEDS

Assessing the learners is the most important aspect of planning when preparing for patient teaching. Nurses are expected to develop and carry out plans for patient teaching that will meet the patient's learning needs in a variety of clinical settings. The nurse in the hospital may be working with a newly diagnosed patient, or the community health nurse may be providing follow-up care for a chronically ill patient who is able to care for him or herself at home. In either setting the ability of the nurse to rapidly and accurately identify the individual's knowledge deficit in a very short time is essential for effective teaching.

A knowledge deficit is defined by Carpenito as "the state in which the individual experiences a deficiency in cognitive knowledge or psychomotor skills that alter or may alter health maintenance" (1983). Data are collected from the patient, family, the medical record, and other health care professionals. Carpenito (1983) guides data collection of both subjective and objective information that is used to determine a nursing diagnosis of "knowledge deficit" (Table 5-1).

The cause of the knowledge deficit should be established in order to properly plan for teaching and write the behavioral objectives. Carpenito (1983) refers to the causal events as etiological or contributing factors.

The contributing factors are divided by Carpenito into three general categories; pathophysiological, situational, and maturational (Table 5-1). Each of these factors must be assessed in order to get a complete picture of the patient's and family's knowledge deficit.

To assess the pathophysiological factors, the nurse will ask questions related to the client's new medical condition as well as any existing conditions. It is important not to assume that the person is managing a chronic illness well just because it was diagnosed many years ago and a treatment regiment was established. The nurse should begin to teach with a good understanding of what the patient knows in order to build upon previous knowledge, to avoid unnecessary duplication, and to present information that is at the patient's level of understanding. Questions such as, "How do you manage your diabetes when you are ill?" or "What changes do you make when you have a flare-up of your arthritis?" will give the nurse an idea of what the patient does to maintain control of an existing medical condition.

For a new condition, it is important to start with what the patient already has been told before giving new information. This can be done by talking with the patient and the physician, as well as the family. Many times a person's psychological reaction to being diagnosed with a chronic disease will make it difficult, if not impossible, to accurately understand the instructions that are being given. The physical effects of the condition itself, such as pain, weakness, or nausea, can further diminish the person's ability to concentrate on the information he or she is receiving. The nurse should consider the person's pathophysiological condition when making the assessment, as well as the situation.

Situational factors will often cause a knowledge deficit to occur. A situational factor can be any event, such as a prescribed medication, a diagnostic test or surgical procedure, that the person will need information about in order to cooperate with the treatment or test and achieve the best possible outcome. Whenever a patient is facing a new test or medical treatment information is needed about what to expect and the most likely response to the experience. Even a test that seems simple from the nurse's perception can

Table 5-1
Knowledge Deficit

Definition

Knowledge deficit: The state in which the individual experiences a deficiency in cognitive knowledge or psychomotor skills that alters or may alter health maintenance.

Etiological and contributing factors

A variety of factors can produce knowledge deficits. Some common causes are listed below.

Pathophysiological

Any existing or new medical condition

Situational

Language differences

Prescribed treatments (new, complex)

Diagnostic tests

Surgical procedures

Medications

Pregnancy

Personal characteristics

Lack of motivation

Denial of situation

Ineffective coping patterns (e.g., anxiety, depression)

Maturational

Children

Sexuality and sexual development

Safety hazards

Substance abuse

Nutrition

Adolescents

Same as children

Automobile safety practices

Substance abuse (alcohol, drugs, tobacco)

Health maintenance practices

Adults

Parenthood

Sexual function

Safety practices

Health maintenance practices

Elderly

Effects of aging

Sensory deficits

Defining characteristics

Verbalizes a deficiency in knowledge or skill

Expresses "inaccurate" perception of health status

Does not perform correctly a desired or prescribed health behavior

Does not comply (noncompliance) with prescribed health behavior

Exhibits or expresses psychological alteration (e.g., anxiety, depression) resulting from misinformation or lack of information.

From Carpenito, L. J. *Nursing diagnosis: application to clinical practice.* St. Louis: J. B. Lippincott Co., 1983. Used with permission.

cause patients to be worried and fearful if they do not understand what will happen. A new medication prescription is an obvious indication for patient teaching. It is important for the nurse to validate that patients understand all of their medications, even those they have taken over a long period of time. It is not uncommon to discover that patients are taking their medications at inappropriate times or that over-the-counter medicines are also being taken that interfere with the therapeutic effect of the prescribed drugs. These are only two examples of what the nurse might discover when the patient's medication use is assessed as part of determining the situational factors that affect their learning needs.

Even positive events, such as pregnancy, availability of new treatments, or acceptance of a donor organ, can lead to new learning needs. When a patient becomes pregnant many teaching needs arise; not only those related to the pregnancy itself, but also with regard to managing any existing chronic condition. For example, the insulin-dependent diabetic needs special care throughout her pregnancy to maintain control of the diabetes as well as deal with the many changes that the pregnancy will bring about. After the birth of the baby, more teaching is needed to prepare the new parents to care for the infant and to adjust to an addition to the family.

It is sometimes assumed that because a person with a chronic condition has been taught once about the disease and its treatment that they will be able to manage it with little teaching from the nurse or physician. Patients will need to be made aware of progress in treatment of their condition. For example, some diabetics will need information about how to manage the new insulin infusion pumps that are now available.

The assumption that people only need to be taught once does not take into account how an individual will vary in the ability to cope with the daily demands of life. Some people will do very well in maintaining control of their condition until they encounter excessive stressors at work or home. When this occurs they become unable to maintain the same control they previously had over their disease condition. They may temporarily lack motivation to continue their daily routines or may use denial to avoid the situation for a period of time. It is important that someone be able to assist the individual during these difficult times and help them re-establish their routines.

Maturational factors also need to be assessed because as individuals mature and reach different stages of life, their teaching needs change. Each different life stage is accompanied by developmental tasks and changing values that will affect a person's learning needs during that stage.

During the early years of life, great emphasis is placed on safety and development. Parents of young children need to be aware of the hazards that their children will encounter and how they can protect them from harm. Parenting is made easier when the parents understand each developmental stage as their children advance and what is to be expected as they go from one stage to the next. For example, diabetic adolescents will be expected to want to exercise their independence but will also have a great need to conform to the pressures from their peer group. For this reason they may disregard their diet restrictions in order to eat out with their friends. The nurse can be helpful to the parents of these adolescents by helping them understand their behavior. The nurse can also assist the adolescents to adjust a diet to accommodate the foods that they want to eat.

Developmental stages are not only limited to the young. As people continue to age, their developmental tasks change. The middle years are characterized by a need to be productive. The nurse planning to teach the young executive needs to consider how much time he or she will devote to personal needs versus career demands. For some individuals, their busy schedules will require some creative planning in order to allow time for management of their treatment. For example, the person with a colostomy needs to plan time in the day for managing the irrigation or emptying routine. The housewife with multiple sclerosis may need to plan for a nap each day to conserve energy.

The developmental tasks of the elderly shift from an emphasis on productivity to adjusting to retirement. Their physical capabilities generally begin to decline with advancing years and there is greater preoccupation with health and finances. While there may be new joys associated with grandparenting, there may also be loss of relationships as friends and spouses die. Rituals and habits provide stability and comfort but become more difficult to change. The adage that "you can't teach old dogs new tricks" has been dispelled through the writings of adult educators such as Malcolm Knowles (1973). Even though it is known that a person can learn at any age, the nurse who is teaching the elderly needs to be patient and understanding when trying to get people to learn new behaviors that will replace old habits.

The nurse should thoroughly assess the factors that contribute to the patient's need for information. At any point many factors may be present simultaneously. The nurse uses the information about pathophysiological, maturational, and situational factors to plan appropriate teaching for the patient.

At each maturational stage the nurse must adapt the teaching strategies to accommodate the developmental level of the client. For instance, the use of play and dolls can be very effective when teaching young children whose language skills are not well developed. Adolescents respond well to the nurse who emphasizes their opportunities for independence and self-care instead of ignoring the teenager and teaching only to the parents. Since middle-aged adults place more emphasis on the practicality of the situation, they will want to know how much time and money will be involved and how this will affect their other time demands. Teaching of the elderly can be very rewarding but the pace should be adjusted to that of the patient.

Defining characteristics are used by Carpenito (1983) to describe symptoms, signs, or other manifestations related to a specific nursing diagnosis (Table 5-1). When assessing that a knowledge deficit exists, the nurse needs to identify the defining characteristics that will validate each patient's learning need. Several possible defining characteristics or indicators of learning needs are included in Table 5-1. The learning need will be apparent when the patient says that he or she doesn't understand something. Families may also express concern about how they will manage their needs when the patient is dismissed from the hospital. Observing how a community manages after a health alert will provide valuable data for the teaching plan.

Another area to assess is the patient's compliance with their previous treatment plan and the current regimen. By determining the degree of compliance, the nurse may detect a knowledge deficit in those patients who fail to comply. It is inappropriate to assume that the patient does not want to cooperate until a thorough assessment of his or her understanding has been completed.

Some individuals will experience a psychological change when they are frightened or depressed about their condition. Their reaction may be justified in some circumstances, but it can also occur needlessly when the patient has a lack of information or misinformation. The fearful, anxious, or discouraged patient and family will need some counseling to alleviate these feelings before teaching can take place.

After describing pathophysiological, situational, and maturational factors that affect

Table 5-2
Focus Assessment Criteria. This assessment is structured primarily
to collect data to determine the person's learning capabilities
and limitations.

Subjective data
1. Determine present knowledge of illness

Severity	Susceptibility to complications
Prognosis	Ability to cure it or control its progression

   Treatment
   Preventive measures
2. What is the pattern of adhering to prescribed health behaviors?

Complete	Not adhering
Modified	

3. What is interfering with adherence to the prescribed health behavior?
4. History of disease
   Onset
   Symptoms
   Effects on lifestyle (relationships, work, leisure activities, finances)
5. Stage of adaptation to disease

Disbelief	Anger
Denial	Awareness
Depression	Acceptance

6. Learning needs (perceived by client, family)
7. Learning ability (client, family)

Level of education	Language spoken
Ability to read	Language understood

8. Ethnic background

Traditions	Health care beliefs and practices
Lifestyle	

Objective data
1. Ability to perform prescribed procedures

Competency	Accuracy

2. Level of cognitive and psychomotor development

Age	Ability to read and write

3. Presence of sensory deficits
   Vision

Problems in focusing	Partial or total blindness
Inability to distinguish colors	

   Hearing

Partial or total deafness	Tinnitus

   Sense of smell (altered or lost)
   Sense of taste (altered or lost)
   Sense of touch

Anesthesia	Paresthesia

4. Physical stability
   a. Circulation/tissue perfusion
      General appearance
      Arterial blood pressure
      Pulse rate and regularity
      Pulse volume (weak, thready, full, bounding)
      Skin (color, temperature, moisture)
      Urine output
      Level of consciousness

Table 5-2 (*Continued*)

---

   b. Respiratory status
       Rate
       Pattern
       Presence of abnormal breath sounds
       Altered blood gases
       Restlessness
       Irritability
   c. Nutritional/hydration status
       Fluid and electrolyte balance (Na, K, urine specific gravity, skin turgor)
       Intake and output
       Weight change
   d. Activity tolerance (good, fair, poor; see *Activity Intolerance* for additional assessment criteria)

---

*From Carpenito, L. J. *Nursing Diagnosis: application to clinical practice.* St. Louis: J. B. Lippincott Co., 1983. Used with permission.

the need for learning, Carpenito identifies focus assessment criteria that are used to collect data to determine the person's learning capabilities and limitations. Important subjective and objective data are outlined in Table 5-2 that will guide accurate assessment for any special considerations to be incorporated into your teaching plan.

PLANNING FOR
THE LEARNING DOMAINS

The overall goals of teaching are to increase knowledge, improve attitudes, develop manual skills, and enhance perceptual abilities. Each of these four aspects of learning can be considered a separate domain or field of learning activity. It is important that nurses consider all four domains when planning any teaching, so that the objectives that are formulated cover all aspects of learning.

Domains of Learning

Cognitive domain
   Knowledge comprehension
   Reasoning
   Processing and recall of information

Psychomotor domain
   Performance
   Skilled movements
   Motor function

Affective domain
   Feelings
   Values
   Attitudes

Perceptual domain
   Awareness
   Comprehension of symbols
   Comprehension of meaning

For some patients, the goal will be to increase the individual's knowledge. Information about medications, disease processes, surgical procedures, treatments, etc., would be related to the cognitive domain, which deals with recall or recognition of information and intellectual skills. The area of learning that involves the development of manual skills is called the psychomotor domain. Learning a new skill or perfecting an old one involves both the understanding of what is to be done and also how to do it. When nurses teach patients new skills, such as how to take care of a catheter at home or how to clean a surgical incision, the patient is learning manual skills. These patients need to learn the psychomotor function to be able to carry out the desired procedure. Psychomotor learning objectives thus must be written to guide this teaching.

There are two other important areas of learning in addition to the cognitive and psychomotor domains already named. These areas are affective and perceptive in nature. Affective learning involves changing beliefs, values, or attitudes in order to bring about new behavior on the part of the learner.

Nurses must be alert to the patients' attitudes so they can influence them to feel positive about all the changes they must learn to make. A very important goal of teaching then is to positively influence individual and family attitudes. Often this affective learning must take place before any cognitive or psychomotor teaching can be effective.

The fourth domain deals with perception, which is one of the most important in order for learning to take place. Perception of sensations of sight, sound, and touch as well as the ability to find meaning in symbols and figures. Perceptive learning is necessary to process information correctly so that cognitive and psychomotor learning can take place. All four areas of learning mentioned will be discussed in greater detail under domains of learning later in this chapter. They are presented initially as an overview to writing learner objectives.

LEARNER OBJECTIVES

Preparing learner objectives is an important part of the teaching process. An objective is a written statement that describes in measurable terms what the patient, family, or group are to learn. Some objectives a nurse might use in patient teaching are listed according to the learning domain for which they were written. It is rare that objectives are written for the perceptive domain as problems in this area of learning must be dealt with before teaching begins.

Psychomotor. The patient will demonstrate self-catheterization, using aseptic technique.
Cognitive. The mother will describe three ways to reduce sibling rivalry.
Affective. The member shares positive opinions about the drug rehabilitation center in community discussion group.

Well-written objectives provide the teacher with many cues to teaching, and direction, as well as outline what the learner will need to do. After the objectives have been written, the rest of the teaching plan can be constructed. The objectives will help in the selection of teaching strategies and methods as well as the content.

There is some controversy as to what is to be written first, the objectives or the content outline. Some teachers prepare the content outline first and then write objectives to divide the content into manageable sections. Others write the objectives first and then prepare the content outline. In most situations it doesn't matter which is written first as long as the objectives and content are directly related.

Measurable objectives are valuable because without them it is very difficult to know what the patient is supposed to learn or to measure the success of the teaching. If the objectives are written in measurable form they will provide the structure for evaluating learning. It has been said in favor of writing objectives, "If you don't know where you are going, you're likely to end up somewhere else!" Writing objectives provide an overview of the entire teaching plan and what is to be accomplished by the learner. In addition, clear objectives that are written on the nursing care plan will allow all members of the health care team to be involved in the teaching. This is of particular importance when there are many persons involved in caring for an individual patient.

Components of Written Objectives

Written objective statements correctly is a challenge that requires practice. A well written objective concisely communicates both what (content) is to be learned and how (action) it will be evaluated. Thus there are two essential components to every objective: an action word (verb and a phrase about the content. The verb used must be specific enough to measure or determine if the behavior described in the objective was accomplished or not. Each objective should describe information to be learned (content) or what the learner is expected to know at the end of the teaching.

Keep in mind that all teaching objectives describe what the learner is expected to do and not what the teacher will do. It is incorrect to have an objective such as "Teach the patient how to administer own insulin," since that describes the nurse's behavior and not the patient's.

In order to measure what the learner knows, the teacher must observe for the specific measurable behaviors or action. For example, if you wanted the patient to know what foods were allowed in a prescribed diet, he or she would have to either name them or select appropriate choices from a list or menu. The verb that is selected for each objective will determine how measurable the behavior will be.

Words such as "understand" or "know" are sometimes used in objectives but they are not specific terms and cannot be measured.

Words to Avoid in Objectives

know	be able to
understand	believe
be familiar with	be interested in
appreciate	enjoy
realize	value
think	feel
internalize	have faith in

How do you know if someone "understands" how to give themselves insulin? The patient could simply say, "Yes, I understand," but never demonstrate the knowledge. It would be better to write "The patient will administer insulin daily." Then to meet the objective the patient must actually administer the insulin. The verb in this objective is "administer." This is measurable by observing the patient giving his or her own injection.

The phrase in the objective describing the content can be very brief or elaborate if detail is necessary for the learner. For example, "Discuss the heart" is quite vague and even though it would be measurable, it is difficult to know what discussion is expected of the learner. It would be better to write, "Discuss how exercise improves circulation through the heart." More about selecting appropriate verbs and content phrases will be discussed under the domains of learning.

Optional Components of
Written Objectives

All objectives should contain a verb and a statement of content. It is also possible to add additional components to an objective that would make it clearer or easier to evaluate. The optional components include a description of the learner, the conditions of evaluation, and a standard of performance.

In most objectives it is not necessary to state who the learner is if that individual is obvious. If several objectives all refer to the same learner it becomes redundant to continually write "The learner will . . ." at the beginning of every objective. Instead, you can write an introductory statement that says, "At the conclusion of the lesson, the learner will do the following" and then follow with the list of objectives, each starting with the desired verb.

When teaching more than one learner, such as a husband and wife, then it becomes necessary to describe each person's expected behavior. For example, the husband may be a diabetic patient who has recently been ordered to take daily insulin. The husband's objectives may relate to the technique of insulin injection, such as "Patient (husband) will describe rotation of sites for insulin injection." An objective for the wife might be "Patient's wife will describe how to modify cooking to conform to the diabetic diet."

The conditions of evaluation and a standard of performance can also be objectives describing complicated tasks or learning situations. The conditions of evaluation describe in detail how the learner will demonstrate that the objective has been met. The statement of performance indicates how well the learner must perform in order to determine that the objective has been achieved.

For example, the objective could read, "Given a menu from a restaurant, the patient will correctly select food that is within the diabetic diet." The statement given of a menu indicates how the patient is expected to demonstrate that knowledge of the foods that are acceptable for a diabetic's diet restrictions. The word "correctly" indicates that he or she is expected to make only acceptable selections from the menu. Anything less would indicate that he or she has not performed to the acceptable standard. Some objectives will specify other standards of performance, such as "three out of four" or "with 100 percent accuracy."

The style of objective that includes conditions of evaluation and performance standards was developed by Robert Mager (1975) and is referred to as a "four-part objective." The opponents to this style of objective believe that by describing the behavior so specifically you limit any possibility of spontaneity on the part of the teacher and learner. It also takes more effort to write the more lengthy objective. For this reason more people seem to choose the simpler form of objective, with only the two essential components of verb and content phrase.

If it is your choice to write the shorter objective it is still a good idea to continually ask yourself as you prepare objectives, "How will I evaluate that the learner has accomplished this behavior?" If the behavior cannot be evaluated the way it is written, choose a more specific verb.

When preparing for teaching, several objectives are needed to describe the desired learned behaviors. Some authors suggest that one write a main objective, sometimes called a learning goal, that is followed by many subobjectives. This is an acceptable method and can be very useful for structuring the teaching plan.

Sample objectives related to teaching diabetic patients are provided in Table 5-3. The essential components have been identified for each objective. Some objectives that contain errors along with a corrected version are included in the table.

Common Errors in Writing Objectives

Whether you are new or experienced at writing objectives there are some common errors to avoid. You want to include only one verb in each objective so that you can measure the learner's behavior accurately. If two different behaviors are described it would be possible for the learner to accomplish one and not the other. If you have an objective that states, "Select foods within the diabetic diet and keep a diary of intake," you have included two different behaviors. The first desired behavior is that the patient can "select" acceptable foods and the second behavior is that the patient will "keep" a diary of the foods eaten. Two separate objectives should be written so that each behavior can be evaluated individually.

Another common error is the habit of writing objectives with double verbs, such as "compare and contrast. . ." or "list and describe. . . ." It is not necessary to have both verbs included because both behaviors can be incorporated into the more complex behavior. For example, in order to "contrast" something you would first need to "compare" it to the other item. The same is true for "describing" something, since you would be listing the items at the same time you were describing them. Only the latter word needs to appear in the objective. For example, stating "The patient will describe the symptoms of an insulin reaction" is better form than "list and describe the symptoms. . . ."

In addition to the errors of word choice mentioned above, there is another common error of format; the "be able to" syndrome. Some writers of objectives will begin each objective with the phrase, be able to, such as "The patient will be able to measure his or her blood glucose." Although this is certainly a desirable behavior, being "able to" does not mean that the person will actually do the behavior that was identified. There is a difference in knowing how to (being able to) test one's blood glucose and actually performing the finger stick four times a day. Keep these errors in mind when writing objectives for the various learning domains (Table 5-3).

Writing Objectives Related to Knowledge Deficits of Learners

When the nurse-teacher begins to write patient teaching objectives, several factors that affect learning need to be considered. The factors that need to be assessed relate to personal, physical, and socioeconomic variables and the basic cause of the learner's knowledge deficit (Pokorny, 1985).

Personal factors include such things as intelligence, developmental level, mental state, past experience with the same or a similar situation, and perceived threat or benefit of taking action. The nurse needs information about each of these areas in order to develop the appropriate level of learning objectives.

Table 5-3
Examples of Objectives

INCORRECT →	The *patient will* ‾learner	*understand* ‾non-measurable verb	*diabetic insulin reaction.* ‾content		
CORRECT →	The *patient will* ‾learner	*describe* ‾measurable verb	*what to do if an insulin reaction occurs.* ‾content		
INCORRECT →	(Be able to) Omit	*name* ‾measurable verb	*the parts of a syringe.* ‾content		
CORRECT →	*Name* ‾measurable verb	*the parts of a syringe.* ‾content			
INCORRECT →	*Appreciate* ‾non-measurable verb	*the benefit of dieting.* ‾content			
CORRECT →	*List* ‾measurable verb	*five* ‾evaluation standard	*benefits of dieting.* ‾content		
INCORRECT →	Teach the patient to administer own insulin. (This is a teacher goal, not a learner objective.)				
CORRECT →	The *patient will* ‾learner	*correctly* ‾standard of measurable performance verb	*measure* ‾verb	*his daily insulin* (under the supervision of the nurse). ‾content	‾conditions of evaluation
INCORRECT →	*List and describe* ‾double verb	*the side effects of each take home drug.* ‾content			
CORRECT →	*Describe* ‾measurable verb	*the side effects of each take home drug.* ‾content			

‾Optional components.

Knowledge Deficit Related to Illiteracy

It is possible for people to complete their formal schooling and still be functionally illiterate. lcNeal (1984) reports that less than 20 percent of the adult population reads at the 5th grade level, and the median literacy level of the U.S. population is approximately 10th grade. In her study, McNeal found that the teaching materials commonly used for diabetic patients ranged from 5.3 to 14.1 grade-level difficulty. A mismatch of written material with the patient's reading ability can account for unsuccessful learning for the patient.

Not only should the printed word be at an appropriate level for the patient to understand, but also the vocabulary used by the nurse. Petrello (1976) conducted a study about how well the patients understood nurses' instructions and teaching. Not one patient in the study could correctly define all of the words or abbreviations used by nurses. The survey was made of 200 hospitalized adults, 50 percent of them high school graduates and 14 percent college graduates. Of the group, 21 percent had some college and 15 percent had only 4–12 years of schooling. Results of that survey indicated that common "nurse words" were not understood by patients. Words such as "hematoma," "secretions," and "post-op" were incorrectly defined by a large majority of those surveyed (see Table 5-4). How often do nurses use those words in their teaching and assume that the patient understands what they mean?

Knowledge Deficit Related to Psychological State (Anxiety)

Another personal factor that can make a tremendous difference in patients' readiness to learn is their mental state or psychological response to their experiences. A patient who has just learned of the diagnosis is usually preoccupied with the impact of that message and not able to accurately process the information that follows. A mother who is told that her child has asthma may be so involved with thinking about what that means she might not be paying attention when the doctor proceeds to explain how to give the asthma medications. When the nurse comes in later, or sees the mother on a return visit, it is important to verify what the mother recalls and that she has the correct information.

Much has been written about anxiety and how it affects people's perceptions and behavior. Peplau (1963) described four levels of anxiety and how the individual is affected in each level. According to Peplau, people who are in moderate to severe anxiety focus on immediate concerns and tend to block out the periphery. They are unable to perceive their environment accurately due to distortion of their perceptual field. This means they are able to see, hear, and grasp less of what is happening around them. Consequently, the messages that are being given when the patient is moderately anxious are often distorted and the patient does not learn what was intended. Many times nurses have discussed the patient who was "taught" repeatedly by the staff and yet has not "learned."

When a person is in a true panic state, no learning is possible at all. Patients must first be helped to reduce their anxiety before the teaching can proceed. It might be that the patient is overanxious or in a state of denial. Whatever the cause, the mental state must be improved before that patient will be able to attend to the learning.

Past experience is another personal factor that influences how the patient learns. If past experiences were positive and the patient learned successful coping methods, there is

Table 5-4
Which Common Clinical Words Puzzle Patients?˙

Words	Correct	Partially correct	Incorrect	Do not know
Abscess	40%	21%	28%	9%
Acute	22	41	34	2
Allergic	96	—	4	—
Anesthesia	89	5	5	—
Bacteria	71	6	19	3
Benign	51	—	24	24
Biopsy	71	4	11	13
Bladder	59	—	39	1
Blood pressure	11	12	71	5
Blood sugar	59	6	23	11
Bowel	40	—	53	6
Buttock	94	—	4	1
Coma	77	—	22	—
Compress	38	31	26	3
Culture	28	48	14	9
Dehydrated	75	3	16	4
Dislocated	76	11	11	1
Elimination	47	2	28	22
Fasting	47	7	34	11
Gastric	42	—	35	23
Germs	57	21	21	—
Hallucination	64	2	29	4
Hematocrit	17	8	6	67
Hematoma	4	21	18	55
Hemorrhage	50	26	21	2
Immunization	76	1	14	8
Impaction	24	9	31	35
Inhalation	64	10	10	15
Intestines	73	5	18	3
Orally	87	—	12	1
Physical therapy	72	24	3	1
Secretions	9	12	51	27
Specimen	72	—	27	—
Spinal	83	—	15	1
Suction	41	11	13	34
Tendon	8	5	79	7
Therapy	70	22	6	—
Traction	19	38	41	1
Urine	79	5	15	—
Vitamin	22	28	48	1
Abbreviations				
CC	64	14	7	14
ECG	67	7	13	12
I&O	13	4	12	70
I.V.	93	1	2	4
OR	78	—	5	16

Table 5-4 (*Continued*)

Words	Correct	Partially correct	Incorrect	Do not know
PO	21	—	17	61
Post-op	50	—	33	17
Prep	85	—	11	3
PT	79	3	7	10
TPR	21	44	12	22

˙From Petrello, J. Your patients hear you, but do they understand? *RN*, 1976, 39, 37–39.
Hospitalized patients' lack of understanding of clinical terms used by nurses is shown by the percentages in this table. The study included 200 adults, 50% of them high school graduates, 14% college graduates, 21% with some college training, and 15% with only 4 to 12 years of schooling. The terms were randomly selected from a list of 92 words and 26 abbreviations frequently used by staff nurses in talking to patients.
Fractional percentages are omitted, so the cumulative figures do not equal 100%.

a greater likelihood that the current learning experience will also be a positive one. If the patient or family is recalling a past experience that was not positive, then the nurse might encounter resistance to learning. However, counseling techniques, such as reminiscing, can be used to guide the family in re-evaluating past experiences that were negative. Affective objectives can be written to guide such activities.

Knowledge Deficit Related to Health Beliefs

The last personal factor to be discussed is the individual's perceived threat or benefit of taking steps to improve one's health. Many such beliefs stem from the communities or societal beliefs. A health belief model predicts why some people are more likely to behave in a way that fosters good health. This model was described by Rosenstock in 1974. It was the subject of a research study by DiMatteo and DiDicola (1982), which hypothesized that people seek and comply with health care practices only under certain circumstances.

Use of the health belief model enables the nurse to structure the teaching to include what the patient is likely to perceive as the threat or benefit associated with certain health practices. For example, a young woman whose mother and two sisters have had breast cancer is more likely to perceive that she is at risk and perform breast self exam than a woman who is not related to someone with this type of cancer. Janice Hallal (1982) conducted a research study that supported the hypothesis that providing information about breast self exam may not produce a change in behavior. If the woman does not perceive that this activity will be of some benefit or if she doesn't feel threatened by the possibility of developing cancer, she may need affective teaching first.

Knowledge Deficit Related to Patient's Physiologic State

Physical factors also play a significant part in the patient's knowledge deficit. These factors may include the presence of acute illness or pain, fluid and electrolyte imbalances, altered nutritional status, lack of endurance, or medications; each of which can alter mental alertness. Other physical factors related to treatments may also interfere with motor abilities and learning.

It should be obvious that an individual in acute pain will not be able to concentrate

on learning new information. If the pain is not relieved, the patient will be so preoccupied with discomfort that he or she will be unable to attend to the information the
nurse or physician is sharing with them. After receiving pain controlling medications the
patient will most likely be groggy and not alert enough to process new information. Some
analgesics will provide the patient with much needed sleep but, at the same time, render
him or her unable to think clearly. In this case, the teaching needs to be carefully timed
between episodes of pain and the hypnotic effect of the analgesics.

Certain electrolyte and nutritional states will also alter the patient's cognitive functioning. The patient may be confused or hallucinatory, or simply too weak to be able to
devote the necessary energy to learning. After the electrolyte imbalance has been corrected, the patient will be better able to concentrate and learn.

If the patient's activity tolerance is significantly limited he or she will find it difficult
to master the needed learning. Patients may lack the physical energy to perform a
psychomotor task, such as a dressing change, or they may lack the mental energy to
concentrate on learning.

Any equipment that is attached to the patient and that restricts movement may be
an additional inhibiting factor. Simply having the intravenous needle placed in the
dominant hand may make even the most simple task difficult, if not impossible. When
patients are encumbered with traction, or other mechanical devices, they are not free to
move about and perform certain self-care procedures, even if they are motivated to do so.
Arthritic changes with advancing age may make fingers less functional for fine motor
tasks. The tactile perception in the elderly may also be reduced so manipulation of small
objects, such as an insulin syringe, can become very frustrating. Nurses must determine
any physical changes that might hamper learning and take steps to alleviate these barriers
when teaching patients and families.

Knowledge Deficit Related to Cultural/Socioeconomic Factors

Socioeconomic and cultural factors may also influence the patient's response to
teaching. These factors can include a language barrier, alternate life style, financial
status, cultural background as related to health practices, and transportation.

The following actual patient example is used to illustrate how several of these factors
influence learning. A woman from India came to the United States for surgical treatment
of an intestinal cancer. The surgeon performed a transverse colostomy and the patient
recovered very well. The nurses, however, were very frustrated because she refused to
take any interest in the colostomy or perform any of the needed care. One nurse discovered through the son's interpretation that in their culture servants attend to the
bodily needs of women of his mother's social status. Thus, the patient had a personal
servant at home who bathed her, combed her hair, and dressed her. The patient expected
that the servant would also take care of the colostomy when she returned to her own
country. For this reason, she felt no need to learn how to manage the colostomy herself,
since she would rely on the servant for this personal service as she did for all others. Once
the nurse realized that the woman felt no need to learn about her colostomy, she turned
her attention to teaching the son, who in turn could instruct the servant. The son
learned quickly and the woman was dismissed to return home a short time later. This
situation illustrates how important it is to consider all of the available information before
begining to do patient teaching.

Knowledge Deficit Related to Readiness to Learn

The most carefully planned teaching will not be effective when the patient is not ready or not motivated to learn or when barriers prevent the patient from learning at a specific time. Nurses who recognize that the patient has a knowledge deficit must carefully determine the appropriate time to teach. Sometimes referred to as "teachable moments," this important time needs to be used to the best advantage. Unfortunately, some nurses do not heed patients' cues that indicate their readiness to learn. Instead, they teach when they have the time, whether the patient is ready or not. When the patient does not learn, or "change their behavior," the nurse becomes frustrated and discouraged because the patient is viewed as uncooperative or difficult to teach. Instead of taking this viewpoint, it is more desirable to determine when the patient is ready and examine the factors that may impede learning.

Knowledge Deficit Related to Domains of Learning

The domains of learning were introduced earlier in the chapter. The three commonly accepted domains of learning are: cognitive, affective, and psychomotor. A fourth domain, called perceptual, has been developed but it is not as widely used as the first three [see page 129]. Not only must the nurse teach in the appropriate domain but also at the appropriate level for the knowledge deficit of the patient, family, or community.

The term "domain" is used to describe a specific sphere of learning. Each learning domain is divided into different levels of behavior, from the simplest to the most complex. The levels of behavior are referred to as a taxonomy because they classify the degree of difficulty in learning. The domains have between five to seven taxonomy levels that are further subdivided to be even more specific. Tables 5-5 through 5-8 show how each of the domains have been divided into multiple levels or taxonomies.

The numbering system developed by the originators of the domains has been included in these tables. Even though nurses rarely attach the code numbers to their patient-teaching objectives, this numbering system may be encountered in the literature. The domains are commonly abbreviated with the first letter of each title (i.e., "C" for the cognitive domain, "A" for affective, and "P" for psychomotor) followed by the corresponding number of the taxonomy level. For example, the analysis level of the cognitive domain could be labeled as "C 4.00".

For the nurse doing occasional teaching it is not necessary to become an expert in leveling, particularly in regard to the subdivisions of taxonomies. It is sufficient to be aware of the various domains, how they can be used to construct appropriate objectives for patient teaching, and how the domains are identified by using an alphabet and numbering system. For this reason, the amount of information presented here about the domains is limited to what nurses commonly would use. For more details, consult the sources named.

When using the taxonomies to construct objectives, first determine what level the learner is expected to function, and then select a verb that represents that level. It is a little like going up a flight of stairs: select the word that describes the highest step or level of learning to be achieved. It is understood that in order to reach the fourth step, for instance, one would have first traversed steps one through three. The "stair-steps" for the first three domains are represented in Tables 5-9 through 5-11.

Table 5-5
Cognitive Domain˙

1.00 Knowledge

    Knowledge, as defined here, involves recall or remembering of information.

    1.10 Knowledge of specifics

        1.11 Knowledge of terminology

        1.12 Knowledge of specific facts

    1.20 Knowledge of ways and means of dealing with specifics

        1.21 Knowledge of conventions (characteristic ways of treating and presenting ideas and phenomena)

        1.22 Knowledge of trends and sequences

        1.23 Knowledge of classifications and categories

        1.24 Knowledge of criteria

        1.25 Knowledge of methodology

    1.30 Knowledge of the universals and abstractions in a field

        1.31 Knowledge of principles and generalizations

        1.32 Knowledge of theories and structures

2.00 Comprehension

    This represents the lowest level of understanding. It refers to a type of understanding . . . such that the individual knows what is being communicated and can make use of the material or idea being communicated without necessarily relating it to other material or seeing its fullest implications.

    2.10 Translation

        Comprehension as evidenced by the care and accuracy with which the communication is paraphrased or rendered from one language or form of communication to another. Translation is judged on the basis of faithfulness and accuracy, that is, on the extent to which the material in the original communication is preserved although the form of the communication has been altered.

    2.20 Interpretation

        The explanation or summarization of a communication. Whereas translation involves an objective part-for-part rendering of a communication, interpretation involves a reordering, rearrangement, or new view of the material.

    2.30 Extrapolation

        The extension of trends or tendencies beyond the given data to determine implications, consequences, corollaries, effects, and so forth which are in accordance with the conditions described in the original communication.

3.00 Application

    The use of abstractions in particular and concrete situations. The abstractions may be in the form of general ideas, rules of procedures, or generalized methods. The abstractions may also be technical principles, ideas, and theories, which must be remembered and applied.

4.00 Analysis

    The breakdown of a communication into its constituent elements or parts such that the relative hierarchy of ideas is made clear or the relations between the ideas expressed are made explicit or both. Such analyses are intended to clarify the communication, to indicate how the communication is organized and the way in which it manages to convey its effects, as well as to indicate its basis and arrangement.

    4.10 Analysis of elements

        Identification of the elements included in a communication.

Table 5-5 (*Continued*)

4.20 Analysis of relationships
Identification of the connections and interactions between elements and parts of a communication.

4.30 Analysis of organizational principles
Identification of the organization, systematic arrangement, and structure which hold the communication together. This includes the "explicit" as well as "implicit" structure. It includes the bases, necessary arrangement, and mechanics which make the communication a unit.

5.00 Synthesis
The putting together of elements and parts to form a whole. This involves the process of working with pieces, parts, elements, and so forth and arranging and combining them in such a way so as to constitute a pattern or structure not clearly present before.

5.10 Production of a unique communication
The development of a communication in which the writer or speaker attempts to convey ideas, feelings, or experiences or all three to others.

5.20 Production of a plan, or proposed set of operations
The development of a plan of work or the proposal of a plan of operations. The plan should satisfy the requirements of a task that may be given to the student or that he may develop for himself.

5.30 Derivation of a set of abstract relations
The development of a set of abstract relations either to classify or explain particular data or phenomena, or the deduction of propositions and relations from a set of basic propositions or symbolic representations.

6.00 Evaluation
Judgments about the value of material and methods for given purposes: quantitative and qualitative judgments about the extent to which material and methods satisfy criteria; use of a standard appraisal. The criteria may be determined by the student or given to hm.

6.10 Judgments in terms of internal evidence
Evaluation of the accuracy of a communication from such evidence as logical accuracy, consistency, and other internal criteria.

6.20 Judgments in terms of external criteria
Evaluation of material with reference to selected or remembered criteria.˙

Bloom, B. S., Englehart, M. D., Furst, E. J., Hill, W. H., and Krathwohl, D. R. Adapted from *Taxonomy of educational objectives: the classification of educational goals: handbook I: cognitive domain.* Longman Inc., 1956. With permission.

THE LEARNING DOMAINS
AND THEIR TAXONOMY LEVELS
The Cognitive Domain

The cognitive domain was the first one to be described. It was the work of Benjamin Bloom and a group of psychologists tha began in the 1940s (Bloom, Englehart, Furst, Hill, and Krathwohl, 1956). The cognitive domain describes knowledge, comprehension, and thinking skills. It begins with the simplest cognitive level, called knowledge, and progresses through comprehension, application, analysis, synthesis, and evaluation (see Table 5-5). These levels denote that in order to perform a higher cognitive function, such as "application," all of the preceding ones must have first taken place. For example,

Table 5-6
Affective Domain˙

1.00 Receiving (attending)
    1.10 Awareness
        Awareness is almost a cognitive behavior. But unlike knowledge, the lowest level of
        the cognitive domain, awareness is not so much concerned with a memory of or
        ability to recall an item or fact as with the phenomen that, given an appropriate
        opportunity, the learner will merely be conscious of something—that he will take
        into account a situation, fact or event, object, or stage of affairs.
    1.20 Willingness to receive
        At a minimum level we are here describing the behavior of being willing to tolerate
        a given stimulus, not to avoid it.
    1.30 Controlled or selected attention
        There is an element of the learner's controlling the attention here, so that the
        favored stimulus is selected and attended to despite competing and distracting
        stimuli.
2.00 Responding
    2.10 Acquiescence in responding
        The student makes the response, but he has not fully accepted the necessity for
        doing so.
    2.20 Willingness to respond
        There is the implication that the learner is sufficiently committed to exhibiting a
        behavior so that he does so not just because of a fear of punishment, but "on his
        own" or voluntarily.
    2.30 Satisfaction in response
        Behavior is accompanied by a feeling of satisfaction, an emotional response,
        generally of pleasure, zest, or enjoyment.
3.00 Valuing
    3.10 Acceptance of a value
        The learner is sufficiently consistent that others can identify the value and
        sufficiently committed that he is willing to be so identified, but there is more of a
        readiness here to reevaluate his position than would be present at higher levels of
        valuing.
    3.20 Preference for a value
        Behavior at this level implies not just the acceptance of a value to the point of
        being willing to be identified with it, but more, a seeking it out and wanting it.
    3.30 Commitment
        Belief at this level involves a high degree of certainty. There is a real motivation to
        act out the behavior.
4.00 Organization
    4.10 Conceptualization of a value
        At this level the quality of abstraction or conceptualization is added. It permits the
        individual to see how the value relates to those that he already holds or to new ones
        that he is coming to hold.
    4.20 Organization of a value system
        Objectives properly classified here are those that require the learner to bring
        together a complex of values, possibly disparate values, and to relate them in an
        ordered fashion with one another. Ideally, the ordered relationship will be one
        which is harmonious and internally consistent.

5.00 Characterization by a value or value complex
    5.10 Generalized set
        A generalized set is a basic orientation that enables the individual to reduce and
        order the complex world about him and to act consistently and effectively in it. The
        generalized set may be thought of as closely related to the idea of an attitude
        cluster.
    5.20 Characterization
        Here are found those objectives that concern the individual's view of the universe,
        his philosophy of life . . . a value system having as its object the whole of what is
        known or knowable.˙

Krathwohl, D. R. *Taxonomy of educational objectives: the classification of educational goals: handbook II: affective domain.* With permission Longman Inc., 1964.

a patient who is functioning at the application level would be able to adjust his or her insulin dosage to accommodate for variations of blood glucose. In order to do this, the patient would first need the knowledge of what insulin is, comprehend the relationship between insulin and blood glucose, and then be able to apply this information to select the appropriate dose.

Examples of verbs that are appropriate for each level of the taxonomy in the cognitive domain are found in Table 5-9.

The Affective Domain

The affective domain also attributed to Bloom and two other associates, Krathwohl and Masia (Krathwohl, Bloom, and Masia, 1964), was introduced in 1948 and appeared in print 8 years later. This learning domain deals with states of feeling and valuing. Behavior is organized related to interests, attitudes, appreciation, and values. The categories of this domain begin with receiving and proceed through responding, valuing, organization, and value complex. If these categories of terms seem an unusual way to describe learning behavior, use Table 5-6 to familiarize yourself with the descriptions of the taxonomy levels. A patient must first "receive" information to learn it. In other words, patients must be interested, have a positive attitude, and eventually "value" the newly learned material so they will indeed act accordingly.

The steps in Table 5-10 provide some examples of acceptable verbs that can be used for writing objectives in the affective domain.

The Psychomotor Domain

The psychomotor domain was added in the early 1970s, several years after the cognitive and affective domains were introduced. The psychomotor domain is associated with physical or motor skills, and the level of behavior necessary to master a specific skill. The taxonomy prepared by Simpson (1972) is included in this text because it seems to be the most applicable for patient teaching. Other authors of psychomotor domains include, Dave (1970), Harrow (1972), and Tuckman (1972).

The categories for the various levels within the psychomotor domain developed by Simpson (1972) begin with perception and proceed through set, guided response, mechanism, complex overt response, adaptation, and origination. Table 5-7 describes each of these in detail. For the patient who is learning a new skill, or perfecting an old one, the

Table 5-7
Psychomotor Domain: A Tentative System*

1.00 Perception
 Process of becoming aware of objects, qualities, or relations by way of the sense organs.
    1.10 Sensory stimulation
     Impingement of a stimulus(i) on one or more of the sense organs.
        1.11 Auditory
        1.12 Visual
        1.13 Tactile
        1.14 Taste
        1.15 Smell
        1.16 Kinesethetic
    1.20 Cue Selection
     Identification of the cue or cues, association of them with the task to be performed,
     and grouping of them in terms of past experience and knowledge. Cues relevant to
     the situation are selected as a guide to action; irrelevant cues are ignored or
     discarded.
    1.30 Translation
     The mental process of determining the meaning of the cues received for action. It
     involves symbolic translation, that is, having an image or being reminded of
     something, "having an idea," as a result of cues received; insight; sensory
     translation; and "feedback."
2.00 Set
 A preparatory adjustment or readiness for a particular kind of action or experience.
    2.10 Mental set
     Readiness, in the mental sense, to perform a certain motor act. This involves, as
     prerequisite, the level of perception already identified. Discrimination, using
     judgments in making distinctions, is an aspect.
    2.20 Physical set
     Readiness in the sense of having made the anatomic adjustments necessary for a
     motor act to be performed, including sensory attending and posturing of the body.
    2.30 Emotional set
     Readiness in terms of attitudes favorable to the motor act's taking place.
3.00 Guided response
 The overt behavioral act of an individual under the guidance of the instructor.
 Prerequisite to performance of the act are readiness to respond and selection of the
 appropriate response.
    3.10 Imitation
     The execution of an act as a direct response to the perception of another person
     performing the act.
    3.20 Trial and error
     Trying various responses, usually with some rationale for each response, until an
     appropriate response is achieved.
4.00 Mechanism
 Learned response has become habitual. The learner has achieved a certain confidence and
 degree of skill. The act is a part of his repertoire of possible responses to stimuli and to
 the demands of situations where the response is an appropriate one. The response may be
 more complex than at the preceding level; it may involve some patterning of response in
 carrying out the task.
5.00 Complex overt response
 Performance of a motor act that is considered complex because of the movement pattern

required. A high degree of skill has been attained, and the act can be carried out with minimum expenditude of time and energy.

5.10 Resolution of uncertainty

Performance of a complex act without hesitation.

5.20 Automatic performance

Performance of finely coordinated motor skill with a great deal of ease and muscle control.

6.00 Adaptation

Altering motor activities to meet the demands of new problematic situations requiring a physical response.

7.00 Origination

Creating new motor acts or ways of manipulating materials out of understandings, abilities, and skills developed in the psychomotor area. [*]

---

[*]Adapted from Simpson, E. J.: The classification of educational objectives in the psychomotor domain. In *Contributions of behavioral science to instructional technology: the psychomotor domain.* Mt. Rainier, MD, 1972. Gryphon Press.

nurse needs to determine what level of behavior will be expected and write the objective accordingly. If the patient is learning to self-administer insulin for the first time, the level of the objective will most likely be "guided response," as in the following example "The patient will imitate the nurse's injection technique into the practice pad." This level implies that the patient is guided through the skill rather than be expected to perform it alone. The next higher level would be "mechanism," where the patient is able to carry out the skill alone and the nurse observes for breaks in technique and reinforces correct procedure.

Samples of verbs that can be selected for the levels of the psychomotor domain appear in Table 5-11.

The Perceptual Domain

The last learning domain is related to perception, which is necessary for all cognitive and psychomotor function. This domain was proposed by Moore in 1970 but has not become as widely utilized as the other three domains. The description of the perceptual domain appears in Table 5-8. It begins with sensation and continues through figure perception, symbol perception, perception of meaning, and perceptive performance.

The perceptual domain involves the ability to respond to both written and verbal symbols, which includes pictures, graphs, words, or numbers. We often falsely assume that the patient will be able to look at a picture or a printed page and be able to comprehend the meaning of the symbols or words that appear there. The nurse should evaluate the patient's ability to perceive information in the initial assessment phase of patient teaching. Any limitations that are discovered can then be incorporated into the teaching plan. For example, extra large print might be needed for the elderly patient with visual impairment. For the deaf patient, a film would be inadequate unless it was accompanied by a printed narrative.

Because information about the perceptual domain is generally applied when consid-

Table 5-8
Proposed Taxonomy of Perceptual Domain *

I. *Sensation*
   Behavior that demonstrates awareness of the informational aspects of the stimulus energy.
   A. Detection and awareness of change. Detection threshold measures in all sensory
      modes.
      1. Ability to specify the attribute that has changed.
      2. Ability to specify the direction of change.
      3. Ability to specify the degree of change.
II. *Figure perception*
   Behavior that demonstrates awareness of entity.
   A. Discrimination of unity; discrimination threshold measures in all sensory modes.
      1. Ability to judge brightness as a property of the stimulus under varying
         illumination.
      2. Ability to judge distance and location of light and sound.
      3. Ability to judge tactile form qualities such as hardness, sharpness, etc.
   B. Sensory figure-ground perceptual organization
      1. Awareness of the relationships of parts to each other and to the whole.
      2. Awareness of relations between the parts and the background, matrix, or
         context.
   C. Resolution of detail.
      1. Response to detail within the sensory (visual and auditory) world.
         a. Ability to judge size as a property of the stimulus at various distances.
         b. Ability to judge shape as a property of the stimulus regardless of orientation.
         c. Tests of field-dependence.
         d. Tests of spatial orientation.
         e. Other.
      2. Response to detail within the sensory (visual and auditory) field.
         a. Ability to discriminate symmetrical figures.
         b. Ability to discriminate asymmetrical figures.
         c. Ability to perceive rapidly successive bits of information.
         d. "Nonsensory" figure-ground segregation.
         e. Other.
III. *Symbol perception*
   Behavior that demonstrates awareness of figures in the form of denotative signs when
   associated meanings are not considered.
   A. Identification of form or pattern and relation of discrete information into visual,
      auditory, and tactile forms; recognition thresholds in all sensory modalities.
      1. Ability to distinguish curves from rectangles.
      2. Ability to distinguish triangles from squares.
      3. Ability to identify letters and digits.
      4. Ability to respond appropriately to gross facial expressions.
      5. Ability to distinguish tones in a musical chord.
      6. Ability to abstract a melody line from its variations.
      7. Ability to distinguish color components of a visual spectrum or composition.
      8. Ability to respond appropriately to verbal directions.
      9. Ability to respond appropriately to written directions.
      10. Other.
   B. Naming classification of forms and patterns.
      1. Ability to recognize faces and identify people by name.
      2. Ability to identify simplications and schematic drawings.

3. Ability to name complex objects, pictures, places, melodies, tastes, odors, etc.
4. Ability to read and comprehend concrete nouns and verbs denoting physical activity.
5. Ability to indicate similarities and differences between visual, auditory, or tactile forms or their representations and to classify them.
6. Other.

IV. *Perception of meaning*
Behavior that demonstrates awareness of the significance commonly associated with forms and patterns and events and the ability to assign personal significance to them; interpretive ability.

A. Mental manipulation of the identified form or pattern.
1. Ability to reproduce forms, tunes, or syllables by memory.
2. Ability to overcome the constancies of brightness, color, size, and shape.
3. Other.

B. Ability to attach significance to a symbol and to relate symbols to achieve a significant synthesis.
1. Understanding of the various parts of speech; comprehension of language.
2. Ability to make simple associations in all sensory modalities; for example, clouds mean rain, smoke means fire.
3. Ability to understand verbal imagery, similes, metaphors, analogies, and other figures of speech—connotative meanings.
4. Other.

C. Ability to attach significance to a series of events occurring over a period of time.
1. Insight into cause and effect relationships.
2. Discovery of new relationships.
3. Ability to generalize, understand implications, and make simple decisions.
4. Other.

V. *Perceptive performance*
Behavior that demonstrates sensitive and accurate observation, ability to make complex decisions where many factors are involved, and ability to change ongoing behavior in response to its effectiveness.

A. Demonstration of a successful analytical or global approach to problem solving in all areas of endeavor.
B. Diagnostic ability with respect to mechanical or electrical systems, medical problems, artistic products, etc.
C. Insight into personal, social, and political situations where awareness of attitudes, needs, desires, moods, intentions, perceptions, and thoughts of other people and oneself is indicated.
D. Demonstration of artistry and creativity in any medium.
E. Other.

Moore, M. R.: The perceptual-motor domain and a proposed taxonomy of perception, *Audio Vis. Commun. Rev.* **18**:379–413. 1970. With permission.

ering all the other three areas of learning, it is rarely separated with objectives that address this aspect of learning alone. For this reason, there is no accompanying list of verbs that represents the levels of this domain.

Although the taxonomies and domains may seem confusing at first, they can be very useful if the nurse will take the time to become familiar with them and to consider which learning domain(s) must be mastered by the patient.

Table 5-9
Steps in the Cognitive Domain*

*1.0 KNOWLEDGE	*2.0 COMPREHENSION	*3.0 APPLICATION	*4.0 ANALYSIS	*5.0 SYNTHESIS	*6.0 EVALUATION
Defines	Distinguishes	Changes	Analyzes	Categorizes	Appraises
Describes	Estimates	Computes	Breaks down	Combines	Assesses
Identifies	Explains	Demonstrates	Compares	Compiles	Compares
Labels	Gives examples	Dramatizes	Diagrams	Composes	Concludes
Lists	Locates	Manipulates	Differentiates	Devises	Contrasts
Names	Paraphrases	Modifies	Discriminates	Designs	Criticizes
Selects	Predicts	Operates	Distinguishes	Explains	Describes
States	Recognizes	Prepares	Identifies	Modifies	Discriminates
	Reports	Relates	Illustrates	Organizes	Explains
	Summarizes	Shows	Infers	Plans	Estimates
		Solves	Outlines	Reconstructs	Justifies
		Uses	Relates	Relates	Interprets
			Selects	Revises	Measures
			Separates	Summarizes	Rates
				Tells	Relates
				Writes	Scores
					Summarizes
					Supports

*Numbers and labels from Bloom, B. S., Englehart, M. D., Furst, E. J., Hill, W. H., & Krathwohl, D. R., 1956.

Table 5-10
Steps in the Affective Domain *

*1.0 RECEIVING	*2.0 RESPONDING	*3.0 VALUING	*4.0 ORGANIZATION	*5.0 VALUE COMPLEX
Asks	Answers	Accepts	Adheres	Acts
Chooses	Assists	Completes	Alters	Discriminates
Describes	Complies	Describes	Arranges	Displays
Follows	Discusses	Follows	Combines	Influences
Guides	Practices	Forms	Completes	Listens
Holds	Presents	Initiates	Defends	Modifies
Sits erect	Reads	Invites	Explains	Performs
Uses	Reports	Joins	Generalizes	Practices
	Selects	Justifies	Identifies	Proposes
	Writes	Proposes	Integrates	Qualifies
		Selects	Modifies	Questions
		Shares	Orders	Revises
			Organizes	Serves
			Prepares	Solves
				Uses
				Verifies

*Numbers and labels from Krathwohl, D. R., Bloom, B. S. & Masia, B. B., 1964.

Table 5-11

Steps in the Psychomotor Domain*

*1.0 PERCEPTION	*2.0 SET	*3.0 GUIDED RESPONSE	*4.0 MECHANISM OR *5.0 COMPLEX OVERT RESPONSE	*6.0 ADAPTATION	*7.0 ORIGINATION
Chooses	Begins	Assembles	Same word list as Guided Response 3.0 (Variation of levels is related to amount of independence and level of skill in performance)	Adapts	Arranges
Describes	Displays	Demonstrates		Alters	Builds
Detects	Explains	Dismantles		Changes	Combines
Differentiates	Moves	Fastens		Rearranges	Composes
Identifies	Proceeds	Fixes		Reorganizes	Constructs
Isolates	Reacts	Manipulates		Revises	Creates
Selects	Responds	Measures		Varies	Designs
Separates	Shows	Mends			Groups
	Starts	Mixes			Originates
	Volunteers	Organizes			Produces
		Sketches			
		Works			

*Numbers and labels from Simpson, 1972

150

Combining the Learning Domains

It is very rare that the domains are separated from each other. Actually, most objectives relate to more than one domain. More commonly, one verb that appears in an objective can represent different levels of learning in two or more domains. An example of an objective that demonstrates the connection between the cognitive, affective, psychomotor, and perceptual domains describes the diabetic patient learning to check his or her blood glucose. Consider the objective "The patient will check his blood glucose daily with Chemstrip." To perform the procedure, the patient uses the psychomotor domain to do the finger stick and place the blood sample in the glucose monitoring device. The cognitive and perceptual domains are needed to read and interpret the results of the test. The affective domain is the one that will influence him to actually do the test on a daily basis.

The domains are also combined in the following example. A patient would have to be functioning at least at the "application" level of the cognitive domain in order to "recall the steps of giving an injection" or "the principles of sterile technique." The actual injection would be considered within the psychomotor domain. The perceptual domain is needed to read the correct amount of insulin in the syringe. The diabetic patient who administers insulin daily is functioning at the highest affective level because the routine has become part of his or her daily life.

Using the Taxonomy Levels

One of the important teaching principles is to start with simple ideas and proceed to those that are more complex. The taxonomies will enable the nurse to correctly select the verb at the level appropriate for each patient. The objectives for each teaching plan will thus be based on the principle of teaching from simple to complex.

Included in the charts depicting the steps of the cognitive, affective and psychomotor domains [Tables 5-9 through 5-11] are verbs commonly used to describe the desired behavior at each taxonomy level. These lists are by no means complete and are not intended to represent the only verbs that can be used in writing objectives. Some verbs appear in more than one level and in more than one domain. For instance, the word "identifies" appears in several places. A simpler level objective could be "identifies the parts of a syringe" where a higher level objective, using the same verb, could be "identifies the relationship between the effects of insulin and exercise on the blood glucose level." The objective writer decides which verb to select based on the intended content and expected level of performance. The verb should convey as accurately as possible what is expected of the learner.

Just as the verb must convey the action, the taxonomy level must represent the patient's level of knowledge. So too, the learning domain for which the objectives are written must reflect the learning needs of an individual or group. If each of these "matches" is not made or if the factors contributing to the knowledge deficit remain, then it is unlikely that learning will take place. It is hoped that nurses will be alert to the causal events or etiological factors that contribute to knowledge deficit and will then plan learning objectives to meet the various learning needs of the patients' families or communities.

Nurses must themselves learn to assess for knowledge deficit and then establish the learning objectives accordingly, as the following teaching plan illustrates.

TEACHING CARE PLAN

Examples of patients with diabetes mellitus have been used to illustrate the content discussed. Because diabetes is a complex illness, it is important to develop teaching plans for these patients by writing specific objectives based on the taxonomy steps in each learning domain. The nurse may be involved in teaching at the time of the diagnosis, during management of problems related to poor control, providing care for diabetic patients who have other health problems, during long-term followup of selfcare, or when complications occur. Assessment of learning needs to document the specific knowledge deficit nursing diagnosis thus must be done.

Because there are constant changes in the medical management of diabetes, the nurse must continually assess the patient's learning needs. Nurses should be aware that when patients are presented with these new advances they may not have a positive attitude toward giving up their old ways. For example, many diabetics still keep their insulin in the refrigerator even though this has been considered unnecessary for over 5 years. They may still follow their old injection rotation pattern instead of adapting to what is currently being taught. The key to getting patients to change their habits is to make it meaningful to them and to first change their attitudes before trying to change their behavior.

Assessment

The first part of this chapter described establishment of the nursing diagnosis of knowledge deficit. Questions about how the patient manages the disease and what affect it has on life style will provide a good background in assessing for knowledge deficit. Asking about the number of times the patient experiences an insulin reaction or the results of urine or blood tests will provide information about the degree to which the disease is being controlled. It is important to include the family members when assessing for knowledge deficit. Parents of diabetic children or adolescents may need teaching in the affective domain related to their attitudes toward allowing the child independence in managing his or her disease (Hoover, 1983). In addition, spouses or sons and daughters of diabetic adults may have knowledge deficits in the cognitive area of potential complications.

There is a variety of well developed assessment tools to test how much diabetics know about their disease and how they have adjusted to it. For instance, there are diabetes knowledge scales (Dunn, Bryson, Hoskins, Alford, Handelsman, and Turtle, 1984) to test the accuracy of what the patient knows about the disease, the Diabetes Assertiveness Test (Gross and Johnson, 1981) to measure coping skills, and the Level of Personal Responsibilities Attitude Assessment System used by the Maine Diabetes Control Project (Anderson, Genthner, and Alogna, 1982), to name a few. More information about assessment tools is available from the American Diabetes Association. These tools would be useful to collect information before a teaching plan is established for the patient. In this way, you can apply the learning principle; that learning is easier if the new information is related to what the person already knows.

Plan

The goals of diabetes management are relief of symptoms: maintenance of normal daily activities; achievement of normal body weight; minimal fluctuations in glucose levels in blood and urine; and minimal complications. Patients need to know what diabetes is and what causes it, how to balance their diet with exercise and insulin, symptoms of problems that need attention, what to do for insulin reactions or when they are ill, and how to minimize the major complications. Plan for objectives in the affective domain that address the fact that not all complications can be prevented. This way the patient is not made to feel guilty if a complication develops that could not have been avoided.

Teaching should be planned for each of the learning domains. In the case of diabetes education, the affective domain is significant because the patients' attitude about their condition will determine how well they will comply with the treatment regimen. Korhonen and his associates (1983) found that the effects of diabetic teaching programs were of limited value if they did not involve changes in attitudes and motivation (Korhonen, Huttunen, Aro, Hentinen, Ihalainen, Majander, Siitonen, Uusitupa, and Pyörälä, 1983). Thus the initial teaching emphasis should be focused on the patient's attitude about having diabetes and what it means for changes in lifestyle and daily activities.

As was discussed at the beginning of the chapter, the individual's tolerance or coping ability will vary at different times in life. The diabetic may be well adjusted to the daily routine of managing the disease until some additional stressor causes him or her to no longer be able to cope in the same manner. For instance, illness, pregnancy, or career conflicts can all add additional burdens to the diabetic's ability to cope. As people advance through various life stages their ability to cope may change. Changes may be made in the treatment regimen, such as changing from oral medication to insulin injections. Physical changes that occur with advancing age may diminish vision and manual dexterity to the point that self injection of insulin may no longer be possible. As a result of these fluctuations, the nurse who is involved with diabetic teaching must be sensitive to the changes that occur and address the patient's concerns.

In planning to teach the new diabetic in the cognitive domain begin with the disease itself and how it will affect the patient. The relationships among diet, insulin, and exercise should be taught so patients know what is likely to cause imbalances. Symptoms of insulin reaction and diabetic acidosis also should be presented so the patient can differentiate between these problems. The diabetic also needs to know what to do when these symptoms occur, as well as what to do if he or she becomes ill. Even if the patient is newly diagnosed as a diabetic, always start by assessing what the patient already knows about the disease and build on that knowledge.

Another important cognitive as well as affective function is the keeping of records that are beneficial for monitoring the blood and urine sugar levels. Most diabetics who are insulin dependent will need to keep daily records of insulin, glucose, and any reactions that occur.

The teaching to be done in the psychomotor domain is related to the daily management of diabetes. The insulin-dependent diabetic needs to know how to administer the insulin as well as how to buy and store the supplies. Information about the rotation of injection sites and signs of local irritation are also important.

The other major psychomotor area for teaching is glucose monitoring, both indirectly through urine testing, and also blood testing. There is a variety of products on the market for glucose testing and it is important to find out what the physician has recommended before introducing a particular product. The perceptual domain is significant when this teaching is being done because the nurse should verify that the patient is able to distinguish the colors of the test tape scale and read the increments.

Implementation

The specific methods selected will vary according to the circumstances of the teaching. Bedside teaching with the diabetic patient who has been admitted for a routine surgical procedure or a formal group course for the newly diagnosed diabetic may be used. The teaching may be best handled on a one-to-one basis, or there may be several people involved, such as the dietician and diabetic nurse clinical specialist in addition to the physician. Use of closed circuit television programs or printed material to present the information and then followup with an opportunity for the patient to ask questions is helpful. The patient may also attend a class or several classes where groups of diabetics are brought together to learn from each other. Whatever the method selected, the nurse needs to be aware of the learning objectives in each domain and be involved in coordinating the teaching and evaluating the results.

Evaluation

Evaluation of learning should be undertaken continuously during the teaching process. By regularly reviewing the objectives and the patient's progress, the nurse will know what additional reinforcement and assistance the patient needs. Continuous evaluation of the diabetic's attitude and degree of compliance with managing their chronic disease is necessary. An important component of evaluation is to carefully document in the chart the patient's achievements and progress in meeting the objectives. This is especially important when several people are involved in the teaching. Many times the objectives must be revised during the process so that they accurately reflect what the patient needs to accomplish or maintain the taxonomy level the patient achieves. Perhaps higher level objectives are needed to describe additional learning once the patient has mastered the lower levels. Evaluation of learning should become a routine part of the nurse's ongoing assessment of the patient. Using each of the steps in the teaching process with a diabetic patient can be challenging as the following teaching plan illustrates.

Mrs. Jackson is a 75-year–old widow who lives alone in her own house. She is able to care for herself with minimal assistance from her daughter, such as shopping trips and transportation to the doctor. She has controlled her diabetes with diet and Diabinase for 20 years. Now she is being switched to daily insulin injections. She is coming to the clinic to learn how to administer her insulin.

REFERENCES

Anderson, R. M., Genthner, R. W., and Alogna, M. Diabetes patient education: from philosophy to delivery. *Diabetes Educator*, 1982, 8, (1), 33–36.

Bloom, B. S., Englehart, M. D., Furst, E. J., Hill, W. H., and Krathwohl, D. R. *Taxonomy of educational objectives, handbook I: cognitive domain.* New York: David McKay Company, Inc., 1956.

Carpenito, L. J. *Nursing diagnosis: application to clinical practice.* Philadelphia: J. B. Lippincott Co., 1983, p. 254.

Dave, R. H. Psychomotor levels. In *Developing and writing behavioral objectives.* Tucson, AZ: Educational Innovators Press, 1970, pp. 33–34.

DiMatteo, M., and DiDicola, D. *Achieving patient compliance.* New York: Pergamon Press, 1982.

Dunn, B. A., Bryson, J. M., Hoskins, P. L., Alford, J. B., Handelsman, D. J., and Turtle, J. R.

Table 5-12
Teaching Plan for Diabetic Patient

Assessment	Plan/Learning objectives Affective	Interventions	Evaluation
Determine how patient feels about switching to insulin from Diabinase.	˙Patient will discuss feelings about needing to take insulin injections daily. (Taxonomy Level A.200) ˙Patient accepts the need for insulin to control diabetes. (Taxonomy Level A.300) ˙Patient will verbalize confidence in own ability to learn to give insulin injections. (Taxonomy Level A.300) ˙Patient will maintain daily records of insulin given, glucose monitoring, and any insulin reactions. (Taxonomy Level A.200)	˙Provide quiet time to ask patient about feelings without interruption. ˙Assess patient's willingness to learn how to inject insulin. ˙Praise the patient for any progress made in learning injection technique. ˙Assist patient to begin a record book to list daily doses of insulin, results of glucose testing. ˙Encourage patient to make notes about any unusual feelings or insulin reactions.	˙Patient will tell the nurse how he/she feels about the change in life now that daily insulin injections are needed. ˙Patient will participate in insulin injection instruction. ˙Patient will tell nurse that he or she believes in own ability to manage daily injections. ˙Patient will show nurse daily records that are complete.

Table 5-13
Teaching Plan for Diabetic Patient

Assessment	Plan/Learning objectives	Interventions Cognitive	Evaluation
Assess patient's knowledge about diabetes and the function for insulin.	˙Patient will complete diabetic knowledge test. (Taxonomy Level C.3.00)	˙Give diabetes knowledge scale to patient with instructions on how to complete it. ˙Suggest someone help read the questions if he or she has trouble with small print, but patient only should answer.	˙Patient will finish the knowledge scale.
Ask patient what he or she knows about the type of insulin he or she has been prescribed.	˙Patient will discriminate prescribed insulin from other types of insulin preparations. (Taxonomy Level C.4.00)	˙Show patient the containers of a variety of insulin products. ˙Provide patient with a list of insulin products available, highlighting the one prescribed. ˙Describe the differences in insulin products.	˙Patient will correctly name and identify the form of insulin prescribed.

Table 5-14
Teaching Plan for Diabetic Patient

Assessment	Plan/Learning objectives	Interventions	Evaluation
		Psychomotor	
Verify what patient has learned about how to prepare the syringe and give injection.	*Patient will inject own insulin using proper technique. (Taxonomy Level P.4.00)	*Assist the patient to prepare and inject insulin dose, providing all equipment at bedside. allow patient to do as much as possible. provide constructive feedback and praise.	*Patient will administer own insulin under guidance of nurse.
Assess how patient tests urine for sugar and acetone.	*Patient will demonstrate proper urine testing. (Taxonomy Level P.4.00)	*Observe the patient's urine testing procedure, checking for: second-voided specimen. ability to read testing tape accurately.	*Patient will test urine properly for glucose and acetone.
Assess patient's ability to test blood glucose.	*Patient will demonstrate proper testing of blood glucose. (Taxonomy Level P.4.00)	*Instruct patient on how to test own blood glucose: perform finger stick. apply blood to test strip. read results.	*Patient will measure own blood glucose accurately.

Development of the diabetes knowledge (DKN) scales: forms DKNA, DKNB, and DKNC. *Diabetes Care*, 1984, 7, (1), 36–41.

Gross, A. M., and Johnson, W. G. The diabetes assertiveness test: a measure of social coping skills in pre-adolescent diabetes. *Diabetes Educator*, 1981, 7, (2), 26–27.

Hallal, J. C. The relationship of health beliefs, health locus of control, and self-concept to the practice of breast self-examination in adult women. *Nursing Research*, 1982, 31, (3), 137–142.

Harrow, A. J. *A taxonomy of the psychomotor domain.* New York: David McKay Company, Inc., 1972.

Hoover, J. W. Patient Burnout and other reasons for noncompliance, *Diabetes Educator*, 1983, 9 (3) 41–43.

Knowles, M. *The adult learner: a neglected species.* Houston: Gulf Publishing Company, 1973.

Korhonen, T., Huttunen, J. K., Aro, A., Hentinen, M., Ihalainen, O, Majander, H., Siitonen, O, Uusitupa, M., and Pyörälä, K. A controlled trial on the effects of patient education treatment on insulin-dependent diabetics. *Diabetic Care*, 1983, 6, (3), 256–261.

Krathwohl, D. R., Bloom, B. S., and Masia, B. B. *Taxonomy of educational objectives, handbook II: affective domain.* New York: David McKay Company, Inc., 1964.

McNeal, D., Salisbury, Z., Baumgardner, P., and Wheeler, F. C. Comprehension assessment of diabetes education program participants. *Diabetes Care*, 1984, 7, (3), 232–235.

Mager, R. F. *Preparing instructional objectives* (2nd ed.). Belmont, CA: Fearon Publisher Inc., 1975.

Pokorny, B. Valadating a Diagnostic Label: Knowledge Deficit. *The Nursing Clinics of North America*, Dougherty, C. (ed.). Philadelphia: WB Saunders, 1985, 641–656.

Moore, M. R. The perceptual-motor domain and a proposed taxonomy of perception. *AV Communication Review*, 1970, 18, (4), 379–412.

Peplau, H. A working definition of anxiety. In S. Bard and M. Marshall, (eds.) *Some clinical approaches to psychiatric nursing.* New York: Macmillan Co., 1963.

Petrello, J. Your patients hear you, but do they understand? *RN Magazine*, 1976, 39, 37–39.

Rosenstock, I. M. Historical origins of the health belief model. *Health Education Monographs*, 1974, 2, (4).

Simpson, E. J. *The classification of educational objectives in the psychomotor domain.* Vol. 3, Mt. Rainer, MD: Gryphon House, Inc., 1972.

Tuckman, B. W. A four-domain taxonomy for classifying educational tasks and objectives. *Educational Psychology*, 1972, 12, (2), 36–38.

6

Planning for Patient Teaching Based on Learning Theory

Sharon E. Hoffman

OBJECTIVES

1. Identify the theorist that provides the rationale for patient teaching plans.
2. Compare and contrast the concepts of the early behavioralists with the cognitive field theorists.
3. Describe the rationale for patient educators to follow a learning theory or model.
4. Develop teaching plans contrasting the approaches used with the child, adult, and elderly with compromised respiratory function.

Patient educators must be well versed in the learning theories used to guide their teaching strategies, research, and evaluation. A thorough understanding of the nature of the learning process and its basic tenets will facilitate freedom to experiment, and initiate improved methods and evaluation of teaching.

This chapter is written with the hope that it will contribute, in some degree, to a long-range sense of direction for patient educators. The chapter will describe learning theories in such a way as to guide readers in constructing and evaluating their own roles as patient educators who optimize learning. Although this chapter is not all-inclusive, a semihistorical approach will be taken, discussing some of the classical theories of learning as well as some of the recent studies of adult learning. The wide range of patient developmental stages that patient educators encounter necessitates a discussion of the pediatric learner, adult learner, and aged learner and their unique needs. But let's start at the very beginning.

DEFINITION OF A THEORY

There are many ideas about what constitutes a theory and it is important for our discussion of learning theories that we look at the variety of uses of the term. Reynolds (1971) describes three common forms of theory as the set of laws form, the axiomatic form, and the causal process form.

PATIENT EDUCATION: NURSES IN PARTNERSHIP
WITH OTHER HEALTH PROFESSIONALS

Set of Laws

One of the most popular and well-known forms is that theory is a well-supported set of laws that can be used to give logically derived explanations. An example of a set of laws with which many people are familiar is Einstein's theory of relativity, which predicts and explains the scientific event of energy. All of the laws in the theory set are supported by empirical research, with all of the concepts used in the laws having operational definitions that include empirical referents.

A set of laws familiar to patient educators is the laws of operant behavior as described by Skinner (1950). Table 6-1 defines the terms used in this set. He presents specific definitions of the concepts of reward, reinforcement, and rate of acquiring a new behavior or learning. The concepts of learning and extinction are defined and then the laws of operant behavior are described using these concepts.

Theories stated in the form of a set of laws can guide classification or analysis, provide predictions and explanations for behaviors, and if defined precisely, may allow for the potential of experimental control. Analysis, prediction, and experimental control are vital to patient education, which at this time suffers from a dearth of research. Each form of theory can be used to guide research in teaching individuals, families, and communities.

The Axiomatic Form

Another idea is that theory is an interrelated set of definitions, axioms, and propositions that give a description of a causal process. Mathematical theories are in this axiomatic theory form and plane geometry can best be described as a set of axioms. Unfortunately the set of axioms and the logical system entailed does not lend itself to social science research as axioms must have the status of laws. That is, only those statements that have the status of a scientific law via empirical research are acceptable, so no hypothetical or unmeasurable concepts exist in axiomatic theory. If the principles of patient education could be empirically validated, these might suffice as axioms for teaching patients. However, at this time, the principles are based in logic and practice, not on scientific law.

The Causal Process Form

The causal process form of theory presents a set of causal statements that describe one or more processes that identify the effect of independent variables on dependent variables. Jean Johnson (1977) has developed a causal process form of theory in identifying, through a series of experimental studies, a new patient teaching process. In several lab experiments and in four major clinical studies, Dr. Johnson has determined that by including sensory instruction in preoperative information, the length of postoperative hospitalization stay and feelings of patient helplessness were reduced significantly. The effect of the independent variable, sensory information in patient teaching plans, on the dependent variable, feelings of helplessness and length of hospital stay, was well documented.

Causal process forms of theory allow hypothetical or unmeasurable concepts to be described, which makes it a very usable form for social scientists attempting to describe social or individual phenomena. Several other researchers have developed hypotheses

Table 6-1
Skinner's Laws of Operant Behavior

FOR EXAMPLE: The Laws of Operant Behavior

The following definitions are important for understanding these laws:

Operant behavior—Any measurable response of an organism, individual, or social system (such as a task-oriented group), that affects or "operates" on its environment, e.g., speech, lever pressing, work activity, etc.

Form of behavior—The actual behavior that is emitted by the organism, e.g., speech patterns may differ, pressing a blue lever is different from pushing a red button, etc.

Rate of behavior—The frequency, in terms of number of actions per unit of time, with which behavior is emitted, e.g., a child saying "daddy" once a minute is emitting behavior at a lower rate than one saying "daddy" ten times a minute.

Reward—Any consequence for the organism that is desirable from the perspective of the organism. Positive rewards increase pleasure and negative rewards reduce pain.

Contingency—The relationship between the past consequences of behavior, its history of rewards from the organism's perspective, and the rate and form of the behavior.

Reinforcement schedule—A particular pattern of contingency, a particular relationship between the occurrence of operant behavior and a pattern of rewards, from the perspective of an observer of the organism-environment system. Reinforcement schedules can be classified into two groups:

Continuous reinforcement—A reinforcement schedule in which every operant behavior is followed by the occurrence of a reward.

Intermittent (partial) reinforcement—A reinforcement schedule in which the occurrence of the rewards is not directly related to behavior in any simple fashion. Rewards might occur after an interval of time (an interval schedule) or after a certain number of behaviors have been emitted (a ratio schedule, referring to the ratio of behaviors to a reward).

Two types of changes in reinforcement schedules are of interest:

Learning—A change from no reinforcement to any type of reinforcement schedule, continuous or intermittent, from the perspective of an observer of the organism-environment system.

Extinction—A change such that operant behavior previously rewarded, with either a continuous or intermittent reinforcement schedule, is no longer rewarded, from the perspective of an observer of the organism-environment system.

Using these concepts, two laws of operant behavior may be stated:

I. An organism will regularly perform the appropriate (rewarded) behavior sooner in a learning situation if a continuous rather than an intermittent reinforcement schedule is introduced.

II. During extinction, an organism will cease to perform behavior previously rewarded sooner if a continuous rather than an intermittent reinforcement schedule was used before all rewards were terminated.

Skinner, B. F. "Are Theories of Learning Necessary?" *Psychological Review*, 1950, 57(4), 193–216.

based on Johnson's work and are using these to test other types of teaching and nursing interventions.

Theory Building

The term "theory" or "theory building" may also be used to signify an untested set of hypotheses or ideas that remain theoretical until they are completely tested. These activities may be referred to as developing models, simulations, or theory building. Theory may also refer to prescriptions about what are desirable social behaviors. Some of our child-rearing theories may fall into this category. The last use of theory is descriptions of events or things that may be vague concepts. This use of the word theory usually provides a taxonomy or a method of organizing or classifying information. These theories may describe a phenomenon and as such refer to a type of categorization but cannot be used as causal statements. The learning taxonomies used by educators will be discussed in the following chapter on learning domains.

Learning theories in this chapter represent several of the ideas about what constitutes a theory. Few are as well-developed as a set of laws and few give statements that are axiomatic in nature. Many of the concepts about learning constitute a method of organizing and categorizing phenomena, they attempt to develop a sense of understanding about the nature of learning. They are not in the strictest interpretation of the word scientific theories, however, they attempt to explain the learning phenomena and as such provide helpful information to the patient educator.

LEARNING THEORY AS A BASE FOR PRACTICE

The relationship between learning theory and the educational practices of a patient educator is the same as that between any science and its application. Even though everything an educator does is colored by the learning theory, there are intervening variables such as the time demands of a patient setting, the resources available, and the external demands. The manner in which the patient deals with illness as well as the physical ability to learn are also important considerations.

The educator may not be able to verbalize the exact theory of learning that is currently being used, however, he or she should be conscious of a pattern of concepts or learning principles guiding the educational decisions that are made. An educator that does not make use of a systematic body of theory is proceeding blindly, using a potpourri of methods without a clear goal in sight and clear parameters to guide the decision making.

Just as there are many definitions and uses of the word "theory," there are also many definitions of learning developed by a variety of psychologists and educators. Bigge's (1971) definition of learning is inclusive and well-accepted by educators.

Learning, in contrast with maturation, is a change in a living individual which is not heralded by his genetic inheritance. It may be a change in insights, behavior, perception, or motivation, or a combination of these.

If we use the idea that theory is a rational plan for action derived from the scientific method, with a defined set of laws or interrelated set of definitions, and propositions; an ideal learning theory, then, would be a series of scientifically based statements that explain why the behavioral change has occurred. Teachers who are well-grounded in learning theory have a basis for making sound decisions that are more likely to bring about a behavioral change. As the sophistication of patient education programs increases, the need for evaluation increases and with added emphasis on efficiency and cost effectiveness, it is important that patient education methodologies are theory based.

EARLY LEARNING PHILOSOPHIES

Nonexperimental psychologies of learning have been present since time immemorial and some of these initial philosophical ideas can still be found among educators. Learning theories as well as many other psychological theories evolved from the study of philosophy. The early philosophers were interested in the mind—how it developed and how it acquired knowledge. Bigge (1971) refers to the most popular of these speculative orientations as mind discipline. Mind discipline disciples believed that education is the process of training the mind or disciplining the mental faculties. Plato's emphasis on mathematics and philosophy as the best preparation to train the mind for any kind of problem-solving, is a form of mind discipline. Information and concepts, as such, are not useful but the training of mental faculties and the development of intellectual powers from within, are what is important. Through the nineteenth century, Latin and Greek were taught as languages not for communication but for mental discipline.

Nineteenth century psychologists believed that to train the mind a person must achieve control over his will, i.e., natural evil impulses. This could be accomplished by pursuing unpleasant work. A teacher's role was to make school work distasteful, difficult, and dull to force appropriate strengthening of the student's will. Knowledge of immediate practical significance was considered of little use if the purpose of education was to discipline the mind and strengthen the will. This philosophy, of course, is the antithesis of current patient education practice. If one finds that rote drill and dull memory exercises are part of a patient education package, regardless of the current technology used to deliver the information, it would be worth investigating the purpose and critiquing the outcomes.

Unfoldment

A second speculative position of how people learn was called unfoldment. The underlying belief was that the individual, as a completely free entity, will grow intellectually without any outside influence. A patient educator ascribing to unfoldment would feel that his role would be the development of a natural environment for the client to "unfold." The patient would learn what was needed by virtue of active self determination. Jean Rousseau (1712–1778) is the philosopher attributed to developing the unfoldment position of learning. His thought was that the mind will naturally unfold without external learning imposed on the organism and that needs which are instinctual are innately present and determine the behavior. The emphasis of this time was on the natural growth inherent in the individual. Both mind discipline and unfoldment were based on the rationalism of Plato and Descartes, who considered that reason was the source of knowledge and that man was born with the ability to reason.

Associationism

A third position about learning, associationism, is based on the assumption that man does not have capabilities that can be developed (as in mind discipline) or have innate ideas that will mature (as in unfoldment). Associationism is based on John Locke's (1632–1704) empiricism, the idea of the *tabula rasa,* or blank tablet, theory of the human mind. Locke and the other philosophers of the day believed that the mind was indeed empty at birth and that all knowledge was derived from the individual sense experience. Locke thought that ideas consisted of associations that originated by copying the original sense impression in the mind and then forming more complex ideas by connecting together these various images. This was the law of association and led to some of the early experiments on memory and learning and the emphasis in modern educational psychology on learning studies.

Considerable attention was given in the 1880s to the laws of association. Psychologists assumed that association formation would vary directly with the vividness of the experience, its frequency, its duration, and its recency. The more recent experimental studies on memory have continued to study these three factors. Twentieth century behavioristic theories are derived from the associationistic ideas of the nineteenth century. Behaviorists such as Thorndike, Pavlov, Guthrie, Hull, and Skinner continued the ideas of the associationism of the previous century.

The first experiments on human memory by the German scientist, Hermann Ebbinghaus (1885) tested memory by association. Edward Thorndike (1898) presented the first experimental monograph on animal learning. These developments had an impact on the learning theories of the twentieth century and are considered by most as the beginning emergence of psychology as a science.

The impact of Locke's work and his conception of the tabula rasa implied that the mind already consisted of ideas, that ideas had to be implanted and connected with other ideas, and that students needed to form proper habits in organizing the information. The shift in education thus moved from mental discipline to habit formation to increase memory. Developments since the early 1900s have refined the associationistic approach, in fact, many memory and learning experiments have accumulated much data about memory. It is apparent that the philosophy of associationism has "set the stage" for contemporary learning theories.

CONTEMPORARY LEARNING THEORISTS

Contemporary learning theories are an outcome of the earlier works by philosophers, physiologists, and other psychologists. Two contemporary learning theories prevail, the behavioristic stimulus-response conditioning theories and cognitive theories of the gestalt-field family.

During the late nineteenth and early twentieth centuries a growing number of psychologists were concerned with making the study of psychology scientific. John B. Watson (1878–1958) who was instrumental in defining the behaviorist position, relied on the reflex (stimulus-response) arc of neurology, and advocated the development of a science of psychology. His focus was observable forms of behavior, using animal models, hence the term, behaviorists. The most notable of these experiments were conducted by the Russian physiologist, Ivan Pavlov (1849–1936). Pavlov's experiments with hungry dogs salivating at the sound of the bell influenced behavioralists in the United States, most notably Thorndike (1874–1949).

Thorndike's principles of learning could be considered associationistic, for he assumed that learning was the process of connecting physical and mental units in various combinations. This concept assumes that specific responses are connected with specific stimuli and that these connections bring about a change within the nervous system. The stimulus response unit (S–R) was adopted as the basic unit to study both simple and complex behavior. In the early twentieth century the emphasis had shifted from the study of the mind as in unfoldment and mind discipline to the study of behavior with special emphasis on learning processes.

Behavioralists

The original stimulus-response psychology of learning was called connectionism, for Edward Thorndike. In Thorndike's earliest writings, emphasis was placed on the bond or connection between the sense impressions and responses, which become strengthened or weakened in the development of habits. The behavioralists began with the assumption that complex learning processes could best be understood by studying the basic or simpler learning units. Thorndike's most basic unit was trial and error learning, learning by selecting and connecting. Thorndike concluded that subjects did not think through problem solving but rather solved the problem by engaging in a series of trial and error approaches until one approach, by chance, was successful. His animal experiments using puzzle boxes scored the amount of time that would elapse before an animal would find a way to escape from a box with a hidden latch or escape route. On successive trials the animal's time of escape would become successively less and the time could be graphed as a "learning curve." Thorndike's hypothesis was that the animal does not "catch on" but learns by repeating the correct response and stamping out the incorrect one. The repetition of situations does not increase the strength of the connection unless the response is rewarded. Responses that are rewarded are strengthened or the connection is made between the situation and how one acts. This was Thorndike's basic tenet for learning, the strengthening and weakening of these bonds or connections and led to the development of his primary principle for learning, the law of effect. This law of effect states that behavior is influenced by its effect on the situation; responses that have satisfying consequences are strengthened, and those followed by discomfort or annoyance are weakened. For example, using this law in a patient education setting, the diabetic patient with the proper skin puncture technique, would receive the nurse's compliments and less pain at the injection site. The behavior of puncturing the skin in the correct manner would influence the satisfying effect on the situation. Thorndike believed that practice is important only because it permits rewards to act upon the connections; in the patient education situation, the repetition of the injection scenario would facilitate the patient's correct puncturing thrusts and the nurse's positive reward.

Transfer of knowledge according to Thorndike's principles could occur if the new situation were closely identified with an old situation so that responses with similar analogies could be used to assimilate the new situation. If the diabetic patient encounters a new syringe, the fact that the injection technique used with the old syringe and the new syringe is similar makes transfer of knowledge more likely to occur. The term understanding could be used in the context of building a body of connections. Thorndike's contribution to learning theory was the behaviorist approach.

The original behaviorists, due to their emphasis on the neural responses of the organism in learning, thought of living organisms as self-maintained machines. Critics of this behaviorist approach reacted to this definition (Bigge, 1971).

". . . the essence of a human machine is described as a system of receptors (sense organs), conductors (neurons), switching organs (brain and spinal cord), and effectors (muscles) attached to levers (bones) plus of course, fueling and controlling organs such as stomach and glands."

This mechanistic approach did not explain ideas, emotions, sentiments, and imagination. The earliest behaviorists thus are thought of as primitive and "mentalistic."

Despite the many criticisms of his work, the seminal impact of Thorndike on successive theorists is immeasurable, for he started researchers on a systematic study of animal and human learning. His greatest contribution to education was his insistence upon measurement in the schools. It is essential that patient educators also insist upon a systematic study of the outcomes of patient teaching.

Pavlov (1849–1936), a Russian physiologist, used dogs in his experiments in his work on the digestive system. Pavlov's basic assumption, like Thorndike's, was that all brain-behavior relationships could be understood as reflex activity. Pavlov determined that a dog would salivate at the ringing of a bell if the bell (a new stimuli) occurred simultaneously with the presence of food and salivation (the unconditioned stimulus). The organism learns to respond to the new stimuli in the same way as the unconditioned stimuli. Eventually the dog salivates at the ringing of a bell even though no food is present. The new stimulus becomes the conditioned one and the response that follows becomes the conditioned response.

Terms such as reinforcement, extinction, and spontaneous recovery can be attributed to Pavlov's experiments and theories. A conditioned response (salivating at the sound of the bell) begins with reinforcement (being fed) that is the repeated following of the conditioned stimulus (the bell) by the unconditioned stimulus (salivating at the sight of food) at the appropriate time intervals. If the reinforcement is discontinued and the conditioned stimulus (the ringing of the bell) is presented alone often enough, the conditioned response (salivation) gradually disappears. This process of gradually diminishing or disappearing is called experimental extinction. If the response (salivation) returns, it is called spontaneous recovery of the extinguished reflex.

It is difficult for patient educators dealing with complex intellectual and affective changes to see how Pavlov's studies have any relevance to their tasks at hand. It is important to remember that it was Pavlov's contention that one needs to investigate the nature of complex learning processes by understanding the most basic forms of the process first. A number of simple conditioned reflexes can be arranged sequentially in chains of stimulus-response associations to form more complex learning processes. This classical conditioning model was seminal in the development of modern day theorists' use of the mechanism of reinforcement.

Conditioning as Components of Learning

Pavlov and his followers conducted 6000 experiments using this classical conditioning model. Most learning theories that followed in the twentieth century emphasized either the instrumental conditioning approach of Thorndike or the classical conditioning of Pavlov or a combination of the two. Thorndike's instrumental conditioning asserted that we learn what produces the most pleasant effects and avoid those behaviors that have unpleasant effects. Pavlov's classical conditioning emphasizes the stimuli as causing the action or the behavior of the organism. Stimuli paired with other stimuli that elicit a response can acquire the ability to also elicit responses, thus controlling behavior. The main differences between the classical and operant conditioning is in the procedure of reinforcement. In Pavlov's classical conditioning, the reinforcement is given before the response is made (e.g., meat powder on the dog's tongue), whereas in operant conditioning, the reinforcer is given after the response is made (praise after the patient uses the correct technique).

During the 1930–1940s three other behavioralists proposed their own interpretations of stimulus response learning, Edwin R. Guthrie (1886–1959) Clark L. Hull (1884–1952), and B. F. Skinner (1904–), all American psychologists. Guthrie proposed the nonreinforcement view of learning. That is, the occurrence of a response in a stimulus situation would be adequate for that stimulus to gain control over the response.

". . . a combination of stimuli which has accompanied a movement will, on its recurrence, tend to be followed by that movement" (Guthrie, 1952).

The association of the stimulus with the response could occur only once and last forever and there would be no need for reward, or need reduction, or pleasure. Guthrie proposed that learning is not extinguished or strengthened as a result of practice but occurs full strength on the first occasion of its pairing with a response. In Guthrie's theory, learning occurs suddenly and happens all at once. This concept is called one trial contiguity conditioning or contiguous conditioning. This does not mean that repetition or practice has no place in learning, but what really happens in practice is that substimuli and subresponses are associated so that practice allows more aspects of the stimuli situation to be paired and responded to. Although a patient learns a new psychomotor skill immediately, repetition will allow additional associations to be formed. The entire psychomotor process, in all its detail, thus will be strengthened by practice.

Guthrie's one-trial contiguity theory initiated the concept of learning processes as involving a variety of stimuli (substimuli) and responses (subresponse) and later theorists have expanded on his views.

Hull's contribution to contemporary learning was called drive-stimulus reduction theory. His theory focused on the individual's internal experiences or drives (for food, air, water, sex, etc.) and the behaviors that were reinforced when the attainment of the goal resulted in gratification or reduction of these drives. Hull's theory described learning as occurring automatically when the organism interacted with its environment. He theorized that some minimal amount of reinforcement is necessary to increase habit strength; that is, for an association to be formed between stimuli and responses (Snelbecker, 1974, p. 73).

Hull's emphasis, unlike the other theorists, was the internal states of the organism that intercede between the stimulus and response. This emphasis on the internal state of the organism led others to characterize his theory as S–O–R, stimulus, organism, and response.

Research is needed to determine how the internal states such a metabolic balance, fatigue level, or emotional stress affect learning theory. Hull's work could guide this investigation by patient educators.

Skinner's contribution to the focus of psychology of the twentieth century is the relationship between the behavior and its consequences; his emphasis is on the reinforcement not on the original causative stimuli. For example, in teaching a patient to give himself asthma inhalant medication using Skinner's operant conditioning theory, learning objectives would be divided into very small units of behavior and reinforced or strengthened one by one. Learning how to manipulate the inhaler would bring about praise and encouragement, reading the calibrations correctly would be rewarded, as would following the correct schedule, etc. Incorrect or inappropriate behavior would not be rewarded. However, feelings or drives or instinct would not be considered in this approach. Skinner considers that the science of psychology predicts and controls only those behaviors that can be observed. His definition of learning would most likely be a change in the probability of the subjects making a response, a change brought about by operant conditioning.

The behavioralists, Guthrie, Hull, Skinner, as well as other less well-known psychologists, were alike in their emphasis of learning as a mechanical treatment of stimuli and responses. Purposive learning or motivation other than that directed by drives was not assumed in the learning process. Patient educators applying Guthrie's contiguous conditioning would have the patient perform in a specified way, and while they were performing that function, provide a stimuli that would be associated with that behavior. Since Guthrie's learning is a sudden, immediate process, the instructor would go on with the next matching of stimulus and response without the need to reward or repeat the process.

The patient educator using Hull's theory of stimulus-response, would make sure that the stimulus preceded the response and because he or she thought that learning does not take place suddenly, another trial would have to occur. Learning, in Hull's theory, necessitates repeated trials to facilitate drive reduction. Reinforcement must occur until the learning is "stamped" in through the repeated trials. Hull's theory also focuses on the adaptation of the organism to its environment, thus, if an internal drive is present, the resulting need provides the stimulus that causes the response. Reinforcement is then part of the survival of the organism and the adapting behavior.

Skinner's operant conditioning would have patient educators devise efficient teaching machines that would bring about response modification through rewards. A home computer could be used using today's technology.

The original behaviorists who would be considered Watsonian behavioralists in that they tended to see learning as a mechanistic model in its pure basic scientific form, are no longer the shapers of contemporary learning theory. The followers of Watson and Thorndike were interested in neural physiology and the physical components of the S–R linkages. The term "neobehaviorists" is now used to describe the behavioralists who are interested in the analyses of purposive behavior rather than the physiological mechanisms behind it. Where historically the behavioralists attempted to identify discrete reactions, today's neobehavioralists are interested in the coordinated behavior of the organism.

Teachers who use behavioralist approaches today tend to mix the learning theories of Thorndike, Guthrie, Hull, and Skinner together, integrating their theories into a synthesis that works for them. This teaching approach requires that very specific outcome behaviors are identified, as well as specific ways to reward and modify behaviors. A behaviorist approach to patient education is that the patient can learn anything he or she is capable of learning if he or she will allow him or herself to be put through the pattern of activity. Each patient is engaged in specified activity that is appropriately conditioned.

Cognitive Theories of Gestalt Psychology

While the behavioralists were concerned with learning studied in stimulus-response atomistic units, gestalt psychologists believed that complex cognitive activities had to be studied in total. The essential point of the gestalt psychologists is that the whole is not merely the sum of its parts. Gestalt is a German word that means pattern or configuration, an organized whole. Gestalt psychologists refer to the totality of one's experiences in a situation. Since they consider learning as a holistic experience, one of the key concepts studied in the learning phenomena is perception. Learning is described in terms of organization of the learner's perceptual or psychological world called "field," thus, the term "Gestalt field studies." Kurt Lewin (1890–1947) is considered the developer of field psychology, the precursor to the cognitive-field learning theories to follow. His twentieth century work was based on the studies of three German colleagues, Wolfgang Kohler (1887–1967), Kurt Koffka (1886–1941), and Max Wertheimer (1880–1943). Lewin and his three colleagues introduced gestalt-field psychology to the United States psychological community in the 1920s.

Lewin's field theory was developed as a theory of motivation and perception, not learning per se. Lewin thought that the basis for psychological behavior was the net effect of the many psychological forces operating within the life space of the individual. These forces would bring about a reorganization of that person's "field." The life space model includes everything that one needs to know about a person in order to understand the behavior; it includes the person and his psychological environment. Lewin's life space model implies that we cannot understand the behavior of an individual until we know the characteristics of both the person and the environment. Lewin formulated laws that predicted relationships between persons and their life spaces. He used constructs, or "invented ideas" to account for phenomena. His theory is in a sense the development, refinement and testing of his construct of the life space model (Fig. 6-1). Lewin's model represents the total pattern of influences that affect an individual's behavior at a certain point in time. Behavior, in this model, is any change in the life space of the individual. It must be understood that life space is the individual's psychological world, the physical

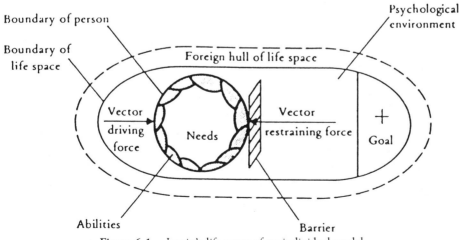

Figure 6-1. Lewin's life space of an individual model.

and social environment in which he or she is interacting. The concept of the individual's perception as well as memories, and sociocultural beliefs are within the life space. This psychological world includes the person's knowledge, beliefs, and abstract ideas, as well as the concrete objects. The following are the major concepts of field psychology as defined by Lewin:

1. Person. A consciously behaving self. Center of abilities and needs. That which a child means when he or she says "I" or "me."
2. Psychological environment. Everything in which, toward which, or away from which a person can make psychological movement—do anything about. Person and psychological environment are mutually interdependent upon one another.
3. Foreign hull of life space. Complex of all nonpsychological facts that surround a life space. That part of a person's physical and social environment which, at a particular juncture, is not included in his psychological environment. Physical and social raw materials. Foreign hull limits behavioral possibilities.
4. Regions. Psychologically significant conditions, place, things, and activities defined functionally as parts of a life space. They have positive or negative valences.
5. Valences. Positive or negative imperative environmental facts. Properties that regions of a life space have if an individual is drawn toward them or away from them. A region that possesses a positive valence is one of such nature that forces correlated with the valence of that region tend to move the person in the direction of that region. A neegative valence means that forces tend to move the person away from that region.
6. Needs. (Person-centered) States of a person which, if they exist in relation to a goal, have a part in determining behavior toward that goal. Correspond to a tension system of the innerpersonal region of a person.
7. Abilities. (Person-centered) Cognitive, capacity to know environment. Manipulative, capacity to affect environment.
8. Tension. Very closely related to, and descriptive of, psychological needs. The state of one system relative to the state of surrounding systems. Either created as a result of opposed forces, or induced by internal physiological changes or external stimuli. The rise of tension is an intention. Release of tension may be achieved either through reaching a goal or through restructuring the life space. The release of tension corresponds to the satisfaction of a need.
9. Goal. A region of valence toward, or away from, which forces within a life space point. Region of life space toward, or away from, which a person is psychologically drawn.
10. Barrier. Dynamic part of an environment which resists motion through it. That which stands in the way of a person's reaching his goal.
11. Force. Immediate determinant of the locomotions of a person. The tendency to act in a certain direction. Its properties are strength, direction, and point of application. It is represented by a vector. The strength of a force is related to, but not identical with, the strength of a valence. The combination of forces acting at the same point at a given time is a resultant force. Force is analogous to, but not identical with, drive or excitatory tendency as used in behaviorism. (Drive, behavioristically defined, is a strong, persistent stimulus that demands an adjustive response.)
12. Cognitive structure. An environment, including a person, as known by the person.

Synonyms are insight or understanding. Has one dimension—clarity (Bigge, 1971).

Lewin felt that learning consisted of four different kinds of changes; change in cognitive structure, change in motivation, change in group belongingness or ideology, and gain in voluntary control of dexterity of musculature. To Lewin, change in cognitive structure meant a development of perceptual knowledge. A change in motivation meant a change in liking or disliking of an activity or aspect of the life space. The change in group belongingness or ideology involves the development of the perceptions of oneself and the individuals in one's surroundings. The last, voluntary control of dexterity, is the development of skill, this too is a change of one's perceptions. All of these changes are, in fact, principally a process of change in the cognitive structure; Lewin's key concept of learning was the change in cognitive structure. In a 1945 publication he wrote,

"A change in action ideology, a real acceptance of a changed set of facts and values, a change in the perceived social world—all three are but different expressions of the same process" (Lewin, 1948, p. 64).

Cognitive field psychologists use Lewin's life space model as a paradigm for thinking about and describing what occurs in reality between the individual and the psychological environment. It is not a picture of a person's absolute existence. The model enables psychologists to characterize learning, thinking, acting, hoping, and dreaming.

The classical gestalt psychologists objected vehemently to the behavioralists excessive concern with rigorous observable research methodologies and their atomistic approach to learning. Instead they preferred to characterize man as capable of seeing meaning and structure in the world around him and able to organize the stimuli in his environment. The phenomenon of "insightful learning," the Aha! experience is basic to all gestalt psychologists and is depicted as perceptual reorganization. Problem solution occurs by developing different ways of perceiving the problem.

Edward Tolman's (1886–1959) theory of purposive behaviorism was a combination of the behavioristic and cognitive theories. Tolman presented a balanced view between the physiological characteristics of the behaviorists theory and the internal cognitive processes of the gestalt psychologists. Tolman combined three competitive theories of learning, the conditioned reflex theory, trial and error theory, and gestalt theory. His writings indicated that learning involves overt observable movements (a behavioralist approach) as well as cognitive operations which are not observable (the gestalt approach).

Emergence of New Instructional Models

It is apparent that not everyone is convinced that a comprehensive learning theory is possible at this point in time. Since the mid-twentieth century, psychologists have concentrated their energies on the development of factual information to produce inductive hypothesis rather than the development of a generalized deductive learning theory. Since the 1950s, the literature is comprised of theoretical models that are more limited in scope than that of a comprehensive learning theory.

Educatioal developments of the 1970s and 1980s have focused on applying scientific methods and principles to the classroom. Programmed instruction, the emphasis on educational objectives, task analysis, educational media, and instructional technology principles are but a few of the developments found in today's educational literature.

Programmed Instruction

B. F. Skinner's learning theory has prompted the development of specific educational objectives that are measurable. His use of operant conditioning theory and techniques applied to instructional processes places emphasis on clearly delineating outcome behaviors. Skinner's model of instruction follows five basic sequencing steps necessary to arrange the contingencies of reinforcement: identifying terminal behavior (specific outcome objectives), initiating the first instance of its occurrence, prompting the behavior, programming complex behavior and sequencing instruction. Programmed instruction is an educational application of Skinner's behavior modification. In the early 1960s this use of programmed instruction was best demonstrated by the use of teaching machines, an arrangement of educational materials allowing the students to make correct responses and then being reinforced when the correct responses were made. In many cases these were in the form of programmed instructional texts that allowed the students to work at their own pace or multiple choice testing devices which informed the students whether or not their answers were correct. Examples of today's teaching machines are computerized instructional units that can be constructed as games that reward the correct answers. Patient education materials can be constructed as programmed instructional units.

Skinner's first programmed instruction was linear, in that all students followed the same sequence of segments, a small piece of knowledge included in each segment. Later programmed instructional units were branching programs in which the students' initial responses determined the route to be followed. The branching programs present more information per frame. Recent developments provide ingenious discovery programs that present a problem followed by a multiple choice question and the need to derive a conclusion, hypothesis, or generalizations.

Following the lead of the programmed instructional movement, learning psychologists continued to develop additional behavior modification procedures that were also called behavioral engineering. Behavioral engineering is characterized by trying to arrange the learning environment so that one gets the behavior one is seeking. These behavioralists recommend using immediate reinforcement for behaviors that gradually approximate the desired educational goals. The goals are described as a contract between the teacher and the student which clearly describes the outcome behavior in a clear, fair, and honest manner. Thus the student and the teacher know the learning goal. In addition, frequent evaluations are conducted to inform the student of his or her progress and provide motivation.

Task Analyses and Taxonomies

One component of the behavioralist emphasis was the need to state the learning task or objective in outcome terms, break down the tasks to be learned into subtasks, and determine the relationship between the prerequisite skills and the order in which they needed to be learned. This emphasis led to task analysis and learning taxonomies. The task analysis enables the instructor to sequence the learning properly so that learning could be more efficient. Robert Gagne (1970) contributed the theory and research to this area of learning. He has arranged different types of learning in a hierarchy of relationships based on the assumption that the higher levels of learning depend on the lower levels. Gagne delineated eight different kinds of learning, each with a unique performance capability. His book, *The Conditions of Learning,* describes each type of learning and the internal conditions or prerequisite skills, attitudes and information necessary for each, as well as the external conditions in the learning situation.

1. Signal learning. The learning that occurs with a general response to a given signal (i.e., the word one learns to describe the color black when shown the color).
2. Stimulus-response learning. A precise response to a discriminated stimulus. The patient educator praises the patient as he or she begins to discriminate between types of breathing responses to produce relaxation.
3. Motor chaining. A chain consists of a sequence of activities which consists of two or more response units. Example: mastering the sequences of psychomotor skills needed to give an insulin injection.
4. Verbal association. Stimulus and response elements are verbal. Example is paired-associate learning.
5. Discrimination learning. The learner is able to make identifying responses to many different stimuli. Example: the patient is able to discriminate between several different inhalers used to deliver asthma medication.
6. Concept learning. The ability to make a common response to a class of stimuli that may differ in appearance. Example: the patient can pick out all foods high in carbohydrates.
7. Rule learning. Learning definitions and rules concerning concepts. This is a higher level abstraction. Example: a diabetic patient who learns the rules for food exchange.
8. Problem solving. Making use of the rules and concepts to generate new concepts to define and resolve a problem. Problem solving in a patient education situation would involve the respiratory compromised patient solving how to adjust to a new work environment.

Gagne's approach to instruction provides guidelines as to how an instructor plans educational objectives and delineates appropriate prerequisites, manages the learning situation to provide motivation, plans and tests instructional procedures, and selects the learning devices, media, and oral and written materials.

Bloom's mastery level of learning is similar in emphasis to that of Gagne as the material to be learned is broken down into small subunits, and the instructional objectives for each are clearly specified. Complete mastery of one of the small subunits is required before the student can proceed to the next unit and an ungraded progress test is given at end of each subunit. In mastery learning time allowance is varied to meet individual students' needs. In describing his concept of mastery learning Bloom (1968) writes:

"Most students (perhaps over 90%) can master what we have to teach them, and it is the task of instruction to find the means which will enable our students to master the subject under consideration. Our basic task is to determine what we mean by mastery of the subject and to search for the methods and materials which will enable the largest proportion of our students to attain such mastery."

Principles of Learning Instructional Theories

While some behavioralists were concentrating on Skinnerian approaches, others focused on specific skills used in concept formation, problem solving, and thinking. The work of these psychologists came to be called cognitive construct instructional theories. The leader of this approach was Jerome Bruner although theorists such as Piaget, Torrance, Ausubel, and others were equally influential in promoting this cognitive perspective. These psychologists were primarily aligned with cognitive studies and developmental theory.

Bruner's model of instruction has four major features: predisposition toward learning, structure of knowledge, sequencing of knowledge, and nature and pacing of rewards and punishments. Bruner states that a theory of instruction must be very specific in providing the conditions and the learning experiences that implant in the learner the desire, willingness, or predisposition toward learning. The structure of knowledge indicates that the body of knowledge must be organized so that it is easily grasped and understood by the learner. The knowledge must be sequenced or presented in such a way as to be effective. A theory of instruction must give the nature and pacing of the positive and negative reinforcements and punishments.

Other constructs attributed to Bruner are readiness and discovery learning. Bruner speaks of learning readiness as the intellectual development of students for the curriculum and the instructional materials. In a patient education setting readiness would be the time when the patient was motivated to learn, had the physical and intellectual energy to learn, and could use the instructional materials. Bruner's theme of readiness characterizes the learning process as that of acquisition of new knowledge, transformation of the knowledge so that it will be useful for the student, and evaluation of the knowledge.

The construct of discovery learning is the antithesis of expository instruction in which the teacher lectures or provides all the educational decisions with the students playing a passive, receptive role. The discovery method requires that the student participate in making decisions about what, how, and when something is to be learned and plays a key role in making these decisions. Bruner discusses four advantages of learning by using the discovery mode: an increase in intellectual potency, emphasis is placed on the intrinsic versus extrinsic rewards, the students masters the process of discovery, and the student is more likely to remember the information. New research into hemispheric learning may shed light on other modes of learning (Dunn, Cavanaugh, Eberle, and Zenhausem, 1982).

Piaget's cognitive-developmental theory is also considered an instructional theory. This Swiss psychologist analyzed the processes involved in the organization of knowledge. He developed a series of developmental stages or age-levels at which children can learn. His stages or phases were divided into four aspects of intellectual growth:

1. Sensorimotor stage (0–2 years)
2. Preoperational stage (2–7 years)
3. Concrete operations stage (7–11 years)
4. Formal operations stage (11 years and above)

Some educators feel that Piaget's developmental observations can assist teachers in developing the structure and sequencing of subject matter in any kind of curriculum. It is important that patient educators are aware of Piaget's stage when teaching children. Educators are aware that all children are not at the same point chronologically in their development.

Each of these theoretical approaches should be studied in depth before being used as the framework for patient education strategies. The references at the end of the chapter list the books that provide a thorough understanding of the application of the various models and theories.

Adult Learning Theories*

The 1970s and 1980s have been a time of research on adult development, which is a broad category for looking at the life stages and life cycles of adults, the ego and personality development of adults, and the moral and cognitive development. This extensive body of literature discusses how adults learn and their stages of readiness to learn during the adult life cycle. Developmental research has been popularized by Sheehy (1976),Levinson (1978), Neugarten (1968), Lowenthal (1975), and others. This research has focused on the life cycles or phases of life (Dinsmore, 1979).

Adult personality or ego development is another area of study and such names as Erikson (1950), Perry (1970), Loevinger (1976), and Kohlberg (1969) can be found in the research literature.

Of the major writers, Malcolm Knowles (1978) is perhaps the best well known. Knowles' andragogy is thought of as a unifying theory although others dispute that any kind of learning theory could cover the diversity in adult learning situations. Knowles (1970) defines andragogy as "the art and science of helping adults learn." In his writings andragogy is differentiated from pedagogy, which focuses on helping children learn. Knowles' four basic assumptions of adult learners are

1. That an adult's self concept moves from one being a dependent personality towards one of being a self-directing human being.
2. Adults accumulate a growing reservoir of experience that becomes an increasing resource for learning.
3. Readiness to learn becomes oriented increasingly to the developmental tasks of social roles.
4. Adults' time perspective changes from one of postponed application of knowledge to immediacy of application.

The work of Malcolm Knowles has generated much discussion in adult education circles. Many of Knowles' critics feel that his description of andragogy is a theory of teaching instead of a theory of learning since it consists of suggestions to assist the teacher in structuring the material presented. Despite the controversy of Knowles' work and the other adult theorists most agree on general principles of learning.

Principles of Learning

Most of early education in the United States was focused on teaching school children to master the three R's and little attention was paid to teaching beyond the walls of the local school house. As the industrial age required faster adaptation to the newest technology, interest in teaching adults increased, yet most of the teaching was conducted in the same style as the elementary classroom. Chairs were all lined up in neat rows, sometimes even fastened to the floor. The learners faced the front of the room and listened to the words of the teacher, with little opportunity for interchange among the students. It wasn't until the late 1960s and early 1970s that the attitudes about teaching adults began to change. Those involved with teaching began to see important differences between the initial formal education of children, referred to as pedagogy, and the education of adults, called andragogy. With the rapid growth of the aging population, a third

---

*section based on material developed by Judith A. Kopper, 1986.

age-related area of teaching has emerged: education for the elderly. Perhaps it is time to ask if a new philosophy is evolving, a philosophy and set of instructional techniques unique to the elderly that could justify a third "gogical" label such as eldergogy (Yeo, 1982).

Eldergogy, * is a specialized approach to education for elders that utilizes strategies or techniques best suited for the aged. Eldergogy takes into account distinct concerns and traits of old age that need to be incorporated into teaching programs.

Billie (1980) makes reference to the third gogy; he refers to teaching the elderly as gerogogy. It is Billie's belief that teaching should be based upon scientific theories of learning. Teaching the elderly proposes a challenge for the patient educator. Meeting that challenge demands that the health care professional work from sound theory derived from an understanding of aging that is appropriate for the person who must learn to adapt because of illness.

When working with the aged, it is important to remember that a 65-year-old person can look forward to several more years of life; thus nurses must counsel and teach as aggressively with the 65-year-old as with the 25-year-old (Jefferies, 1985). Elderly persons have strong desires to learn; this has been expressed by senior citizens attending the Elderhostel programs. The Elderhostel programs attest the fact that elders can learn. This program is based on the assumption that retirement does not mean withdrawal (Ingalls, 1980). These positive assumptions about aging need to be used in patient teaching. Other valid assumptions about teaching the child versus the adult follow.

Assumptions About Learners Used in Patient Teaching

Most education is based on several assumptions that are not relevant to the adult who has already left school and entered the job market. Child learners are a captive audience for the teacher since children were required by law to attend school up to a certain age. For this reason there is little attempt to entice learners to come to class since the child really had no choice but to attend school on a daily basis. Nurses involved in patient education may need to develop creative ways to entice adult learners to attend their classes. Since adults do not have mandated forms of education they will often seek out an educational offering or course that will fill a particular need (Dinsmore, 1979). In this way, adults are self-directed in their educational pursuits. For example, expectant parents may seek a class on how to prepare for childbirth.

Another assumption about child learners is that they will comply with the requests of the teacher out of respect for adult authority as well as perhaps fear of unpleasant consequences for disobedience in school. This phenomenon does not hold true for adults, since many of them are older than their teachers and, in some cases, have had much more experience in the work world. Nurses must keep this in mind when teaching patients because most adults will not accept what is said without discussion. Most adult learners, including patients, expect to obtain information that will be useful to them and will usually not hesitate to challenge a teacher. The wise teacher will capitalize on the experience of the adult learners and allow ample opportunity for patients to learn from

---

*Eldergogy information based on material developed by George Ann Eaks, BSN,RN, Diabetes Clinician, 1986.

each other. In many instances, patients are well informed about their condition. Patients might not sit quietly and listen to a nurse "teach" them about a disease or condition they understand better than the nurse since they have lived with it for many years. It is important that the nurse is able to provide information that will be useful to the patient.

As mentioned above, adults are usually interested in a particular subject area and will find a way to learn the desired information. Adult learners are usually not willing to devote the time and money to taking classes that do not fit their needs. Because adults generally pay for their own education, they are more likely to insist on quality for their investment. In many circumstances, such as weight-loss classes or smoking cessation clinics, patients pay a fee. It is predicted that individuals will have to pay for patient education in the future as a result of cost reduction efforts.

A significant difference between the education of children and adults is the time with which the learning is to take place. Children come to school daily and have many hours of repetition in which to master the subject matter they are expected to learn. Adults, on the other hand, are more problem-oriented and wish to have immediate application of what they need to learn. Adults have too many other ways to spend their time than doing needless repetitions of a lesson. Time also becomes an important factor for the nurse who is trying to do patient teaching. Patients do not stay as long in the hospital and need to know how to manage their own care prior to dismissal. The short period of time available for teaching requires that the nurse is well prepared to make the most of the opportunities that present themselves. Factors that influence the patient's readiness to learn point out how crucial it is to conduct the patient teaching during the "teachable moments."

Some adults and many elderly want to and are able to learn at their own pace. For those individuals, programmed self instruction or computer-assisted learning may be well accepted because they can proceed at a speed that is comfortable. With early discharge from hospitals, self instructional take-home learning packages are essential. Some adults will find this type of independent learning very appropriate but others will find it frustrating. A patient who has not become comfortable with computers, for instance, might be immobilized if faced with a computer-assisted instruction program. The key, obviously, is to match the learning method to the person's preference.

There are many things that have been learned about teaching adults that can be and should be applied to younger learners as well. One obvious application of some of the research on how people learn is the change in the appearance of school classrooms. No longer are the desks bolted to the floor in neat rows in most elementary classrooms. Rather, the chairs and tables are arranged in clusters with opportunity to rearrange the room to serve the purposes of the teacher and to facilitate learning in groups. The following section will present several principles of learning that can be applied to learners of any age.

Almost any text on teaching will provide a list of principles of learning that are to be used by the teacher in planning how to accomplish the behavioral objectives. The 12 principles that have been included in this chapter are an amalgamation of those from a variety of sources and can no longer be identified as the work of any particular author. When nurse-teachers follow these principles they increase the likelihood that the patients will indeed learn what is expected. It is helpful to try to relate the teaching strategies the nurse selects to at least one of these 12 principles.

Principles of Learning

1. Perception is necessary for learning.
2. Learning, because it is considered a change in behavior, is threatening. Therefore, learning takes place more readily when threats are at a minimum.
3. Learning is more effective when it is in response to a felt need of the learner.
4. Learning is made easier when material to be learned is related to what the learner already knows.
5. Learning is facilitated when the material to be learned is meaningful to the learner.
6. Active participation on the part of the learner is essential if learning is to take place.
7. Learning is retained longer when it is put into immediate use, than when its application is delayed.
8. Periodic plateaus occur in learning.
9. Learning must be reinforced.
10. Learning is made easier when the learner is aware of his or her progress.
11. Organization promotes retention and application of learning.
12. Accountability for learning rests with the learner.

In some cases several principles can be applied to the same learning situation (Smith, 1978). The brief explanation that follows below illustrates how these principles are used to teach patients in various age groups.

1. Perception is necessary for learning. The principle that perception must occur before a person can learn is directly related to the perceptual domain discussed in Chapter 5. When this principle is violated learning can not take place. For example, there may be times when nurses try to explain something to a deaf patient who was not wearing a hearing aide. Perhaps the nurse will try to teach a patient who was unable to see because their glasses were on the bedside table or were too smudged to see through.

    Teaching children can be a particular challenge if they are too young to perceive what they are expected to do and how they should behave. There are many creative ways to adapt teaching to fit the perceptive capabilities of any patient. Use of a multisensorial approach—seeing, hearing and handling the material—benefits perceptional learning for all age groups (Crigler-Meringlola, 1984; Thomas, 1982).

    Older learners need space to help the eyes in coding and de-coding (Doak, 1983; Kim, 1981; Miller, 1984; Oswald, 1985). Thus, the use of large black print on non-glare paper, with ample white spaces between letters is essential.

2. Learning, because it is considered a change in behavior, is threatening. Therefore, learning takes place more readily when threats are at a minimum. Learning for the elderly is enhanced in familiar surroundings such as the patient's home (Crigler-Meringlola, 1984; Thomas, 1982). Use of conversational style and terminology that best fits the generation being taught decreases anxiety and threat (Doak, 1983; Thomas, 1982).

    In order to reduce threats in the learning environment, the nurse who teaches patients should keep in mind the relationship between anxiety and readiness to learn. Patients who perceive that the task that they are trying to learn is very dangerous will encounter more difficulty in the learning process. Psychomotor tasks related to dialysis, or use of oxygen, for example, can be very frightening to an inexperienced person and the family.

Threats can also be psychologically induced by the nurse-teacher if care is not taken to ensure that the teaching environment is calm and conducive to learning. If the patient is given the impression that the nurse has only so long to devote to the teaching and the patient had better "get it" the first time, anxiety and time pressure may preclude learning. When children are faced with the frightening experience of being in the hospital or having something done to them by the nurse or physician, they will benefit from efforts made to reduce the threat. For example, spending a few minutes to prepare a child on what to expect when a laceration is sutured will make the child less frightened. This will probably save time overall, if the child cooperates with rather than fights the physician. For the elderly, design sessions that are self-paced and short, in which the patient has control over the session (Alford, 1982; Kim, 1981; Miller, 1984; Oswald, 1985).

3. Learning is more effective when it is in response to a felt need of the learner. A "felt need" is a knowledge deficit that is recognized by the learner and produces some action on the part of the learner to obtain the needed information. For example, a child swallows a hazardous substance at home and the mother immediately calls the Poison Control Center to find out what to do.

    After the nurse completes the assessment of the patient's learning needs there may be several areas that are considered to be knowledge deficits for the patient. Those that the patient also recognizes will clearly receive the majority of the patient's attention, and it is those learning needs that should be attended to first. For patients who do not recognize that they have other knowledge deficits, the nurse should begin by raising the patient's interest in the subject before trying to teach in that area.

4. Learning is made easier when material to be learned is related to what the learner already knows. To plan teaching that builds on what the patient already knows, the patient's level of understanding and cognition should be determined during the assessment phase of establishing the nursing diagnosis (Palmateer, 1985). This data needs to be continually validated and updated because patients are exposed to many different sources of information.

5. Learning is facilitated when the material to be learned is meaningful to the learner. This principle is similar to the previous one, but the meaningfulness to the patient can be from several sources. According to the health belief model discussed in the previous chapter, the patient will seek information if a risk is perceived or benefit from the change is perceived. The nurse can be instrumental in helping patients recognize when they are at risk and identify how the learning can be meaningful to them.

6. Active participation on the part of the learner is essential if learning is to take place. In order to actively involve the patient in learning, all of the domains (cognitive, psychomotor, affective) should be considered. In the cognitive area, active participation requires concentration and mental activity in order for learning to take place. Affective learning also requires active participation. The first level in the affective taxonomy refers to "attending." For the learner this means such a simple thing as staying in the room to listen to instructions. For the nurse this means turning off the television set so both the patient and the nurse will not be

distracted during teaching. Nurses sometimes assume that the patient is always ready to attend to what they wish to tell them. Family teaching sessions can be nonproductive because the spouse was attending to the patient and not to what was being said. Sometimes this lack of attention is obvious but other times more covert.

The importance of active participation in the psychomotor domain is obvious. Most people are unable to master a physical task without the opportunity for direct experience and practice. Someone cannot be expected to be able to play par golf merely by reading a book. The same need for practice applies to any skill that patients need to learn.

7. Learning is retained longer when it is put into immediate use, than when its application is delayed. Since it is difficult to remember information that is not used, effective patient teaching should provide ample opportunity for practice. There may be several tasks the patients need to learn before they are ready to manage on their own. As each one is taught, it is a good idea to allow the patient to perform the skill rather than have the nurse do the procedure. Some hospitals provide a means for patients to take their own medications or family members to carry out treatments before dismissal. In this way, the nurse can observe that the patient administers the medications at the prescribed dosage schedule. Diabetic patients should be given the opportunity to continue to administer their own insulin while hospitalized. However, even when the patient is giving his or her own injections the nurse can observe the technique and give constructive feedback. Any time that the learner has the opportunity to apply new information immediately it will be retained longer.

8. Periodic plateaus occur in learning. You can expect patients to learn rapidly at some times but to level off and learn less at other times. This phenomenon refers to the plateaus that can occur while learning something new. Remarkable progress is made initially and then a plateau is reached when there is no noticeable improvement. A variety of factors may account for this. Both the nurse-teacher and the patient should not be discouraged if there are periods of time when little progress is evident.

9. Learning must be reinforced. This principle identifies the need to continually plan how to reinforce the new learning as well as what was previously learned. In other words, for behavior change to take place, the patient will need rewards such as praise and recognition of accomplishments. By periodically reviewing what has been taught and providing regular periods of practice, the new skills can be reinforced and are more likely to be retained and eventually become habit for the patient.

10. Learning is made easier when the learner is aware of progress. Learning by patients, families, and also groups will be enhanced when they realize that they have gained new information, improved their skills, or achieved positive attitudes. Even though patient education is not a formal class with a grade attached, the learner wants to know how he or she is doing during the learning experience. Praise needs to be used regularly but judiciously. People can become very tired of hearing "good job" over and over. The nurse-teacher needs to plan to provide feedback to patients at regular intervals.

11. Organization promotes retention and application of learning. When teaching is carefully designed and well organized the learner is more likely to remember what is taught and use the information. The taxonomies of the learning domains can be

useful to apply this principle as they can serve as a guide to plan learning from simple to complex. The time taken to organize the teaching into a logical order from the simplest ideas to the more complex tasks will enhance the learning. The taxonomies will help in selecting appropriate verbs to describe the learner behavior that is expected at the desired level of complexity. (see Chapter 5)

12.   Accountability for learning rests with the learner. The patient or group is indeed ultimately responsible for learning or changing their own behavior. This principle is probably the most important and yet one of the most difficult for new nurse-teachers to accept. The old saying, "you can lead a horse to water but you can't make him drink" helps illustrate this point. Even the most dynamic teacher with the fanciest slides and most explicit objectives is going to be unsuccessful if the patient does not assume responsibility for his or her own learning. The job of the teacher is to provide information in an easily assimilated manner and identify any barriers that may interfere with the patient's ability to learn.

THE ROLE OF THE BEDSIDE NURSE
AND LEARNING THEORIES

The role of the bedside nurse in patient education has been clarified by the 1975 American Nurses Association document entitled *The Professional Nurse and Health Education*. This document speaks of the professional nurse's responsibility for "teaching the patient and family relevant facts about specific needs and supporting appropriate modification of behavior." In addition, the Joint Commission on Accreditation of Hospitals (JCAH) places emphasis on teaching and its documentation.

In fulfilling the role as a professional registered nurse the bedside practitioner needs to be aware of the various learning theories and teaching principles. Without a theory to provide guidelines for the teaching decisions to be made, a nurse can at best provide a potpourri of methods. Perhaps the most significant part of a teaching plan is the agreed upon outcomes. What behaviors should the nurse look for to "know" that the patient has learned (Smith, 1978). Learning theories provide the framework for planning the strategies and learning outcomes.

Observation and documentation of learning outcomes are often overlooked by nursing staff. Patient education for some is incidental instruction without the benefit of followup or evaluation. Observation of outcomes must occur to determine if the learning objectives were met, what strategies should be repeated or revised, and how the learning can be reinforced. Documentation has to occur to meet professional nursing standards. When care is not documented and is therefore not retrievable for comparison with the audit standards, the obvious assumption is that patient education was not done. In addition, knowledge of results is essential to effectively implement and support policy decisions about patient education. Without the observation and documentation efficacy will never be proven.

Observation and documentation assist with the nursing research studies on patient education that are needed by the profession: studies on readiness, methodologies, cost effectiveness, impact on preventive behaviors, and implementation policies. The necessity to show that this specific course of action, patient education, has an impact on discharge rates, return rates, chronicity, and disease is essential. Well-developed hypotheses should be tested about this health care delivery mechanism in order that the allocation of resources for patient education can continue.

Learning theory issues will continue to play an important role in patient education decisions. When nurses can identify the learning theory or model, demonstrate its efficacy and document the outcomes, patient education will be considered an important part of everyone's care plan. As patient education moves from an experimental step to a well defined delivery model of patient care, these decisions will be even more imperative. The following care plan illustrates the decisions made for teaching an elder, adult, or a child with the same medical problem.

TEACHING CARE PLAN: ADULTS AND CHILDREN
WITH COMPROMISED RESPIRATORY FUNCTION

The ultimate goal in teaching either an adult or child with compromised respiratory function is to motivate these individuals and their families to take responsibility for their own care, and to build confidence in their ability to manage. No matter what specific pulmonary disease is diagnosed, these persons typically need skills in selfcare for medication inhalation, clearing airways, avoiding infection, and controlling any factors contributing to the illness. The adult who has lived with the illness must be mindful of preserving as much pulmonary function as possible while the child must be conditioned to maintain good health practices that ensure maximum ventilatory capacity. To reach these goals, the nurse must use the steps of the teaching process and keep in mind the unique concerns and developmental levels of the adult and child.

Assessment

Assessment of the learning needs of respiratory patients should begin by encouraging them to describe their illness and how they manage their care. The child could be asked "when you have trouble getting your air inside, what do you do to make it better?" Of course, the child's parents are queried in addition, and because difficulty in breathing is such a universally frightening experience, it is best to ask the adults' significant others to describe the patient's reactions and coping patterns in caring for themselves. Deconditioned persons of any age may need just as much emotional support and physical assistance as the child during acute respiratory difficulties.

The nurse can assess the patient and families' perception of the illness and their attitudes toward selfcare by listening to these descriptions. Assessment data can also be obtained from the medical record, physician colleagues, and respiratory therapists.

A complete picture of the patient's pulmonary status, medical therapy and the families' basic strengths for dealing with the disease must be ascertained. If the family of an asthmatic child needs psychological counseling to avoid emotional strain or the wife of an incapacitated patient with emphysema is angry because of the patient's smoking, then referral to counseling would be made prior to initiating the teaching plan. Discharge planning would begin with referrals to cystic fibrosis parent support groups or I Can Cope lung cancer family groups as needed.

Planning

To plan learning objectives for the elder, adult or child with pulmonary disease, the nurse needs to contemplate the advantages and disadvantages of behavioral theories versus cognitive field theories as a base for the teaching plan. In either case, the learning necessitated by the pulmonary patient's disease process is very vast, so building on knowledge already possessed and beginning with what knowledge is desired as the adult educators suggest is important.

For the pulmonary patients to manage their illness knowledge of respiratory anatomy and physiology and ability to recognize pulmonary symptoms is needed. They also need psychomotor skills in the administration of inhalants and in the use of mucus draining procedures. Most important is the need for a positive attitude to control factors that initiate exacerbations of the disease and coping with disease limitations. Objectives to guide the nursing interventions implemented for each of these topics should be written in terms of the cognitive style and developmental level of each adult or child.

Implementation

The actual implementation of the teaching plan will be influenced by the internal and external factors impinging on the patient at the time of instruction. Many of the interventions used to teach the child will be visual. Pictures of psychological stress situations that precipitate asthma attacks are available for pulmonary patients. Illustrations of factors to avoid (overfatigue, crowds, allergens, and occupational hazards) are often used with adults. A video cassette series on learning to breathe better, clearing airways and building endurance, was developed by the Encyclopedia Britannica Educational Corporation in 1980. The American Lung Association has also developed patient teaching materials for both the child and adult asthmatic as well as chronic obstructive lung disease.

But even visual aids will not enhance learning if used at a time when the adult or child is too anxious and hypoxic to learn or while they deny that their respiratory problem is chronic. The nurse must be cognizant of the best time to initiate interventions as well as the best timing to provide feedback and reinforcement.

Evaluation

Evaluation of learning depends on the objectives that were established. If the objectives were realistic for the person's age and the interventions incorporated sound learning constructs or concepts then, most likely, the patient's behavior will have changed. If learning is not apparent then the patient education team must judge what has gone awry. Was the assessment of learning needs inaccurate? Were learning objectives mismatched to patient needs? Was the major learning intervention inappropriate for the patient's learning abilities, or is the person's pulmonary condition deteriorating? Whatever the reason for poor learning outcomes, the evaluation step of the teaching process should guide the nurse to change the plan.

The following teaching plan was developed to help contrast the differences in approaches to a elder, child and adult suffering from bronchitis (Tables 6-2, 6-3, and 6-4).

Table 6-2
Teaching Plan for Adult and Child with Bronchitis

Assessment	Plan/Learning objectives	Interventions	Evaluation	Learning Theory/Principle
		Affective		
Patient reveals fear of breathlessness through rapid speech, tachycardia (*adult*)	Patient discusses fear of breathlessness with nurse (*adult*)	Nurse uses active listening and referral to patient support group (*adult*)	Patient has openly talked of breathlessness and has normal variation in speech and heart rates with dyspnea (*adult*)	*Cognitive field theory* Need to decrease tension as defined by Lewin. Learning for the patient is an interactional process whereby the patient attains new insights into his fears.
Parents describe child's nightmares about "choking" (*child*)	Child makes positive statements at bedtime about ways to stop the "choking" feeling if it comes (*child*)	Nurse uses dolls and play therapy and instructs parents on positive imagery to enhance child's confidence (*child*)	Child awakens with dyspnea and sits up, leans forward, saying "I can help myself" (*child*)	*Learning Principle* Learning is more effective when it is in response to a felt need of the learner.
Patients, significant other or care takers describe frustrations and fears of declining respiratory function (*elder*)	Patient, significant other or care takers accepts limitations of aging and illness (*elder*)	Nurse points out the strengths and abilities of the patient while realistically describing limitations (*elder*)	Patient admits limitations due to breathlessness but describes continued activities and self-actualization (*elder*)	Learning takes place more readily when threats or anxiety are at a minimum.

Table 6-3
Teaching Plan for Adult and Child with Bronchitis

Assessment	Plan/Learning objectives	Interventions	Evaluation	Learning Theory/Principle
		Cognitive		
Determine knowledge level regarding inflamed bronchial tree and excess mucus (*adult*)	Patient describes factors causing bronchial irritation and inflammation (*adult*)	Discuss pamphlet entitled "Facts about Bronchitis" (*adult*)	Patient avoids nonhumidified environments, stops smoking (*adult*)	*Cognitive Field Theory* Lewin—Life Space Model changes in cognitive structure (a development of perceptual knowledge).
Ask if parents recognize the early signs of excessive mucus and inflammation (*child*)	Patient and child point to bronchial irritants on illustrated handout (*child*)	Use illustrated handout/hand draw some irritants the family states cause their child's irritation (*child*)	Child points to dog, paint can and other irritants on illustration and says he will "stay away from those" (*child*)	Bloom's model of instruction—Knowledge should be organized and sequenced. *Learning Principle* Learning is made easier when material to be
Determine the terms used by the patient to describe his or her condition (*elderly*)	Patient lists activities or factors in the environment that result in "shortness of breath" (*elderly*)	Use large print pamphlet to illustrate common bronchial irritants (*elderly*)	Patient lists factors in their home that cause "shortness of breath." (*elderly*)	learned is related to what the learner already knows. Perception is necessary for learning.

185

Table 6-4
Teaching Plan for Adult and Child with Bronchitis

Assessment	Plan/Learning objectives	Interventions	Evaluation	Learning Theory/Principle
		Psychomotor		
Does patient utilize diaphragmatic breathing? (*adult*)	Patient demonstrates diaphragmatic breathing (*adult*)	Videocassette describing breathing exercises (*adult*)	Patient initiates diaphragmatic breathing using correct procedure (adult)	*Theory* Gagne—motor chaining The patient links diaphramatic breathing immediately when reacting to the stimulus of bronchial irritation. The diaphram muscle contraction and subsequent deep breathing provides the reward of relaxation. (See Gagne, *Conditions of Learning.*)
Can you breathe by using your tummy? (*child*)	Child causes the hand of his parent that is resting on his upper abdomen to go up and down during breathing (*child*)	Parents and child are given demonstrations in diaphragmatic breathing (*child*)	Child demonstrates diaphragmatic breathing with and without hand resting on his abdomen (*child*)	
Does patient recognize changes in respiratory system due to aging? (*elder*)	Patient describes curvature of the spine or other normal aging processes that impact breathing (*elder*)	Demonstrates breathing exercises appropriate to functional capacity (*elder*)	Patient demonstrates chest movement by placing hands over diaphragm during exercise (*elder*)	*Learning Principle* Learning must be reinforced. Active participation on the part of the learner is essential if learning is to take place.

BIBLIOGRAPHY

Alford, D. Tips for teaching older adults. *Nursing Life.* 1982, 60–63.

American Nurses Association. *The professional nurse and health education.* Kansas City, KS, 1975.

Bigge, M. *Learning theories for teachers* (2nd ed.). New York: Harper and Row, 1971.

Billie, D. A. Educational strategies for teaching the elderly patient. *Nursing and Health Care,* 1980, 256–263.

Bloom, B. S. Learning for Mastery. UCLA Evaluation Comment, 1 (2), 1, 1968.

Crigler-Meringola, D. Making life sweet again for the elderly diabetic. *Nursing 84,* 1984, *14* (4), 62–64.

Dembo, M. H. *Teaching for learning: Applying educational psychology in the classroom.* (2nd ed.). Glenview, IL: Scott, Foresman & Co., 1981.

Dinsmore, P. A health education program for elderly residents in the community. *Nursing Clinics of North America.* December 1979, 14, (4), 585.

Doak, C. C. Communicating with the elderly. *The Diabetes Educator,* 1983, 9, 45–47.

Dunn, R., Cavanaugh, D., Eberle, B., and Zenhausern, R. Hemispheric preference: The newest element of learning style. *The American Biology Teacher,* 44 (5), 1982.

Erikson, E. H. *Childhood and society.* New York: Norton, 1950.

Estes, W. *Learning theory and mental development.* New York: Academic Press, 1970.

Gagne, Robert. The Conditions of Learning (2nd ed.) New York: Holt, Rinehart and Winston, 1970.

Guthrie, E. R. The psychology of learning, (rev. ed.) Harper & Row, New York, 23, 1952.

Hildegard, E., and Bower, G. *Theories of learning.* Englewood Cliffs, NJ: Prentice Hall, Inc., 1975.

Hill, W. F. *Learning: A survey of psychological interpretation* (3rd ed.). New York: Harper & Row, 1977.

Huckabay, L. M. *Conditions of learning and instruction in nursing.* St. Louis: C. V. Mosby Co., 1980.

Jefferies, M. B. Diabetes education and the older patient. *The Diabetes Educator,* 1985, *11,* (2), 34.

Johnson, J. A better way to calm the patient who fears the worst. *R.N.,* April, 1977, 47–53.

Kim, K. K. and Grier, R. Pacing effects of medication instruction for the elderly. *Journal of Gerontological Nursing,* 1981, 7 (8), 464–467.

Knowles, M. S. *The modern practice of adult education: Andragogy versus pedagogy.* New York: Association Press, 1970.

Knowles, M. D. *The adult learner: A neglected species* (2nd ed.). Houston: Gulf, 1978.

Kohlberg, L. Stage and sequence: the cognitive-developmental approach to socialization. In D. A. Goslin (Ed.). *Handbook of socialization theory and research.* Chicago: Rand McNally, 1969.

Lefrancois, G. R. *Psychological theories and human learning: Kongor's report.* California: Wadsworth Publishing Company, 1972.

Levinson, D. J. *The seasons of a man's life.* New York: Knopf, 1978.

Lewin, K. *Resolving social conflicts.* New York, Harper and Row, 1948.

Loevinger, J. *Development: conceptions and theories.* San Francisco: Jossey-Bass, 1976.

Lowenthal, M. F., Thurnher, M, Chiriboga, D. *Four stages of life: A comparative study of women and men facing transitions.* San Francisco: Jossey-Bass, 1975.

Miller, L. V. Educating the geriatric diabetic. *The Diabetes Educator,* 1984, 10, 67–69.

Neugarten, B. L. Adult personality: Toward a psychology of the life cycle. In B. L. Neugarten (Ed.), *Middle Age and Aging.* Chicago: University of Chicago Press, 1968.

Oswald, S., and Williams, J. Optimizing learning in the elderly: A model. *Lifelong Learning,* 1985, 9 (1), 10–27.

Palmateer, L. M., and McCartney, J. Do nurses know when patients have cognitive deficits? *Journal of Gerontological Nursing,* 11 1985, (2), 6–15.

Perry, W. G., Jr. *Forms of intellectual and ethical development in the college years.* New York: Holt, Rinehart and Winston, 1970.

Rankin, S., and Duffy, K. *Patient education: Issues, principles, and guidelines*. Philadelphia: J. B. Lippincott Co., 1983.

Redman, B. K. (Ed.). *Issues and concepts in patient education*. New York: Appleton-Century-Crofts, 1981.

Reynolds, P. D. *A primer in theory construction*. Indianapolis: The Bobbs-Merrill Company, Inc., 1971.

Sheehy, G. *Passages: predictable crises of adult life*. New York: Dutton, 1976.

Skinner, B. F. Are Theories of Learning Necessary? *Psychological Review*, 1950, 57 (4), 193–216.

Smith, C. "Planning, Implementing and evaluating learning experiences for adults" *Nurse Educator*, Nov-Dec, 1978, 31–36.

Smith, C. "Principles and implications for continuing education in nursing," *Journal of Continuing Education in Nursing*, March-April, 1978, 25–28.

Snelbecker, G. *Learning theory, instructional theory and psychoeducational design*. McGraw-Hill, New York, 1974.

Thomas, K. P. Diabetes in the elderly. In A. R. Van Son (Ed.) *Diabetes and Patient Education: A Daily Nursing Challenge*, 1982, (pp. 115–127). New York: Appleton-Century-Crofts.

Yeo, G. "Eldergogy": A specialized approach to education for elders. *Lifelong Learning: The Adult Years*, 1982, 5 (5), 4–7.

7

Implementing Use of Learning Resources in Our Technological Age

Brian H. Kaihoi

With Teaching Plan by
Mary Jean Brown and Lucie McCallum Black

OBJECTIVES

1. Illustrate implementation of patient education through the use of learning resources.
2. Define the advantages and disadvantages of implementing print, audio, video, projected media, telecommunications, and computer learning resources.
3. Discuss the ramifications of borrowing, purchasing, developing and copyrighting learning resources.
4. Develop a teaching plan for infant stimulation that uses a variety of learning resources.

This chapter is about technology, specifically educational technology and how it can be applied to situations where patients are trying to learn. The word technology alone can generate strong reactions for many people, both positive and negative. Some people are excited by new gadgets and new ways of doing things. Others are distrustful of new things that often turn out to be less useful than the salesman said they would. Still others just do not want to change their way of doing things, just on principle. I do not wish to be the overzealous salesman, and I hope you bring to this chapter a healthy skepticism with a strong dose of desire to do the best for your patients.

TOOLS FOR EDUCATION

In this chapter we will look at how specific educational technology has developed in our world of technology, and how it fits in our technological society. We will look at ways to evaluate technology for usefulness. Skills will be developed for deciding when a given tool is appropriate to use and when it is not. We will look at the tools currently in wide use and evaluate their strengths and weaknesses. We will also look at the near future and make some guesses as to what will be available for us to use.

This chapter will not show you all there is to know about any of the technologies at our disposal. There are many books and programs that are available to do that. You will not learn exactly which piece of equipment to buy or what works in all situations. You will not be told that someone is a poor educator because he or she does not use a certain piece of technology.

Patient teaching involves structuring the situation to the best advantage of the patient. The professional needs to exercise solid judgment as to what will be best for this patient. In order to make good decisions, you need to have the best information available, and have the skills yourself to compare and analyze. This chapter will give you the information and skills you need to start making good decisions about the use of educational technology for your patients.

The effective educator possesses many skills. Working with people, assessing learning situations and readiness, and arranging content are some examples. The physical implements of our trade as educators are in a toolbox that can be labeled "Educational Technology." The effective educator is able to use these tools that will make information more clear, understandable, and concrete.

We know that people learn at different rates and with different modalities. Because of this, it is very difficult for one educator to meet all the learning needs of a patient. Technology can be the bridge that will make an educator successful in the task of making sure that learning takes place. The proper use of tools can provide the content in a variety of modalities, at varying rates, at any time of the day, with exact repetition, and in some cases with built in feedback and reinforcement.

DEVELOPMENT OF TECHNOLOGY

Technology is a powerful word producing a powerful image. The term brings to mind pictures of microchips, landing on the moon, wonder drugs, artificial hearts, and a world of information at our fingertips. Before patient educators can effectively use the vast world of technologic aids for teaching, they must come to grips with their own feelings and biases regarding the use of technology, and the "gadgets" themselves.

Patient teaching tools are developed because someone recognizes a need, decides to do something about the problem instead of ignoring it, and accepts the responsibility of the educator to help the learner learn. To develop an effective tool, the educator must make sure that it works for the teacher and the learner, and that it is cost effective in terms of time and money. The tool must also "fit" socially, aesthetically, and physically in the intended environment. Our technology of education may very well irritate one patient, and be tolerated very well by another.

The job of the educator then, is to find technology that works, both with groups and individuals. We must realize that not all of our tools will work equally well with all of our patients. We must exercise good assessment skills and be willing to adapt and change to meet the individual needs of our patients. We must know what is available and how to use it.

LEARNING RESOURCE CENTERS: TECHNOLOGY DEVELOPERS

If you are working in a situation where you have access to a Learning Resource Center (LRC), or something like it, you have access to a great support service. The LRC most likely has equipment that you can use in your teaching, but more importantly, it will have staff who are concerned with making you successful in your teaching. An LRC will likely have instructional designers who can help plan an education program that will take into account what is known about learning theory. There will also be media specialists who can help you with the design or selection of instructional programs, and library specialists who can help you find information and illustrate how to put this information into a format that is understandable.

The LRC exists to help teachers solve educational problems. The staff of the LRC will be aware of technology that is currently available, and as situations are presented to them, they will be able to help find educationally sound ways to use technology to improve instruction for patients.

To effectively deal with the LRC, nurses must learn some of the language of technology that experts use. This is the same as learning medical terminology in order to work effectively in the health care field. Good communication between the patient educator and the learning resource specialist is essential for development of effective instructional material.

Technological Change

Three factors must be present in order for any technology to be effective. These factors are technical feasibility, economic feasibility, and social/political feasibility. These factors and their relationships are illustrated in Figure 7-1. All three factors must exist simultaneously.

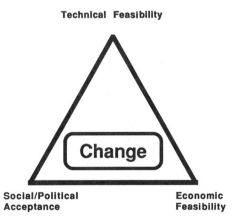

Figure 7-1. The three necessary ingredients for any change or innovation to be successful are technical feasibility, economic feasibility, and social/political acceptance. If any one of the three components is missing, the change will not take place.

When looking at technological change in education, the three issues of technical feasibility, economic feasibility, and social/political acceptance must be addressed. These issues are important as you decide to use a particular technology with your patients, or as you try to decide if a technology that is new on the market will be useful to you as you teach. These factors fit if you are looking at the technology for yourself, a small group, or society as a whole.

Technical Feasibility

The first issue to address when looking at something new, is whether or not the project is technically feasible. Some of the questions to raise are obvious, and some are more subtle.

Technical Feasibility Questions

1. Do I have the technical expertise to operate the technology?
2. If not, can I get the expertise?
3. Does the technology do the job that I want done?
4. Is there professional support available?
5. Is repair service available?
6. Is there enough equipment on the market so that replacements can be purchased?
7. Will the equipment fit in the patient room or other space that is available?
8. If not, can construction or renovation be done?

The hardware—software questions and the related technologies questions are especially critical for educators to ask. It is very easy to buy hardware (physical pieces of equipment) that works well and is exactly what is needed, only to discover that there is very limited software (programs) that will run on that type of equipment. When looking at technical feasibility, it is important to make sure that the whole project is feasible, hardware and software. If the intent is to develop original programs and not purchase them, then the hardware is all that is necessary to be concerned with. If however, the intent is to purchase programs, it is necessary to be sure that both hardware and software that work together are available.

Economic Feasibility

The second question to address is economic feasibility. This item approaches the need for cost effectiveness. Sample questions related to the economic feasibility of a project or program are listed. To answer the questions, educators must have a clear idea of the task at hand, what is to be accomplished, and be able to measure the outcomes of teaching the learner.

Economic Feasibility Questions

1. If not feasible, can the dollars be obtained through the budgeting process or outside benefactors?
2. Will the technology be used enough to justify the cost?
3. Can the same job be done with technology that is less expensive?
4. Will the technology allow the learners to learn better or faster in a way that can be measured easily and converted to dollars?

5. Will this technology allow more learners to use the material?
6. What is the expected "down time" (nonoperational due to malfunction)?
7. How can I cope when the technology isn't working?
8. How much labor will be saved by using this technology and what is the dollar value of that labor?

There are several ways to get answers to the economic questions. Accounting, finance, and personnel departments can help supply some dollar figures. It can be very helpful to describe the problem to two or more suppliers and see if they recommend the same solutions. Professional publications and personal contacts with people in other institutions who are working on the same problems can be very valuable. Once a technology has been chosen, the final step is to try working with a pilot group of 5–10 patients. The pilot study will show if the technology economically gives what you expect and the learners get what they expect.

Social/Political Acceptability

The third issue is whether or not the technology is socially and politically acceptable. This issue is probably the hardest to deal with, and is probably the most crucial. Some of the questions to ask in this regard are listed.

Social/Political Feasibility Questions

1. Will the patients be willing to use the technology?
2. Is the "look" of the new technology going to scare off patients, like computer phobia?
3. Will the administration back it, or is it too new to be accepted?
4. Will the technology put people out of a job, including educators?
5. Is there a way to use the technology that will not make the learner feel that they are interacting with a cold machine?

This third question becomes very crucial, because many technological advances have come on the market, and people have not been willing to use them. This fact makes it extremely important to conduct pilot studies when you are trying to implement something new. It is important to not only look at what learners learned from the session, but how they felt about doing it. This "feeling" will largely determine whether people will use the tool in the future, and how anxiety, boredom, and other negative factors will affect learning.

There is a technology on the market that meets the technical, economic, and social acceptability criteria just discussed. This tool is easy to produce and is relatively inexpensive to reproduce. It allows learners to progress at their own pace as well as actually input into the system and will keep that input on file. It is easy to use and requires little or no training for the learner. It is portable and does not require a power outlet in order to operate. It can be programmed by the teacher to provide immediate feedback for correct and incorrect answers. Believe it or not, the new technology that I am describing is a patient teaching pamphlet! Print technology is the most often used so those teaching patients should learn all they can about appropriately developing such materials.

PRINT LEARNING RESOURCE MATERIALS

Print media are the most often used of the tools available to the patient educator. Possibly because it is so common, we often take it for granted and do not necessarily use good judgment when we produce or purchase materials. If you are involved in producing materials for patients, you will probably be involved with professionals who have skills to assist in producing a worthwhile and useable product. However, you as the patient educator have a responsibility to be conversant with their vocabulary and be able to provide advice and direction to them about the things that you know: your patients.

There are several factors to be considered when looking at printed material. These include readability and cost. Readability refers to the ability of the reader to decifer the symbols on the page, understand what is being communicated, at what speed and with how much effort. Cost is an increasing reality in health care, but the least expensive alternative in a given situation is worthless if our patients cannot or will not use the material. This section will provide you with information that will help you make informed choices about printed material that will be good for patients.

The issues of readability and cost, apply to any media where the patient is expected to read. It doesn't matter whether the patient is reading from a TV set, a computer screen, a slide or overhead transparency projected on a wall, or a pamphlet. The principles discussed in this section regarding print media apply to all reading that patients must do. As each specific educational technology is discussed, there will be specific suggestions to help patients comprehend the material. However, since printed material is the most common teaching tool, the general concepts regarding readability and cost will be introduced here.

Typewritten Versus Typeset

One of the most basic differences in printed material is whether it is typewritten or typeset. With the advent of word processors and sophisticated computer printers, the differences between these two methods of producing copy are becoming less noticeable, but they are still worth mentioning.

The major difference between typewriting and typesetting is spacing, that is, the amount of space that is given to each letter. Most typewriters give the same amount of space to an "i" as they do to a "w." This allows you to count the spaces accross the page and know exactly how many characters will fit in one line. Typeset is proportionally spaced, meaning that an "i" takes up considerably less space than a "w." Proportional spacing is more costly than equal spacing. Some typewriters and word processors will give you proportional spacing, but they are generally more expensive than equal spacing machines. Some machines say that they provide proportional spacing, but in fact all they do is put more or less space between the words in a line to make the right hand edges line up. This kind of spacing can be particularly difficult to read. Proportional spacing looks more professional and gives the impression you took more care producing this material. I do not think that many of us would think very highly of a text book that looked like it came off someone's typewriter.

Another obvious difference between typewritten and typeset is the variety of type-styles available for use. Although new typewriters and word processors with sophisticated printers can provide a great deal, typeset generally comes in a greater variety of styles and sizes, and provides more flexibility in putting print down on a page.

For the purposes of this chapter, the terms and procedures that are described will be referring to typeset. The principles that are discussed can be applied to typewritten material, however.

Type Terms

Printers and typesetters have their own language for measuring and describing type. A review of the following terms will help as you talk with printers and designers of patient education material.

Point, Pica

The term "inches" can be used for both horizontal and vertical measurements, but the terms "point" and "pica" are more commonly used in measuring either direction. A point is the smallest measure of type, approximately $\frac{1}{72}$ of an inch. A pica is about 12 points, so there are approximately 6 picas to the inch. Points are discussed later under size of type.

Serif, Sans Serif

All type styles can be divided into two basic categories—serif and sans serif. Figure 7-2 shows samples of various type styles. Serif type has little hooks and feet on the letters. Sans serif type is plain, without hooks and feet.

Family

There are literally hundreds of type styles. A given style of type comes in many shapes (italic, bold, regular, light, condensed, elongated, shadowed, outlined) and sizes. Any particular type style with all of its sizes and variations is called a type family. Figure 7-3 show several examples of variations within one type family. When trying to distinguish one type family from another, it is often helpful to look at the e, a, y, and g as they tend to be the most distinctive from one family to another.

Weight

A given letter of type can require different amounts of ink, so type can vary as to how "bold" or "solid" it is. Figure 7-4 illustrates the variety that is available.

Proportion

Type can also be pushed together or extra space can be inserted. This results in type that is condensed or expanded. Figure 7-5 is an illustration of how this effects the look of one particular type.

Size

The size of a given type is given in points, and is measured from the top of the the the highest letter to the bottom of the lowest letter. For instance, a type size could be measured from the top of the upper case "A" to the bottom of the lower case "p." Figure 7-6 illustrates the difference in point size. For practical purposes remember, the bigger the number, the bigger the type.

X-Height

X-height refers to the height of the lower case letter "x" of that typeface. The X-height is usually 50–60 percent of the point size of the type. Refer back to Figure 7-5 and

Serif Type Styles

ABCDEFGHIJKLMNOPQRSTU
WXYZ 1234567890   Baskerville
abcdefghijklmnopqrstuvwxyz

ABCDEFGHIJKLMNOPQRSTU
WXYZ 1234567890   Bookman
abcdefghijklmnopqrstuvwxyz

Sans Serif Type Styles

ABCDEFGHIJKLMNOPQRSTUV
WXYZ 1234567890   Futura
abcdefghijklmnopqrstuvwxyz

ABCDEFGHIJKLMNOPQRSTUV
WXYZ 1234567890   Helvetica
abcdefghijklmnopqrstuvwxyz

Figure 7-2. This figure shows some samples of serif and sans serif type styles.

Light	*Light Italic*	Light Condensed
Book	*Book Italic*	Book Condensed
Bold	***Bold Italic***	**Bold Condensed**
Ultra	***Ultra Italic***	**Ultra Condensed**

Light Condensed Italic	Outline
Book Condensed Italic	Outline Shadow
Bold Condensed Italic	**Contour**
Ultra Condensed Italic	ITC Cheltenham

Figure 7-3. This figure gives an illustration of a family of type and of some of the possibilities of varying the face of the type.

196

Avant Garde Extra Light   Avant Garde Medium

Avant Garde Demibold   Avant Garde Bold

Figure 7-4. This figure shows the difference in the amount of ink that can be applied to one size of type. This is called the weight of the face.

Helvetica Regular

Helvetica Bold Condensed

Helvetica Compressed   Helvetica Ultra Compressed

Figure 7-5. This illustrates the concept of proportion with type. Notice how the height of the type does not change, just the horizontal distance.

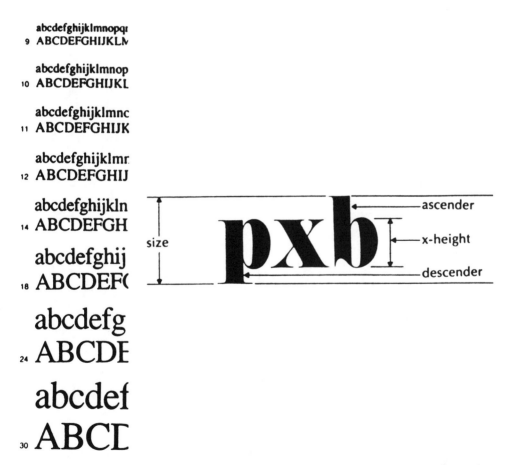

abcdefghijklmnopqr
9 ABCDEFGHIJKLM

abcdefghijklmnop
10 ABCDEFGHIJKL

abcdefghijklmnc
11 ABCDEFGHIJK

abcdefghijklmr
12 ABCDEFGHIJ

abcdefghijkln
14 ABCDEFGH

abcdefghij
18 ABCDEF(

abcdefg
24 ABCDE

abcdef
30 ABCL

size — ascender — x-height — descender

Figure 7-6. This figure shows how type size is measured: from the top of the ascender to the bottom of the descender. Also shown are different sizes of type and their point measurements.

197

notice that the X-height (or height of the lower case "a" for that matter) does not change when type is condensed or expanded. This measure is not terribly important, except that type faces with a high X-height tend to be somewhat easier to read than type with a low X-height.

Leading

The space between lines of type is called "leading" (rhymes with heading). The normal leading is 1 point unless specified otherwise. Some of the factors that can affect the amount of leading that is used in a particular document are listed.

Factors That Affect Leading

1. X-Height. Typefaces with a high X-height tend to be somewhat easier to read than type with a low X-height. But higher X-height can also require greater leading between lines because the set type appears more crowded than types with lower X-heights.
2. Vertical stress. This refers to the emphasis, or stress, of the vertical lines in a given type style. The stronger the vertical emphasis is, the greater the need for added leading.
3. Serif. The presence of serifs helps to create a horizontal flow and aid reading. The absence of serifs generally requires more leading so that the eye does not skip lines as easily.
4. Length of line. Additional leading helps to some degree to offset the problem of an overly long line of type. However, if the type is drastically too small for the length of the line, it would take so much added leading that it would really make more sense to increase the type size or decrease the line length.

Readability

Now that some of the terms have been explained, we can move on to see how these things affect readability.

As mentioned earlier, the idea behind this concern for the mechanics of print is to keep cost down, and most importantly to make the material as readable as possible. For our purposes, that is for those of us who are not in the printing business, a good rule of thumb to keep in mind is that readability goes down as we depart from "normal." When you are producing materials, keep an eye out for the other materials that are produced by other people, especially professional publishers and material producing companies. In the next sections, you will find other "rules of thumb" and descriptions of "normal."

Selecting Type

As mentioned earlier, there are many type styles to choose from. Selecting type is important from the standpoint of the ease with which it can be read, and also for the mood it creates. If you are in doubt as to the readability of a type as opposed to the mood it creates, choose readability over any other factor. There are vehicles other than type selection through which visual interest can be created.

The ease with which a type can be read is important. Many of the "caligraphy" styles that are currently popular are extremely difficult to read especially in paragraph form. Do not assume that because "they" are using "a lot of this typeface" that "they" are right. There are fads in type just as there are in clothes. The readability of a particular type can be checked, just as the content copy is checked for accuracy and clarity before it is used.

To develop a type test, select material which is not familiar to the reader. Ask a number of people to read a selection of copy, perhaps 300–500 words, and then tell you know they felt about reading it, whether their eyes moved smoothly, if they tired, or if they skipped lines. Then ask a few simple questions about the copy to see if the material was comprehended.

Readers may not know it, but they are affected by the "mood" of the type they are looking at. In the extreme, for instance, readers of patient education material about amputation would be discouraged by use of a frivolous-looking type. On the other hand, material for expectant parents set in Gothic and heavy type would not encourage the parents to see their situation as "happy."

Sans serif type often looks cleaner, neater, and more modern than serif type. However, serif type is easier to read, especially in block or paragraph form. Your eyes use the little hooks and feet as anchors to keep on track and stay on the correct line. If sans serif type is used, it generally requires that another point of leading be used to make it more readable.

LONG BLOCKS OF COPY SET IN ALL CAPITALS BECOME MUCH MORE DIFFICULT TO READ BECAUSE THE READER IS DEPRIVED OF THE NATURAL TENDENCY TO USE A FLOWING EYE PATTERN TO WHICH TRADITIONAL UPPER AND LOWER CASE HAS ACCUSTOMED HIM OR HER. For this reason, never use all capital letters for patient education materials unless it is for a short heading.

The same thing is true of the use of bold type, italics, script, heavily expanded, and extremely light type. Occasional use of these styles is certainly a good idea, but overuse can be detrimental to the intent to increase readability. Whenever the reader loses the normal eye pattern, he or she has to constantly backtrack to pick up something that was missed in the initial passage over the copy.

Color

The color of the ink and the paper stock is an often overlooked item that affects readability. Using colored ink and paper can certainly make a printed piece look more attractive and professional. It is very important, however, that you remember who is going to look at the material and where they will do it. Older persons have altered color perception, meaning that color combinations that are very attractive to a 20-year-old person may not at all be attractive to a 70-year-old. Older persons tend to prefer subdued colors, almost "dusty tones." A certain percentage of younger people are also color blind. Color blind people literally may not be able to read some patient education materials because of the color combinations that are used.

Where a piece is read, and consequently under what kind of light can be a big issue. If you have ever picked out paint in a store and then realized that it looked very different when it got to your walls at home, you have experienced the light issue first hand. You need to pick out colors and papers under as nearly the same lighting conditions that your readers will have. Light intensity is a related issue. Most offices have more light in them when materials are being produced than the readers will have as they read the material, whether they are in their own homes or in a hospital bed. This can affect readability very negatively.

Paper Stock

The paper that is used for the printed material can also affect readability. Besides color, a basic difference in paper is whether it is coated or not. Coating is a process that usually makes the paper more "glossy." This glossy coating can make the material harder to read because of reflected light, although the type itself tends to be more crisp on coated stock.

Reader Assessment

It is particularly important to remember who is going to read the material as you make choices. Are your readers going to be older persons so you cannot assume 20/20 vision even with correction? Are your readers going to be in the hospital where they may or may not be wearing corrective lenses even if they have them? Are two or more people going to be trying to read this material at the same time, such as a spouse?

Several things are known about readers that need to be considered, especially for hospitalized patients. The first fact is that as the reader ages, vision deteriorates. As a person ages, the rate at which vision deteriorates increases also. This means that even though a patient has regular eye exams and corrective lenses, eyesight may have changed significantly since the last exam. We also know that some groups of people correct their vision as they age, and others do not tend to do so. The people that tend to take care of their vision are professionals and support personnel for professionals. The groups that tend to not take care of their vision include housewives and househusbands, retirees and blue collar workers, especially those who work outdoors a great deal.

Knowing the age and economic background of the patients who are going to read the material that you produce can have a great impact on the choices that are made for the mechanical aspects of the finished product. Knowing the average age of the patient population that is in the hospital is important. It makes no sense to produce materials that cannot be read.

In summary, a commonly used formula for optimum readability for corrected eyes is 10 point type with 1 point leading, serif type face. X-height of 50–60 percent, black type on white or off-white paper, on uncoated stock. Knowing the patient population that will be using the materials that you develop will help you make wise choices as you alter this formula.

Reading Level

It has been shown that the readability of patient education materials is affected by many mechnical things. The content of the piece is also certainly important, but the words used to explain the topic can make it understood or ignored. The words that you choose will determine the reading level necessary to comprehend the material. The complexity of the vocabulary, both medical and otherwise, should be carefully considered when producing materials or purchasing them.

There are several tests that can be performed on the material to determine the exact reading level needed to comprehend the material. The professionals that you are working with will probably have their own favorite tests. The basic way that they work is to take samples of the text and count the average syllables per word, the number of words per sentence, the difficulty of the words, or the words per paragraph. The score is then compared to a table and a reading level is determined, such as 8.5. This would mean that someone in the middle of the eighth grade should be able to comprehend the material.

One readability formula that is quite easy to use is the SMOG Index (Journal of Reading). The SMOG formula is quick to perform and assures a 90 percent comprehension (i.e., a person with a tenth grade reading level will comprehend 90 percent of the material rated at that level) and is relatively reliable and respected. Table 7-1 lists some possible SMOG scores and shows how they can be related to publications.

Table 7-1
SMOG Score and Interpretation

Grade level (score)	Level of style	Typical magazine
6–7	Very easy	Comics
8	Easy	Pulp fiction
9–10	Average	*Readers Digest*
11–13	Fairly difficult	*Atlantic Monthly*
14–16	Difficult	Academic magazines *Psychoanalytic Review* *Child Welfare*
17+	Very difficult	Scientific, professional magazines *Music Educator Journal*

Many formal readability scores come out placing the material at the comprehension level of upper elementary and junior high school. This may seem low to you, but the national average reading level is not that high. Most newspapers are written for the sixth grade reading level. This fact should reinforce the idea that you need to know your audience and their abilities.

Many individuals read well beyond the fourth to eighth grade levels, yet when a person is using health-related materials, they are probably reading topics generally foreign or potentially threatening to them. Thus, the lower grade reading levels can be useful to present the complicated and often fear-arousing aspects of health care information. After the patient and family have had time to accept the illness, after they have had basic information on the topic, or when they begin asking more detailed questions, the higher reading level materials may be appropriately used.

One practical method for checking the appropriateness of material for a particular patient is to check the patient's comprehension of one paragraph or section of the material. For example, the nurse could explain that this material is used to help teach patients about their illness. This nurse could then ask the patient to read the first paragraph and explain, in his or her own words, what that section says. The patient's response can be judged for accuracy, completeness, and any fear-arousing or anxiety-producing notions picked up from the reading. The nurse can then ask the patient if the material was clearly written and there would be any benefit from reading the remainder of the sections.

Another easy way to be certain that a particular piece of printed material is at the appropriate reading level is to have the patient tell his or her family what was learned. If the patient can convey the information to others it is apparent that he or she has learned from the materials. The nurse can then ascertain the family's understanding and inquire as to their interest in reading the material themselves.

Besides checking the overall reading level of the material, individual words or terms that may be foreign to the patient must be identified ahead of time. For example, the newly diagnosed diabetic will not be familiar with the term "U100" nor will the mother seeking nutrition information for her infant necessarily recognize the phrase "basic food groups." Both of these terms represent information that these individuals can eventually master. However, in the first introduction such unfamiliar or complex words should be defined for the patient who is given the material to read.

Layout

Another factor that affects readability is the layout of the material. If you are working with people who produce pamphlets regularly they will have specific recommendations as to the layout you should use for your particular material. General guidelines are to keep the material in logical order, use illustrations wherever possible, keep paragraphs short, move from front to back, don't split items or columns like a newspaper, and use headings and subheadings.

Cost Effectiveness

Cost is another consideration in printing. The cost per piece of a given pamphlet goes down as you buy or print more. The cost of using a full service printer will be greater than using an "instant printer," and typeset will be more costly than typewritten. But there will be quality differences with each of these choices that are proportional to the cost differences. It costs more to use colored inks and the cost goes up as you use more than one color of ink. Many other factors will effect the cost of the product and you will have to decide what image and effect you want to project. A reliable printer or other vendor of printing services can be a very valuable help in finding ways to get the best product for the money, especially if you do not have access to a professional within your own institution. Often you will not have the luxury of deciding on the budget for your project, but will rather have the task of getting the best product for the amount you can spend per patient.

The search for cost effectiveness can lead to some unusual solutions to rather complicated problems. It has been said that a picture is worth a thousand words. Sometimes a $5 picture can be worth $1000 in patient teaching.

Photographic Prints

Pictures can speak very eloquently and be very cost effective. Photographic prints, like the ones you get after developing your vacation pictures, can be a valuable teaching tool. For instance, we use a photo album to teach pediatric patients preoperatively. The pictures show a child what happens when he or she goes through the admission process with his or her family, meets the staff, goes to surgery, and recovers in his or her room. There are minimal captions with each picture, and the child is allowed to keep the album for a period of time after the admitting nurse explains it. The child can then review and explain things to his or her family. This type of tool is very effective.

The same principle of using a photo album is used with adolescent bone marrow transplant patients. These patients meet many people from various disciplines in the course of their rather long hospitalization, so the photo album of all the various activities and the respective care givers (including pictures of all the staff) is a very reassuring tool for the patient.

For our adult renal patients, photos are used in a different way. These patients are dismissed with what seems like a truckload of different medications that must be taken at home on a variety of schedules. To help in the learning process for these patients, we have a photo album with pictures of all of their medications, and in the case of tablets and capsules, the pictures are larger than actual size. These photos are used by the nurses as they teach the patients about their different drugs, how to recognize each by shape and color, and when to take each one.

Video Learning Resources

Printed material may be the most common teaching tool that is used with patients, but television is by far the most used "teaching" tool used by industry in general when they wish to convey a message to the general public. Patient educators are starting to take advantage of this popular device, and hopefully will find ways to use it that are as effective as print.

Because this technology is used so much and in such quantity, it has become relatively inexpensive. Virtually every home has a TV set, and home type videotape recorders have become common. In our society, people are becoming more accustomed to receiving information over the television and health educators are starting to use this media extensively for in-patient teaching as well as for home teaching.

The next sections will discuss the many types of video tools that are available to the patient educator. Illustrations will also be given for the ways in which different video programs can be used.

Video Formats

Video tape recorders come in several formats, most of which are mutually exclusive, in that a tape recorded in one format is not able to be played on a machine of another format. The common commercial (home) types of videocassette recorders (VCRs) are Beta and VHS, the former being patented by the Sony Corporation and the latter by the JVC Corporation. Beta and VHS are both recorded on tape that is ½-inch wide, but the information is put on the tape in two very different ways. There is not a noticeable difference in the picture quality of the two formats on the TV screen, but they can't be used interchangeably. Tapes for the Beta and VHS machines come in different lengths, the most common of which will allow the recording of 2 hours of material. Some VCRs allow the speed of the tape to be varied, so that a tape that normally records 2 hours, can be used to record 4, 6, and even 8 hours of material.

The most common format for videotape in business, including hospitals and clinics, is the ¾-inch U-Matic format. This type of tape is ¾ inch in width and comes in a cassette like Beta and VHS. U-Matic recorders are made by many manufacturers, are generally more expensive than ½-inch machines, and have more features that allow good editing and a more stable picture. There are other industrial (business) formats of tape, including 1- and 2-inch open reel tape. However, these formats are not normally used outside of television stations and video production firms.

As the technology of video improves, more and more hospitals and other businesses will probably convert to the ½-inch formats of tape. The main reason will be cost, in that very good picture quality is coming from the smaller, less expensive machines.

Video Cameras

Video cameras have followed the lead of all other electronic devices in the last 10 years: they are smaller, more reliable, easier to use, and less expensive. Cameras come with many different types of features, pick-up tubes, lenses, and accessories. It is not important to discuss them here, but you should know that the market is changing so fast that price alone is not a good judge of the quality of the picture. Most cameras have automatic features that make operation of the camera as simple as operating a 35-mm still camera for taking family snapshots. When purchasing a camera, it is important to see the pictures from each on monitors, side by side, and then to actually operate them yourself.

Video cameras have become inexpensive and easy enough to use that there are many new uses for them in patient education, besides formal television productions. Many families like to videotape the delivery of their children to show siblings and other relatives. Patients who are learning to use crutches or braces can be taped and shown the playback immediately so they can critique themselves. Visitation of patients in isolation can be improved by using video cameras and microphones instead of putting a whole group into isolation gowns.

Video Discs

A new concept in video recording and playback equipment arrived on the scene a couple of years ago. Video disc technology is new, but it promises to make some major contributions to education. A video disc is very similar to a record album in size and appearance, except that the video disc is shiny silver in color.

There are two basic types of video discs: laser and capacitance. In both types the pick-up device does not touch the surface of the disc and consequently there is no wear of the surfaces. This makes the picture quality of the disc image extremely good, and allows it to stay sharp without the normal deterioration in quality that one would expect with tape because of wear on the tape. As a matter of fact, if a videotape machine is left in the pause mode (that is the same picture is kept on the screen and the tape is not moving, and the heads are reading the same piece of the tape), it can actually wear a hole right through the tape, although this would take some time. On the video disc, however, the disc can play the same picture "forever" without wear to the disc or the image pick-up device.

The other advantages of the video disc are its ability to store large amounts of information and to get to any particular piece of information in a hurry. At the present time, a video disc can store 50,000 images. In practical terms, that means that an entire set of the *Encyclopedia Britannica* can be stored on one disc. From a speed standpoint, the disc can find any one piece of information in 3 seconds or less. The reason for this speed is that the information is encoded digitally, and each image has a number. As the disc spins, the pick-up head passes over each spot on the disc rather quickly. The storage statistics I referred to are for still images. If the disc is being used for storing "moving pictures", then a disc will hold about 60 minutes of information. An advantage of the disc is that it will store still pictures, moving video and screens of text information all on the same disc.

A more recent adaptation of video disc technology has been the use of video discs and computers that are connected together and called "interactive video." This system uses a computer to solicit information from the learner; after analyzing the input the computer directs the video disc player to show certain segments of the disc, and then ask the learner for input. Basically this system uses the computer to hold the program sequence and uses the video disc player to store segments of the disc, and then ask the learner for input. Basically this system uses the computer to hold the program sequence and uses the video disc player to store segments of video to be shown as well as text. Programs that are made using this technology are very effective, but at this point, are quite costly.

Screen Readability

One issue that must be addressed when using video is the same concern that we have with all forms of visual communication—readability. When text information is placed on the screen, can the patient read it? The problem is that everyone who sees the screen will be at a different distance from the it. Therefore, the size of the type that appears on the screen is very important. Also to be considered is the visual acuity of the patients, whether or not they will have vision correction and whether or not corrective lenses will be worn when they watch the screen. Another complication is that regular television screens do not have good resolution, that is, the picture is not particularly sharp compared with a computer monitor.

When showing a video program to a group, a good rule of thumb is that for every inch of screen size, people can watch from one foot away. For instance, with a 19-inch TV set, people should be able to see from 19 feet away. This rule assumes that the amount of text on the screen is limited to about eight lines of type and five words per line. To see what will fit on a screen, watch a few commercials on TV and see how much information is placed on the screen at once.

Video Distribution

Another advantage to video technology is that because the signal is electronic, it can be transmitted to many places in many ways. A video recorder can be placed on a cart with a TV set and taken into a patient's room. The signal can also be placed on a closed circuit TV system and sent to all of the rooms in a hospital from one VCR. The signal can be placed on a satellite and sent literally anywhere in the world. The signal can also be placed on videotape and the patient can take it home and play it then, or anytime in the future.

We use VCRs on carts that go to patient rooms to play entertainment programs, especially movies. Many of the long-term patients, such as burn victims, enjoy the movies that are available from the hospital and those that can be rented from outside vendors. The more actuely ill patients do not have the attention span or the interest for movies.

We also use VCRs on carts that nurses move into patient rooms to show particular programs and teach patients. Our closed circuit system plays programs for patient teaching on one channel that is received on all the TV sets on the walls in the patient rooms. These teaching programs cover topics like diabetes, heart disease, presurgical exercises and routines, and breast self examination. (Closed circuit systems will be discussed in more detail in a later section.) We also have video cassettes that demonstrate exercises for pregnant women that are available for sale to patients that wish to have them. This trend of information provided directly to the patient to use in the home is likely to increase.

When patient education programming is placed in the hands of patients it is especially important to be sure that the technology that is being used is "socially and politically" acceptable to patients, otherwise they will not use it. For certain patient groups, playing a videotape in their own homes is a common experience. For other patient groups, the videotape in the home is a new experience and they will require support, both technical and emotional, to use the material.

Video for Therapeutic Entertainment

Video can be used for instructional purposes as we have seen, but it can also be used for entertainment. The entertainment value of TV should not be underrated. Several studies have shown that a positive mental attitude has a positive effect on healing and wellness. The value of laughter has also received media attention. With careful attention to selection of the right kind of program, a hospital closed circuit TV system can be used to show motivational programming, and entertaining and humorous programs. These programs can also be sent home to patients. Wouldn't it be interesting to have prescriptions for watching humorous TV programs?

TV Commercials as Teaching Models

One of the most effective teaching tools that has ever been used is the television commercial. These short "programs" are very effective in getting people to change their behavior and alter their attitudes. Health educators can take some lessons from these "programs." The producers of the commercial are very careful to do a detailed analysis of the intended audience. The program content is chosen very carefully, a great deal of attention is paid to the way that the information is presented, messages are simple and direct, the message is repeated many times in a variety of ways, the message is reinforced by many media, and the result of the commercial is measured to determine its impact.

Telecommunications

Putting signals out over the TV broadcast airwaves is only one way to transmit information from one place to the other. In our information society, we as patient educators will have to become more skilled at using other media and other ways of communicating.

Telecommunication, by definition, is to take information and turn it into electrical energy that can be sent to another place and turned back into a form that makes sense to the receiving person. As our patients are in the hospital for less lengthy stays, and as they come from further away, we are going to need to use telecommunication to get our job done. Telecommunication strategies will allow us to get the message to many people at the same time and will also let us get that message to a wide variety of places at great distances.

Telephone

The telephone is a tool that is used daily, and it is a tool that can be put to good use for patient education. The American Cancer Society has recognized this, and has a toll-free number that can be dialed to request short, taped messages about various kinds of cancer. The Minnesota Dental Association has a similar service with messages about dental care and disease. Some hospitals also have a call-in service with messages about various topics. This type of service is not terribly costly, and can be operated by someone with minimal medical background, because the messages contain all the content. This type of service can be a good source of referrals.

Audio Teleconference

Audio teleconferences are another potential use of the telephone for instruction. In this case a person or group on one end of the line is able to hold a conversation with a person of group on the other end of the line. The equipment involved is such that everyone in a given location can sit around a table or in a classroom setting and not have to hold a telephone receiver; a central microphone and speaker can do the job. This type of set-up could be especially useful if a particular speaker could not be physically present for a class, but could still give the information and answer questions. Several speakers in different locations can be involved in this arrangement at the same time, and if things are worked out ahead of time, even slides or other projected material can be shown while the person is speaking.

One particular patient education setting where audio teleconferencing is useful is when the group that needs to be together is small, but spread out over distance and travel is difficult, such as spinal cord injury patients and rehabilitation teams. With audio teleconferencing, patients can talk to each other, share tips for better living, and provide emotional support for each other. Rehabilitation specialists can share their expertise with patients who are not even in the institutions where they work. Patients can be in their own personal environments and still communicate and be served.

Broadcast Radio and Television

Commercial broadcast radio and television have a mass audience, but generally are too expensive for health educators to use on a regular basis. There are always public service spots that can be used, but regular programs are infrequent, except for the call-in variety. A recent variation of broadcast TV is called ITFS (instructional television fixed service).

ITFS is a low power TV station that can broadcast for only a few miles from its source. This type of signal can be picked up on a regular TV set in a home, and could be used by local health education providers if their patients were concentrated in a particular area. To set up an ITFS station requires a license from the Federal Communications Commission in Washington, DC and quite a bit of equipment and technical expertise. However, an institution that is serious about reaching a group in a local area may want to consider this option.

Cable Television

Another television option is cable TV in areas where this is available. By law, cable companies must provide channels for members of the community to use to put on their own programs (this is called public access programming). Health education can be placed on the cable system and picked up in any home that is attached to the cable. Some cable companies are particular about programming that "advertises" for an individual institution, and rightfully so. Public access channels are not intended for advertising. Purely educational programs will be aired, however.

The advantage of this option is that it is inexpensive to distribute programs. The disadvantages are that purchased programs may or may not be licensed for cable distribution. Production of television programs is relatively expensive; you may not be able to be sure that anyone is watching, and unless you set up call-in phone lines, there is no way for someone who is watching to ask questions.

Closed Circuit Television

Closed circuit television has been used in institutions for many years and continues to be a cost effective alternative for program distribution. In this situation, television programs are played in one place and sent over wires to other locations, such as the patient rooms. In most systems, the programs are sent to all of the locations at the same time. A variation of this is to have individual sets turned on to the appropriate channel by a computer as the patient requests the program, so that only certain patients see a particular program at any given time. This type of system is similar to the type that is in place in many hotels, whereby the customer is charged for a movie in the room a particular channel is turned on or a button pushed for a movie.

When closed circuit systems are used it is important to make sure that programs are available when patients need to see them, which usually means playing them many times in a day or week. Another important point to remember is that patients need to know when the program is available and they need followup by health educators to make sure that learning occurred and to answer any questions.

Satellite Broadcasting and Receiving

Satellite broadcasting is another new entry into the communication arena. This type of broadcasting allows programs to be sent up to the satellite from one location on earth and then be sent back down to earth and picked up in any number of other locations. Because there are many satellites and many channels per satellite, there are a great number of programs that can be carried at one time. Traditional satellite programming is still quite expensive and this vehicle is not used extensively by individual institutions for sending health information. Many institutions do use the satellites for receiving information, however. The American Hospital Association has a good resource booklet *Purchasing a Satellite Receiving Earth Terminal,* that is very helpful in this regard.

There are several health networks that broadcast at the present time over satellites. One such network, Lifetime, a for-profit company located in New York, is picked up and transmitted by several cable companies and hospitals. Other networks market their programming directly to hospitals and clinics, who pick up the programs on their own satellite dishes (earth stations) and send the programs (both health related and entertainment) to their patients. This kind of patient education can be cost effective compared to producing the programs yourself, but the programs may not be acceptable to your institution or patients. Screening of programs becomes very important for these reasons.

A new type of satellite system is being developed, called direct broadcast satellite (DBS). The sending process for this system is very similar to regular satellites, but the receiving end of the process is different. Regular satellite signals require a rather large and expensive earth receiving station: about 10 feet in diameter and costing $20,000 for a good signal at an urban hospital. DBS on the other hand will need a receiving system that is about 18 inches in diameter and costing about $200. This will make DBS affordable to a great many people and may make it possible for a given institution to send programming to all of its patients, no matter where they may live in the world.

Video Teleconferencing

Video teleconferencing has found a place in education in the last 10 years. Many staff development programs and nursing continuing education programs are now presented by use of video teleconferencing technology. The American Hospital Association (AHA) has had success with an ongoing series of video teleconferences on topics that are of interest to various groups within a hospital setting. AHA sends teleconferences virtually every month, and institutions pay for and receive only those conferences they want. Teleconferencing technology is particularly good for getting information to a wide variety of people who are located in diverse locations, but who need to receive current information without the cost and time of traveling.

Teleconferencing allows video and audio information to be sent by satellite, microwave or ground telephone line from one place to another. One version of teleconferencing is video and audio that is sent from one place to the other. Another case would be for the second location to be in contact with the first location by regular telephone (as in the case of call-in questions). In still another variation, video and audio can be sent both ways by satellite. One type of video conferencing involves sending still pictures, such as slides or textual information over the telephone lines along with voice. This type of conferencing is much less expensive than sending moving video images.

PROJECTED LEARNING RESOURCES

Projected media are probably the best known of all the audiovisual formats. This category includes slides, movies, overhead transparencies, and computer outputs and video that can be projected onto a screen. While projected media are most often used with groups, there are ways to use this very effective tool with individuals.

Projection Surfaces

When you project anything, you have to have something to project it on, so screens were invented. There are many types and sizes, but they can be thought of in two categories, front and rear. With front projection, the projector and the audience are on the same side of the screen. With rear projection, the projector is on one side of the screen (usually hidden from the audience) and the audience is on the other side.

There are three basic types of front projection screens; matt, lenticular and beaded. The beaded screen gives the brightest image, but the poorest viewing as people move off to the side of the screen. Matt screens are less expensive, not as bright, but have the best viewing from the sides of the screen. Lenticular screens are in the middle for both criteria.

One of the common questions in regard to screens is location and size. We have all been to presentations where someone's head was in the picture, which is a common problem if the screen is not located high enough. Many presentations are also made where the information presented on the screen was too small to read from the back of the room, or the seating is so close to the screen that it was difficult to grasp the whole image at once.

As a general rule of thumb, a screen size and room size relationship should be arranged so that the closest seat is located at a distance that is twice the height of the projected image (2H), and the furthest seat is located eight times the projected image height from the screen (8H). To avoid obstruction of the screen image by the seated audience, the ceiling height should permit the bottom edge of the image to be located at least 4 feet above the floor. There are certainly exceptions to these rules, but it is a good basis from which to start and will eliminate most projection size problems.

Location of the screen in the room will greatly affect the view. In a square room, more people will have a good view if the screen is in the corner of the room. In a rectangular room, the viewing is best when the screen is on the short wall.

The size of the screen will determine how big the image can be, and the size of the image and the distance to the furthest viewer will determine how well the material can be seen or read. You know from doing eye checks using the Snellen Eye Chart that characters must be of a certain size to be read by a person with normal vision from a certain distance. The same is true with projected media, but the situation is complicated by the fact that people are viewing the image from different distances. To make sure that material can be seen, you need not ask the person in the front, but rather the person in the back. If the person in the back can't read it, perhaps it shouldn't be used.

Projection with Room Light

The biggest advantage for most projected media is that many people can be in one place and see the image at the same time. The information can then be explained to many people at a time. The biggest disadvantage from a teaching standpoint, is that projected media used with a group, with the exception of the overhead projector, must be used with the lights lowered or off. This condition causes the teacher to lose audience eye contact. Very few patients, especially frightened or apprehensive ones, will ask questions when in the dark. The overhead projector should be used in a room with the lights on. This characteristic of the overhead projector makes it a particularly good tool to use when you want to encourage group discussion.

Slide Presentations

Slide presentations, especially those that are accompanied by an audio tape that advances the slides automatically along with the narration, can be very effective with groups as well as individuals, and they are relatively inexpensive to produce and purchase. There are several manufacturers of small, portable projection boxes that take a slide tray on the top, and an audiocassette in the side. (Kodak, Bell and Howell, and Singer are examples. Your audiovisual equipment dealer may have other sources.) The image is produced on a square screen on the front of the unit (or by opening a small door, can be projected on the wall for a group) and the audio comes from a speaker in the unit or it can be heard through headphones. The units are portable and will easily fit on the patient's bedside or overbed table. The units can also be placed on small carts and moved from room to room. The advantage for us is that the patients can start and stop this equipment on their own, and individual programs can be changed and new slides inserted at little cost as procedures change.

Projection Resources

Because projected media are so commonly used and relatively inexpensive, there is a great deal of equipment on the market and there are many resources to help in producing this type of material. One of the best sources of technical information about equipment, projection and producing materials is the Eastman Kodak Company in Rochester, NY.

Three of Kodak's publications that are especially helpful are *Audiovisual Projection*, number S-3; *Legibility—Artwork to Screen*, number S-24; and *Effective Lecture Slides*, number S-22. There are many other pamphlets that are helpful and they are all listed in Kodak pamphlet number L-5, *Index to Kodak Information*. This index can be obtained free of charge by writing Eastman Kodak Company, Department 412L, Rochester, NY 14650. As of this writing, many of the pamphlets listed in the index are available free of charge in quantities of one.

Computer Learning Resources

No technology has turned us into a technological society more than the computer. Our lives would be changed dramatically if for some reason the computer ceased to be in our world. Although the computer has been used extensively in other industries, it is only recently being seriously applied in education.

Hardware

Every computer has three parts, and Figure 7-7 shows graphically how they relate. In a desktop micro computer like the Apple IIe or the IBM PC, these parts are all housed together in the same chassis. In larger "mainframe" computers the three components may be located in very distant places, sometimes thousands of miles apart. The three parts are an input device, a central processing unit (CPU), and an output device. An input device can be a keyboard, a computer touch screen, a tape drive, a floppy disk drive, a joystick

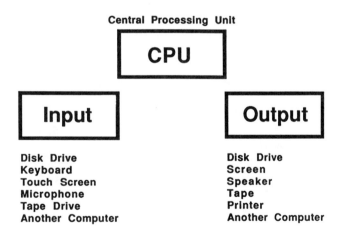

Figure 7-7. The three basic parts of any computer are the input module, the central processing unit (CPU), and the output module. Many different devices can be used for the modules, such as a keyboard, screen, disc drive, or printer.

control, or any number of other things. The CPU is the part of the computer that actually does the "thinking." The output device can be a computer screen, a printer, a floppy disk drive, or a speech synthesizer.

Software

A computer program is a set of instructions that tell the machine when to get input, how to think about it, and what to do with the results of the thinking. The machine itself is actually quite dumb, and it only will do what the programmer tells it to. Sometimes we wish that the machine would do what we are thinking, but it actually does exactly what we tell it to.

Computer software that is purchased or developed by educators is just a set of instructions to the machine so that it will ask for information from the learner at the right time, analyze the information in a certain way, and provide certain information back to the learner in a certain way. Software varies in its complexity, and also in how much knowledge about the computer and programs is necessary to get the desired results from the machine. Another characteristic of software is that for the most part, programs that run on one type of computer will not run on another computer. It is very important to know what computers will work with a given program before it is purchased.

Teaching Options with Computers

The state of computer technology gives the educator many options for teaching. The machine has the ability to store large amounts of information, use and display pictures as well as text, and change the presentation depending on the input of the learner. Computer teaching can be designed so that the learner can control the pace of the instruction, a particularly useful characteristic for dealing with adults.

Because the machine can ask questions and analyze the responses, the machine can actually do an assessment of the learner and alter the content, pace, or examples provided. Computers can also be set to control other pieces of equipment, such as slide projectors and video projection equipment. Computers can also be programmed to keep track of the learners that use it and provide reports to the educator of concepts that were learned, speed with which the content was learned, and where reinforcement is needed.

Computer Problems

The problems with computers are numerous, but slide projectors had their problems when they first came out too. The major problem with computers is cost, which is substantial at this time. Computers are expensive to purchase and program, so that to justify using an educational program, one needs to be able to amortize the cost of the program over many patients.

The majority of computers use a screen to present information, and keyboards to get information. The problem with screens is readability. Can the patients see the information on the screen, and can they read it and make sense of it? Although it is true that computers can be built to use almost any type of input device, the majority of commercially available computers use a keyboard to get input. If this is true for a patient teaching tool, then the educator must take into account whether the learners are able to use the keyboard and whether the process will be intimidating. Developments in the computer field for the next several years will likely deal with the problems of getting the machine to work with a human being in a way that is more natural and flexible for the person, such as voice input, and do it in a way that is cost effective.

Computer Applications

Many people and companies are working to produce patient education materials that use the strengths of the computer to best advantage. Because computers can accept data from many sources and then decide which course of action is appropriate, computers are good at assessment type projects. For instance, there are several programs on the market that will ask a patient for the food items that were eaten in a certain time period, and the computer will calculate the calories consumed and other nutrient information. Other programs help diabetics keep track of information that is helpful to them in managing their disease.

Another way that computers can be put to good use is providing educational material to patients during times that would otherwise be considered "wasted." At least one company is producing health instruction software that is designed to be used in physician's waiting rooms. In this case the computer can provide information on a wide variety of topics and may very well prompt the patient to ask more appropriate questions of the health care provider. The educator in this situation can concentrate on providing the specific instruction that is needed, and not spend so much time providing redundant information.

A third example of using computers to monitor the instructional process and control several pieces of equipment is being developed. Under this proposed system, hospitalized patients will be provided with a credit card size piece of plastic with their name on it and some holes punched in it. In the case of a new mother on the Obstetrics unit, the nurse would instruct the patient to insert the card into a small box next to the bedside telephone when she is ready to look at some programs that might be helpful to her as she takes care of her new baby. The nurse would tell the patient that she would be back later to answer any questions and help in any way.

When the new mother puts the card in the slot, several things happen. First, the computer that is attached by telephone to the box activates the room television set to a certain channel. The computer will know that this patient is a new mother and that she has not watched any of the programs in the series that has been arranged. The sequence of programs would include instructions for bathing and feeding infants, carseats, infant development, and other topics.

The television image will be provided over the hospital closed-circuit TV system from a video disc machine so the image will arrive quickly, no matter which program the patient wishes to see. The programs will ask the patient to dial a hospital telephone number that will tie her into the computer. As the program progresses and asks the patient for responses to questions, the patient will touch the appropriate button on the telephone and the response will be recorded and analyzed by the computer. The telephone buttons can also be used by the patient to select which program she wants to see, much like a menu choice.

This type of computer-assisted instruction can have several advantages for the nurse. If the hospital has computer charting, the education computer can log what programs were viewed and when. In addition, a computer printer located on the nurses station can, at the end or begining of each shift, list the programs that each patient has used, which content questions were answered correctly and which concepts were reinforced. The printout can even list areas on which the patient would like more information or help.

This third example of how computers can help the instructional process is a predecessor to systems that will be developed to allow people available access to the vast amount of health information that is available in their own homes. There is now and will continue to be a great deal of activity in this area of technology. Even with all the new technology that is available, there are still things that we can learn about the tools that we have had for a long time.

Audio Learning Resources

Audio technology has been around for a long time and exists in primarily three forms at this time: tape, disc, and radio. Audio has not been used a great deal for patient education except in cases where the patient is blind or has some other serious visual or motor disability. However, this is a significant technology that has some real application in a patient care environment.

Radio

Radio has a large impact on all of our lives, but it is not used very heavily for health care teaching. This is probably due to the commercial nature of radio and the mass markets that it usually appeals to. There are a few health teaching programs on public and private radio stations, but these usually fall under the category of "community service" or "talk shows" and are not now used as consistent vehicles for patient teaching. One use of radio that should be given more consideration by patient educators is radio that is particularly sent to people who are blind or physically handicapped.

These radio stations are generally publicly supported or supported by private foundations. They broadcast information and read materials over the air on a particular frequency that is only received by specially tuned radios that are available from the sponsoring agency. Since these radios can be a major source of information for a special group of patients, we should be looking more carefully at using this vehicle.

Audio Disc

Audio discs have also been on the market for a long time, and I expect that there are very few people reading this book who do not have a favorite album. Traditional records are made by placing a groove in a piece of vinyl. As a stylus is moved along the groove and rubs against ridges in the groove, a signal is produced and sent to amplification equipment that makes the sound audible. This recording system works quite well, but has the disadvantage of wearing with age. As the stylus and the groove wear, the fidelity of the recording deteriorates, and eventually is unuseable. A new type of disc has arrived on the market, known as the compact audio disc.

The compact audio disc is different in that there are no grooves, and the "stylus" does not actually touch the record surface. It is a very similar technology to the video discs described earlier. There are currently two types of these compact discs; one uses a laser to reproduce the sound, and one uses a capacitance device. The major advantage of this new disc is that the fidelity does not deteriorate over time because of wear, and the original fidelity is superior because of the production techniques. The disadvantage is expense. As is true with all new technologies, the compact disc is relatively expensive, but it is also true that as more of a given technology is available to the general public, the costs generally go down. This has been true of the compact disc and will certainly be true in the future.

Audio Tape

Audio tape has been around for a long time as well. The three ways that audio tape are largely used are in the cassette, 8-track, and reel-to-reel formats. Reel-to-reel is not used very much anymore by the general public. The 8-track was very popular in the 1960s and 70s, especially for use in automobiles for playing commercially prepared tapes, mostly music. Today the 8-track tape is used very seldom. The most popular tape format today is the cassette. Cassettes are small, portable, inexpensive, require inexpensive hardware to be used and consequently are very popular. Cassettes also hold good possibilities for patient education.

Cassettes are used by the blind to get information. Cassettes can be made quickly and inexpensively, and they can be duplicated quickly. (In a high-speed cassette duplicator, a 60-minute cassette can be reproduced in about 1 minute.) Cassettes can be particularly effective when they are used in conjunction with a booklet or other media.

Patient educators might do well to use an idea that the Kodak Company uses. Kodak sells cassettes to be used in the darkroom by photographers developing pictures. The Kodak cassettes give step by step instructions for each process, and play music while a given process is timed out. This way the process is explained as well as timed, so that each step is done in the right order and takes the correct amount of time.

This technique could also be used with patients who need to perform time critical procedures, such as testing blood sugar or mixing hyperalimentation solutions.

Another approach to cassettes is to use them with a speech compressor, a device that will play back a cassette at varying speeds and adjust the audio so that the speaker does not sound like Donald Duck or Alvin and the Chipmunks when it is played at high speeds. We know that people can listen at a much higher rate of speed than they can speak, and we know that people tune out an audio presentation when they are not required to work hard enough at listening. When the content is easy or boring, the speech compressor provides a good solution. This author personally likes to listen to spoken material on a speech compressor at a rate of 1.8 times normal, and comprehension of the materials is not reduced. This means that I can listen to a 60-minute audio cassette in only 34 minutes! That is a significant savings to me.

Copyright

Copyrights become thorny issues for many people who are in the business of education. It is a double-sided issue on which educators find themselves on both sides at different times. We will look at copyright from both sides and try to get some perspective.

Purpose of Copyright

The copyright law has one main purpose: to prevent the copyright owner from losing income. With this purpose in mind, educators have a logical base from which to make decisions about what constitutes copyright infringement and what does not. If you are using materials that are copyrighted and have any question as to the legality of your use, seek the advice of an attorney. I will relay to you the basic principles of the copyright law, and how this translates into practice on an everyday level.

Without the copyright law there would be little incentive for anyone to produce good educational materials. Making a good product takes time and energy, and in our society that means that we should expect some reward, be it financial or the recognition of others of our work. The copyright law protects this basic right. As educators, we sometimes rebel against the need to get permission to use materials, especially when the need to use the material is so obvious to us. If we do not support the principles of the law, however, very soon there will be no material that is worthwhile for us to use. Our own incentive to produce material will certainly be diminished because we would not have any way to protect our own material from misuse and stealing, much less protect any income we might get.

Copyright as a Law

The copyright law under which we are presently operating was passed by the United States Congress and signed into law by President Ford and took effect on January 1, 1978. As is true for all laws, "it's never for sure until it has been tried in the Supreme Court." There have been several lawsuits concerning the new law, and undoubtedly there will be several more. The significant points for us to remember are twofold.

First, it is important to note that the copyright statute is Federal. Therefore, copyright infringment is prosecuted on the Federal level, and is not the jurisdiction of local, county, or state authorities. Changes in the law are initiated at the national level through federal legislators. It also means that provisions of the law are in equal force from state to state. If it works in one place, it will work in all places.

Secondly, as a law, copyright protection can be waived or altered by a contract or binding business agreement. This means that even though the law provides that someone may not use your copyrighted material without your permission, you can sign a contract that takes that right away from you. In court, the contract will take precedence over the law because you signed away your rights.

Copyright and Non-Print

The area of non-print copyright has been the most active in recent years. The advent of video tape recorders and satellite dishes has raised new issues for Congress and the courts to deal with. Some significant decisions have been reached already.

The Supreme Court of the United States has ruled that videotaping material that you are receiving legally in your own home is legal. You may view this tape in your own home as often as you wish and keep the tape for as long as you wish. What you may not do is take the tape to your hospital or clinic and use the tape for educating or entertaining your patients, unless you meet certain requirements.

The use of material recorded off the air for educational purposes is covered by a set of guidelines for off-air recording that was developed by a congressional committee and read into the Congressional Record. The basic provisions of the guidelines state that material can be taped and used for a limited number of times in a classroom setting for a period of 10 days after the original broadcast. The tape may then be kept for an additional 35 days, during which time the program may not be shown to groups. During this time you are presumably writing to the copyright owner for permission to keep the program permanently. The copyright owner may give you permission to keep it and use it at will, or may require you to pay a fee for keeping it, or may require you to purchase a new copy of the program, or may forbid you to use the program at all. There may be further restrictions on specific items such as showing the program over closed circuit television. Most agreements forbid the making of copies of the program. However, many can be obtained through purchase or borrowing.

OBTAINING TEACHING MATERIALS

Materials that are going to be used for patient education can be obtained from several sources. Materials may be purchased, borrowed for free or for a fee, or produced. Sometimes it is tempting to produce the materials that are needed in order to make sure they are exactly right. However, production of materials is very costly in terms of time and money, and production strategies are not covered in this chapter. It is more realistic from a time and cost standpoint to review carefully the steps that will insure that materials which are purchased or borrowed will meet the needs of the patients.

Evaluating Materials

Before purchasing or borrowing teaching aids the nurse should review the materials from an overall point of view so that format and visual appearance can be judged. The size of the type, use of photographs, clarity of diagrams, organization of the content, and the eye catching or interest-attracting features should be critiqued.

Next, the content presented in the material must be critiqued. Materials may contain either too much or too little of what is appropriate to convey to the patient. These problems can be overcome either by indicating to the patient what materials should be read or by supplementing the materials with more detailed information.

Do not use pamphlets that contain information that is incorrect, obviously outdated, or in conflict with the therapy or suggestions that the patient has received. Patients do have the right to know about and understand conflicting points of view relative to their therapy. However, these issues should be explained by the medical staff. It would be confusing and disheartening to be presented with materials that vary from what is being carried out.

Patients might also respond negatively to educational materials that conflict with their personal values. For example, pamphlets that have photographs depicting an elderly man using a walker might insult the arthritic gentleman who prefers to use a cane. Or providing a new mother who has chosen to bottle feed, with a nutrition pamphlet from the La Leche League that encourages breast feeding may cause her embarrassment and distress. These examples indicate the need to assess the values of patients and their families before distributing materials to them.

Sources of Materials

Due to increasing costs, health care teaching materials or aids may be shared by several hospitals in the community. Check to see if there are local networks for developing materials or for sharing what has been successful in other locales. For example, hospitals may unite with industrial nurse groups to develop teaching materials for the cardiovascular patients seen in acute care and then rehabilitated for return to work. There are many other local and national sources from which patient education materials can be obtained.

Nursing journals commonly have sections devoted specifically to reviewing the latest audiovisual and print materials related to health care. Television production companies that produce documentaries or health related programs often make the videocassettes or transcripts of these programs available for public use. Health care agencies, both public and private, may have health educators and learning resource centers which have materials to purchase or borrow.

State public health and local community service agencies, visiting nurse associations, hospice centers, family counseling and mental health services, health maintenance organizations or offices and vocational rehabilitation centers are examples of agencies that may provide health-related materials.

Industries and corporations are also calling upon doctors, occupational nurses, pharmacists, nutritionists, and gerontologists to assist them in developing health education materials for their employees. Some excellent brochures designed to help families maintain their health or enjoy successful rehabilitation are available from these groups.

Organizations established to support research or services for persons with certain illnesses are also excellent sources for teaching materials. These agencies include American Heart, Cancer, Dental, Diabetes, and Lung Associations, among many.

There are a number of societies established to provide services for people with specific ailments that also provide educational resources. Local chapters of these groups are listed in the telephone directory. Such societies include the Arthritis Foundation, Alcoholics Anonymous or Alanon, Center for Drug Abuse and Chemical Dependency, Battered Women's Shelter, Birthright, Councils for the Blind, Hearing Impaired or Physically Handicapped, La Leche League, Ostomy and Larengectomy Clubs, Poison Control Centers, Paraplegia Foundations, Planned Parenthood, Reach to Recovery, Rapeline, Weight Watchers or TOPS (Take Off Pounds Sensibly), and Senior Citizens Organizations.

Many support, recreation, and safety oriented agencies also abound with health teaching materials. These include YMCA, YWCA, Red Cross, Boy and Girl Scouts, 4-H, Gray Panthers, Parents Without Partners, Association for Retarded Citizens, local park and recreation departments, chambers of commerce, and consumer protection agencies.

The Federal government is another source of print and audiovisual health education materials. The Health and Human Services Department has numerous divisions supporting health education. The Federal Consumer Information Center produces catalogs available from the Consumer Information Center, Pueblo, CO 81009. These catalogs list federal publications under various health-oriented categories. Some of the categories in the *Consumer Information Catalog* include health and child care, food, diet, nutrition, diseases, common ailments, drugs, medications, housing, and recreation.

A majority of the materials described in the federal catalogs are free of charge while most of the rest are available at minimal expense. Many of the agencies previously described also have catalogs of their educational materials, which can be obtained by telephoning their local offices.

The above listing of sources of health related teaching materials is by no means complete. Possibly the best place to start in searching out such materials are local public, medical, or hospital libraries. Local or state universities and colleges have departments with interest in and materials for health education. Many Chambers of Commerce of cities and towns keep lists of local clubs and churches involved in health education. Also local clinics may have materials with the particular perspective and content you wish to teach the patient.

Audiovisual materials can also be borrowed but a drawback of this is that it may be very costly. On the other hand, many films are available free of charge from organizations or government agencies. Free audiovisual materials are often widely used and must therefore be scheduled in advance. Remember when borrowing audiovisual materials it is necessary to have the equipment to display them, the cost of mailing or handling, and the resources to replace them if lost or damaged.

Consideration must be given to the cost, equipment, scheduling and necessary man-hours for their use before borrowing learning resources. If none of the materials available for borrowing is appropriate then the nurse may wish to pursue the development of the materials through other routes.

Technology holds many promises for the patient educator who wants to use all of the resources necessary to ensure that patients learn. But our technological society provides many traps that can cause teaching to be ineffective. There are many tools available to the educator, both print and non-print. The task of the patient educator is to choose the tools that are really effective and use them to their best advantage.

This chapter has provided a brief overview of educational technology that is commonly available today, as well as possibilities for the near future. Besides knowing what tools are available, patient educators must supply a healthy dose of creativity, common sense, and cost consciousness when deciding what to use and how. This chapter has provided some guidelines and criteria for making the choices and the applications of educational technology to patient education. The following teaching plan that uses a variety of learning resources illustrates individuals, families, and community group instruction in infant stimulation.

TEACHING CARE PLAN: INFANT STIMULATION

Mary Jean Brown and Lucie McCallum Black

Infant stimulation is the art and science of providing pleasing sensory stimuli for the newborn (Ludington-Hoe, 1985). Throughout the last five years there has been a proliferation of articles and information in the lay media on this topic. Professionals are responding to these expressed learning needs by providing a variety of classes, books, articles, videotapes, and suggestions for pleasing stimuli for infants. Teaching individuals, families, and community groups how to appropriately utilize these learning resources is both a challenge and an opportunity. Health care providers, parents, grandparents, and day care providers all need instruction to fully engage in infant stimulation, which has an impact on infants in the first year of life.

Parents have known for a long time what pleases and comforts their babies and scientific research reinforces and builds on what most parents have known about their babies sensory capabilities and preferences. Table 7-2 describes the capabilities of the newborn and their preferences in terms of the six senses. Parents, however, can be taught infant stimulation strategies to provide a pleasing variety of sensory input for their babies. The use of infant stimulation enhances parents' self-confidence in caring for their children and helps them recognize their care is based on scientific research.

Assessing

The teaching emphasis in the past has been on the physical care of the newborn. Today, assessment needs to also include the parent's beliefs and knowledge about their baby's capabilities, states, and cues.

Table 7-2
Sensory Capabilities and Preferences of the Newborn

Visual (sight)	Auditory (hearing)
Has visual acuity within 10–13 inches. (Fantz, 1962) Prefers black and white (Fantz, 1963) Prefers geometric shapes (Hainline, 1962)	Hears acutely at birth. (Dunkle, 1982) Prefers heartbeat (Salk, 1983) Able to discriminate mom's voice in first two weeks of life. (Gorski, 1979)
Tactile (touch)	Olfactory (smell)
Sensitive to stroking (Rice, 1979) Discriminates different fabric textures (Ludington-Hoe, 1983) Prefers skin to skin stroking (Rausch, 1981)	Sense of smell is well developed. (Crook, 1981) Can differentiate mother's odor of breast milk. (McFarlane, 1975) Can differentiate between pleasant and noxious odors. (Crook, 1981)
Gustatory (taste)	Vestibular (motion)
Needs nonnutritive sucking (Anderson, 1979) Can detect breast milk or formula	Can appreciate changes in position and movement. (Weeks, 1979)

Observation and questions concerning the mother's physical well-being will enable the nurse to determine mother's readiness to discuss infant stimulation at that time. Watching the interactions between the baby and family members provides the nurse with opportunities to comment on family actions that could have relevance to infant stimulation. For example, while a mother holds her baby, the nurse might suggest bringing the baby closer so that the mother's face is within baby's visual field, to aid baby in the identification of her parents.

Assessment also includes questions about the types of learning resources the parents would be able to use when seeking information about infant stimulation. Some parents or community groups such as La Leche League might have video or tape players so they could utilize these sources of information about infant stimulation. For instance, videotapes best illustrate infant states and cues. Motor activity in infants and changes in temperament can be easily depicted via videotape. Developing videotapes is an extensive project for the teacher and learning resource person to undertake. Learners gain much and respond well to high quality video presentations so the effort is well worthwhile. Also assess to determine if the individuals or group being taught has access to cassette tape players. Audiotapes can be used to illustrate speech and nonspeech sounds. Tapes of classical music and *in utero* sounds are used to illustrate prenatal and postnatal auditory stimulation. The infant responds well to the music of Vivaldi, Mozart, Brahms, and Murooka. Tapes of family voices talking, singing, or reading simple stories are fun to do and useful during periods of short separation between baby and family.

Learners must also be assessed to determine if they have toys that can be used as audiovisual forms of stimulation for their infants.

Audiovisuals/Toys Useful for Infant Stimulation

- Black and White Schematic Face (drawing)
- Black and White Panda Bear
- Black and White 8/10 Glossy Picture of Parents
- Scraps of Material (i.e., velvet, satin)
- Mirrors
- Pre-recorded Music
- Scented Books
- Infant Carriers
- Black and White Geometric Shaped Mobile
- Parents/Siblings Wear Black and White Clothes
- Black and White Sheets

Many of these items listed can be found or made in the home. Black and white toys are not readily available in toy or department stores at this time. The creation and development of appropriate toys provides an excellent opportunity for the involvement of siblings and other family members in the infant stimulation process.

In addition, to learning resources the person needs to have the ability to judge the "state of consciousness or state of the newborn" (Brazelton, 1973).

Brazelton (1973) identified infant sleep and awake states. There are two sleep states (deep and light) and four awake states: drowsy, quiet alert, active alert, and crying. There are appropriate stimuli that are most acceptable to the infant in each sleep or awake state.

The parent's identification of the quiet alert state is critical to their ability to provide successful infant stimulation. Quiet alert is when the newborn is most ready to be stimulated. Infants give nonverbal cues and it is essential to be able to interpret the baby's signs. Baby's cry and cues are the method of communication with the caregiver. Parents need to take cues from their baby.

Cues that Babies Give

Baby says, "I like this stimulation" by
    Pupils dilate
    Eyes widen
    Seems to look at source of stimulus
    Smile
    Sucking slow
    Spreads toes and fingers
    Reaches toward caregiver
    Grasps
    Motor activity slows
Baby says, "I'm being overstimulated" by
    Frowning—facial grimace
    Yawning
    Cough Sneeze
    Hiccup
    Avoid eye contact
    Eyes squeezed closed
    Pull away
    Cry (but this may also be hunger, anger, pain)

Planning

The infant stimulation instructor must plan for cognitive, psychomotor, and affective information to be taught. The teaching plan lists many of these objectives. The learners need to identify infant states and cues, as well as have an understanding of brain growth in the first year of life as it relates to sensory stimulation. These content areas are complicated and based on well-founded scientific knowledge that has been organized into four levels for teaching.

To ensure quality control it is strongly advised that all people who teach infant stimulation become infant stimulation certified instructors. When planning a program, time for obtaining certification must be allotted. The certification process requires that the participant attend Infant Stimulation Education Association Levels I through IV Infant Stimulation Seminars and be accepted for admission into the Teacher Training Institute, approved by the National Education Association (Ludington-Hoe, 1984). The candidate must submit a course syllabus, parent evaluations, marketing approaches and a certification examination within a two-year period. Notification of certification will be sent from the Infant Stimulation Education Association.

The basic content for classes can be drawn from the Infant Stimulation Education Association seminar attendance and syllabus and instructor's own expertise. This content is appropriate for anyone interested or involved in the care of the infant (i.e., preadoptive parents of newborns, grandparents, older siblings, health care providers, high school and college classes, organization members and day care providers: institutional, church, and home. Content is designed to fit into any number of sessions depending on the identified objectives and needs of participants.

Implementing

The method of implementation is limited only by the infant stimulation instructor's time, imagination, and financial resources. Both group and individual classes are equally applicable formats.

The physical environment of the class must be conducive to parents special needs. Parents may be either pregnant or have newborns with them. Consider a variety of seating arrangements (floormats, desks, easy chairs) factors: moderate temperature of the room, time and length of class, number of breaks during class, the noise level and the lighting in the room. Lecture, demonstration, question and answer and use of audiovisual and reading materials are all appropriate teaching methods for groups learning about infant stimulation (Auerbach, 1980). Careful planning can enhance the learning environment.

Individual classes are applicable for the parent of the newborn who has not attended a class or who requests postdelivery instruction. Instruction can be offered by certified instructors in the hospital or home setting by the community health nurse. The teaching methods employed in individual sessions are brief lecture, demonstrations, and questions and answers which usually pertain to a particular newborn. Group or individual instruction will rely heavily on lecture and discussion. However, many learning resources should be employed. The following resources and strategies have been used effectively at the bedside and in groups learning infant stimulation.

Lecture/Discussion

Discuss each sense as it corresponds to the family's interaction with the newborn. Review each of the six senses and expand upon the learner's knowledge base. One of the major goals is for the parent to easily recall each of the six senses and select appropriate stimuli, toys, and techniques for infant stimulation.

Slide Presentation

Reinforces lecture content with slides that can be written words, drawings, or photographs. Instructors might consider having slides of toys that class participants have made, recommended toys, pictures of the newborn's environment, and opportunities for sibling involvement. The instructor needs to determine the content which is best represented visually. A slide presentation with an audio tape could be used in a new mother's room to present basic materials.

Overhead Projectors

Overheads are used to support and emphasize lecture material and inject humor with cartoons. During brainstorming sessions the instructors can write participants' input on the overhead projector to encourage discussion. Use of a variety of colored pens can stimulate the visual sense. Remember to display one or two ideas per transparency so that the adults are not overstimulated!

Flip Charts

The flip chart can serve as group memory of ideas generated during discussion or brainstorming sessions. Also, chart paper can serve as a pictoral outline for lecture. The charts should be colorful. visually simple, and contain few ideas per page. Flip charts are also an innovative method for conducting evaluation. Participants are given the opportunity to write brief comments on flip chart pages labeled "Things We Liked," Things We Didn't Like," "Things That Need Change."

Chalkboard

Chalkboards are used similar to the flip charts. This method helps the instructor focus the attention of the participants on one or a main idea. Chalkboards are inexpensive and readily available in most settings.

Bulletin Boards

The many uses of the bulletin board make it a fun tool for the instructor as well as opportunity for involvement for a whole community. It can be used to post announcements, class brochures, mail order catalogs, and class rosters. Pictures of all class participants, both parents and babies are posted. Parents are encouraged to bring pictures that are expressions of important class points they've incorporated in the home setting.

Mail Order Catalogs

Catalogs offer another avenue for obtaining appropriate toys for the newborn. Parents can look at these for further examples and ideas for creating homemade toys. Some mail order catalogs may have video or audiotapes for infant stimulation advertised.

Handouts

Due to the quantity of information those learning infant stimulation receive, handouts are necessary. A booklet of the handouts that corresponds to the lecture and discussion topics will decrease paper shuffling and provide a reference at home. Handouts might include:

- Philosophy of Infant Stimulation
- Class Goals and Objectives
- Class Outline
- Class Bibliography
- Infant States, Cues and Senses
- Class Evaluation
- List of Community Resources.

In addition a gift certificate for friends can be handed out for future classes to generate interest in future classes.

It is important to remember the copyright law when preparing your class handouts. Authors must be credited when used in your handout materials.

A photo release for any slides, photographs, or videotapes that are used in class must also be obtained and on file prior to use. When writing to obtain a release remember to describe the expected audience and the educational purpose for use of the materials. In addition, your signature, date and class time are essential components of a legal release form.

Resource Table

Appropriate pamphlets, magazines, toys, video or cassette tapes, records, and books can be displayed on a table in the classroom. This allows easy accessibility to the latest literature and infant stimulation materials during class breaks. Table 7-3 lists the costs related to the learning resources selected.

These selected methods and learning resource materials are most appropriate for teaching infant stimulation. The instructor needs to create an atmosphere that is conducive to the learning of the sensory modalities. Adults need to be reminded of how they experience life through their own senses. The instructor should attempt to create a heightened awareness and appreciation for a sensory world by utilizing a number of teaching methods and learning resources, and repeatedly pointing out that this instruction is sensory stimulation.

Table 7-3

Potential Costs Related to Learning Resources Selected

1. Room availability and/or rental.
2. Material costs.
   A. Toys
      1. Purchase available toys.
      2. Design and develop toys.
   B. Slides
      1. Film (purchase and development)
      2. Slide projector
      3. Carousel
      4. Purchase nationally marketed slides
   C. Videotape
      1. Video cassettes
      2. Video cassette recorder
      3. Video camera
      4. Purchase nationally marketed video tapes
   D. Audiotape
      1. Tape cassettes
      2. Select and obtain original music
      3. Tape recorder
   E. Audiovisual Technician
      1. Photograph/develop slides
      2. Record/develop/edit film
      3. Record audio tape
   F. Overheads
      1. Overhead Projector
      2. Transparencies
      3. Overhead pens (variety of colors)
   G. Flip Charts
      1. Easel
      2. Flip chart paper
      3. Variety of colored pens
   H. Chalkboard
      1. Chalkboard
      2. Eraser
      3. Chalk
   I. Bulletin Board
      1. Bulletin Board
      2. Pushpins
      3. Construction paper
   K. Mail Order Catalogs (Cost per catalog.)
   L. Handouts (secretarial support, xerox costs.)
   M. Resource Table (Purchase of books and pamphlets.)
   N. Infant Stimulation Certified Instructors Preparation
      (Attendance of Infant Stimulation Seminars I, II, III, and IV.)

In the infant stimulation classes, adults are self-motivated and ready to learn. They want feedback on what they've learned and tried with their babies. The class is structured yet personalized and informal according to the number of sessions and learner's needs (Smith, 1978). As each sense is discussed, appropriate toys and techniques are demonstrated and then these items are passed among the participants. They are encouraged to play and practice with these toys. However, babies are the best resources for illustrating and reinforcing lecture content. By focusing on the baby's behavior learning is enhanced. Babies are also the best source of evaluation data to determine if the adults have indeed learned infant stimulation appropriately.

Evaluating

Observing the parents' or caregivers' stimulation of their infant is probably the most essential element of evaluating this topic. Do the parents, siblings or grandparents recognize the babies quiet-awake state? Have the appropriate learning resources (videotapes, books, handouts, etc) been used by those studying infant stimulation? Are the learners selecting the correct toys, music, and touch techniques to use with the baby?

As a result of their instruction in infant stimulation the family should provide appropriate stimulatory toys and techniques for the newborn. For example, black and white geometric figures for the visual sense, head-to-toe and bilateral stroking for the tactile sense, speech and nonspeech sounds for auditory sense, avoidance of noxious odors for the olfactory sense, encouragement of hand-to-mouth activity for the gustatory sense and a variation of linear and rotary movement for the vestibular sense. Parents get excited when they can see their infant respond with a smile, increased attention span (at birth 4–10 seconds), increased reaching out behavior and/or quiet behavior in response to voice and music. Baby's positive responses reinforces the parent's behaviors. Parents repeat actions when they receive positive feedback from their newborns. The parent's increased knowledge and actions helps convince the parents that they are their baby's reason for living, they are their baby's best stimulators. In the postpartum recovery period these parents might have a small black and white object for baby's crib, play prerecorded classical music, provide a variety of textures for their baby, any of which demonstrate their commitment to infant stimulation (Ludington-Hoe, 1984). These parents take a more deliberate and knowledgeable role in the provision of stimulation for their baby and present observable evaluation data of successful learning.

Different methods of evaluation can be utilized for group instruction. Utilize both verbal and nonverbal feedback from the participants. Questions, comments, body language, and written evaluation forms will aid the instructor in evaluating the learner's comprehension level. The learning goals for the group and the individual instruction are the same and the instructor should evaluate the group or individual's knowledge, application, and internalization of infant stimulation.

The following teaching plan illustrates the benefit the Jimenez family received from their instruction on providing visual stimuli (Tables 7-4, 7-5, and 7-6).

During her pregnancy Mrs. Jimenez, her husband, and 11-year–old daughter attended a 4-week infant stimulation community group class that was taught by an infant stimulation certified instructor. At the last class the family requested a follow-up visit in the hospital after their baby's delivery. Mrs. Jimenez delivered vaginally a full-term female named Juanita.

Table 7-4
Teaching Plan for Infant Visual Stimulation

Assessment	Plan/Learning objectives	Interventions	Evaluation
		Cognitive	
Assess knowledge of principles of infant stimulation.	Describe at least two appropriate stimuli for visual stimulation.	Discuss with parents various stimuli.	Older sibling responded to verbal and nonverbal positive reinforcement with increased ideas for her new sister's visual stimulation.
Determine if family owns black and white toys or checkerboard pattern. Ask if family has video player at home to review infant stimulation tapes after discharge.	Describe infant eye contact during the visual stimulation.	Verbalize positive reinforcement for recalled stimuli.	Parents remembered that holding baby close aided in increased attentiveness and tracking.
		Interject ideas for other stimuli during discussion.	
		Discuss rationale for visual stimulation.	
		Discuss principles of infant stimulation as they relate to the visual sense.	
		Use videotape of parents and siblings providing visual stimulation.	

Table 7-5
Teaching Plan for Infant Visual Stimulation

Assessment	Plan/Learning objectives	Interventions	Evaluation
		Affective	
Demonstrate/verbalize emotional responses toward baby while stimulating infant.	Parents will state that they are their baby's best stimulator.	Observe parent and infant actions and responses to each other.	Dad holding baby and comments how pretty she is, just like her sister.
Ask about family's interest in joining a support group for infant care.	Parents express security in their ability to give appropriate infant stimulation to newborn.	Comment on baby's positive responses to parents stimulation.	Mom reaches over to pat Dad's hand.
		Reinforce parent's positive verbal and nonverbal behaviors.	Mom states the baby prefers us over all others.
		State how baby responds best to parent (i.e., baby looks at parent when speaking, (not towards nurse).	Parents state they'd enjoy an infant support group because they can share how to provide visual stimulation.

Table 7-6
Teaching Plan for Infant Visual Stimulation

Assessment	Plan/Learning objectives	Interventions	Evaluation
		Psychomotor	
Assess utilization of appropriate stimuli (checkerboards, geometric shapes) for visual sense.	Provide pleasing stimuli for the visual sense.	Discuss baby's awake state.	Mother held baby within 8–12 inch visual field and was pleased with positive comments made by nurse.
Ask if there is a quiet environment at home where visual stimulation can take place.	Readies environment (room lighting, noise, etc.) for visual stimulation.	Reinforce mother holding baby in the en face position and within the newborn's visual field.	Mother showed 11-year-old sibling how to hold infant in the *en face* position.
		Comment on infant's attention span and quieting behaviors.	Mother identified quieting behaviors of infant.
		Give mother a black and white checkerboard for the hospital crib.	
		Use mail order catalogs to point out what items are appropriate for visual stimulation.	

229

TEACHING PLAN REFERENCES

Anderson, G. C. Nonnutritive sucking in the preterm infant, *J. Obstetric, Gynecologic and Neonatal Nursing,* 1979, September/October, 345–350.

Auerbach, A. *Parents learn through discussion: Principles and practices of parent group education.* New York: Robert E. Krieger Publishing Company, 1980.

Brazelton, T. B. *Neonatal behavioral assessment scale.* Philadelphia: J. B. Lippincott Co., 1973.

Cantor, M. The roles and responsibilities of continuing education in nursing. *The Journal of Continuing Education in Nursing,* January/February 1977, Vol. 8 (1),16–25.

Crook, C. Functional aspects of the chemical senses in the newborn period. *Developments in Medicine and Child Neurology,* 1981, 23, 247–259.

Doyle, M., and Straus, D. *How to make meetings work.* New York: Playboy Press, 1976.

Dunkle, T. The sound of silence. *Science 82,* April 1982, 30–33.

Fantz, R. L. Maturation of pattern vision in infants during the first six months. *Journal of Comparative and Physiological Psychology,* 1962, 55, 907–917.

Frantz, R. L. Pattern vision in newborn infants. *Science,* 1963, 140, 296–297.

Gorski, P. A., Davison, M., and Brazeton, T. Stages of behavioral organization in the high risk neonate: Theoretical and clinical considerations. *Seminars in Perinatology,* January 1979, 3 (1), 61–72.

Hainline, L., and Lemerise, E. Infant's scanning of geometric forms varying in size. *Journal of Experimental Child Psychology,* 1982, 33, 235–256.

Ludington-Hoe, S. *How to have a smarter baby.* New York: Rawson Associates, 1985.

Ludington-Hoe, S. Syllabus: Infant Stimulation I, II, III, IV, 1984.

Ludington-Hoe, S. What is infant stimulation? *Infant capabilities and appropriate stimulation.* Reprint. Handout, Infant Stimulation Education Association for Levels I, II, III, IV, 1983.

McFarlane, A. Olfaction in the development of social preferences in human neonates. In *Parent infant interaction, Ciba Foundation Symposium* 1985 33, 103–113.

Rausch, P. Effects of tactile and kinesthetic stimulation on premature infants. *JOGN Nursing,* (January/February 1981), 10, 34–37.

Rice, R. D. The Effects of the Rice sensorimotor infant stimulation treatment in the development of high risk infants, *Birth Defects,* 1979, 15 (7), 7–26.

Salk, L. The role of the heartbeat in the relations between mother and infant. *Scientific American,* 1973, 220, 24–29.

Smith, C. E. Planning, implementing and evaluating learning experiences for adults. *Nurse Educator,* November/December 1978, 31–36.

Weeks, Z. R. Effects of the vestibular system on human development, Part 1. Overview of functions and effects of stimulation. *AJOT* (June 1979) 33, 376–381.

REFERENCES

Audiovisual Projection, Pub. No. S-3, Rochester. NY: Eastman Kodak Company, 1980.

Characteristics of Rear-Projection Screen Materials, Pub. No. S-73. Rochester NY: Eastman Kodak Company, 1977.

Effective Lecture Slides, Pub. No. S-22. Rochester, NY: Eastman Kodak Company, 1982.

Legibility—Artwork to Screen, Pub. No. S-24. Rochester, NY: Eastman Kodak Company, 1983.

Materials for Visual Presentations, Pub. No. S-13. Rochester NY: Eastman Kodak Company, 1977.

Planning and Producing Slide Programs, Pub. No. S-30. Rochester, NY: Eastman Kodak Company, 1981.

Purchasing a Satellite receiving Earth Terminal. Chicago, IL: American Hospital Association, 1983.

Cipolla, C. M., and Birdsall, D *The technology of man.* New York: Holt, Rinehart & Winston, 1979.

McLaughlin, H. SMOG grading—A new readability formula", *Journal of Reading*, May 1969, p. 639.

Rybczynski, W. *Taming the tiger*. New York: The Viking Press, 1983.

Strachey, J. *Civilization and its discontents*. New York: Norton, 1962. Translation of same title by Sigmund Freud, 1929.

BIBLIOGRAPHY

Cable Network Sees Strong Reception From Health-Concious Americans. *Modern Healthcare*, 1982, *12*(9), 72.

Displays and Exhibits, Part 17. *Journal of Continuing Education in Nursing*, May–June 1981, 35–37.

Films and Videotapes, Part 15. *Journal of Continuing Education in Nursing*, January–February, 1981, 34–37.

It Won't Work . . . . Common Problems of Audiovisual Equipment, Part 6. *Nursing Times*, January 1981, 120–121.

Media Handbook, Chicago, IL: American Hospital Association, 1978.

Visual materials, Part 16. *Journal of Continuing Education in Nursing*, March–April 1981, 31–33.

Archibald, M. Closed-circuit TV: tuning in to health. *Dimensions in Health Service*, July 1984, 23–24.

Bailey, C. S. Gillspie, and Hubbard, K. The State of the art in A/V education. Dimensions in Health Service, March, 1982, p. 24.

Billie, D. A. The dilemma of patient education. *Nursing Administration Quarterly*, 1980, 4(2), 87–95.

Braak, L., and Cate, M. Collaborative research promotes patient teaching. *Nursing Administration Quarterly*, 1980, 4(2), 97–100.

Bronzino, J. D. *Computer applications for patient care*, Addison-Wesley Publishing Company, Reading, Massachusetts,

Cardone, J. The value of a hospital CCTV system. *Educational and Industrial Television*, 1980, *12*(12), 35–37.

Carlberg, S. Technical video's not so tough. *Journal of Training and Development*, February 1985, 97–100.

Carver, J. Effective use of the overhead projector. *Canadian Nurse*, July–August 1982, 54.

Clark, F. E. Teacher commitment to instructional design: the problem of media selection and use. *Educational Technology*, May 1981, 9–15.

Daynes, R., and Butler, B. *The videodisc book*. New York: John Wiley & Sons, 1984.

Dale, E. *Audiovisual methods in teaching*, (3rd Ed.). New York: Holt, Rinehart & Winston, 1969.

Doughty, S. Educational inservice guide. *Nursing Management*, January, 1984, 56–77.

Erickson, C. W. H., and Curl, D. H. *Fundamentals of teaching with audiovisual technology*, New York: Macmillan, 1972.

Evans, M. The use of slides in teaching—a practical guide, *Medical Education*, May 1981, 186–191.

Farace, J. Ten steps to better slide shows. *Training*, July, 1984, 52.

Faris, J. P. How to use films in training. *Training and Development Journal*, May 1984, p. 108.

Farrell, J. Hints for developing orthopaedic patient education tools. *Orthopaedic Nursing*, July–August 1983, 2(4), 21.

Ford, D., and Griffin, J. Closed circuit TV. *Nursing Management*, January 1983, *14*(1), 19–21.

Garman, L. W., Lockwood, D., Helms, B. G., and Hiss, R. G. Development of a guide to recommended audiovisual materials on diabetes. *The Diabetese Educator*, 1984, Winter, 45–47.

Ginsburg, B. H. A computer program for the diabetic patient. *Diabetes Patient Management*, March–April, 1984, *11*(2), 35.

Gustafson, M. Poster presentation—more than a poster on a board. *Journal of Continuing Education in Nursing*, March–April 1981, 28–30.

Hilt, N. E. A case for the sound-slide program. *Orthopaedic Nursing*, July–August 1983, 2(4), 20.

Hortin, J. A. Using media with adult learner-innovative and practical suggestions. *LifeLong Learning*, September 1982. p. 15.

Hurlburt, A. *Publication design*, (Revised Ed.) Van Nostrand Reinhold Company, New York, 1976.

Kenny, M. *Presenting yourself.* New York: Wiley and Sons, 1982.

Kinflrnrthrt, C. P. Intaeractive video, 1984. *Applied Video Technology*, 1984.

Logsdon, T. *Computers and social controversy.* Potomac, MD: 1980. Computer Science Press.

Lyons, C., Krasnowski, J., Greenstein, A., Maloney, D., and Tatarczuk, J. Interactive computerized patient education. *Heart and Lung*, 1982, July–August, 11(4), 340–341.

McRobie, G. *Small is possible.* New York: Harper & Row, 1981.

McVluarag, E. Developing an effective patient teaching program. *AORN Journal*, September 1981, 34(3), 474–479.

Morra, M. E. How to plan and carry out your poster session, *Oncology Nursing Forum*, 1984, March–April, 52–57.

Overmann, M. H. Analyzing and selecting audiovisual materials. *Nurse Educator*, Winter, 1984, 24–27.

Pace, P. W. et al. Producing video cassette programs for diet instruction. *Perspectives in Practice*, December 1981, 689–692.

Pask, G., and Curran, S. *Micro man*, New York: Macmillan Publishing, 1982.

Rose, S. N. Barriers to the use of educational technologies and recommendations to promote and increase their use. *Educational Technology*, December 1982, 12–15.

Schoen, D. C. Types of audio-visual materials: an overview. *Orthopaedic Nursing*, July–August 1983, 2(4), 18–20.

Smith, J. New and tested ways to use slides for effective training. *Training*, May 1982, p. 41.

Soderstrom, R. M. Slides making or breaking your speech. *Journal of Continuing Education in Nursing*, February 1981, 57–64.

Spindler, C. E. Audiovisual preoperative teaching for the total hip patient. *Orthopaedic Nursing*, January–February, 1984, 3(1), 30–40.

Stewart, P. H. Utilizing slides in the learning experience. *Nurse Educator*, July–August 1981, 9–11.

Stimson, G. V. Obeying doctor's orders, a view from the other side. *Social Science and Medicine*, 1974, 88–97.

White, J. V. *Mastering graphics.* New York: R. R. Bowker Company, 1983.

Witt, G. A. Six media guidelines for memorable training. *Training*, May 1982, p. 7.

Zauher, J. Hospital CCTV—more than patient education. *Educational and Industrial Television*, 1981, 13(6), 56–59.

8

Evaluating Patient Education—A Vital Part of the Process

Dorothy A. Ruzicki

OBJECTIVES

1. Discuss the value of evaluation.
2. Give an example of each of the following types of evaluation: individual, program, needs assessment, formative, summative, outcome, process.
3. Explain how cost data can be used in evaluating patient education programs.
4. Describe the basic steps involved in planning an evaluation.
5. Give examples of an evaluation question, its evidence, criteria and techniques for collecting data.
6. Develop a sample evaluation action plan.

Evaluation is a vital part of the patient education process, both in teaching individual patients as well as in developing effective patient education programs. We take an in-depth look at what evaluation is, why it matters, and the kinds of evaluation that can be undertaken. Specific steps involved in planning, conducting, analyzing, and reporting an evaluation are described. Most importantly, this chapter translates the seemingly for-midable task of evaluating into a realistic and manageable step-by-step process.

The importance of evaluating the patient teaching process cannot and should not be underestimated. It is only through evaluation that patient educators can determine if their programs and interventions have been effective. It is only through evaluation that patient educators can demonstrate their accountability for what they do. It is particularly important to justify teaching, with the increasing competition for scarce health care resources.

What is evaluation and why is it important? Simply stated, evaluation is an assess-ment or judgment of worth or value, derived by comparing evidence against specified criteria (Boyle, 1981). Everybody evaluates, although usually without awareness of the process or the criteria they use. Try buying a pair of new shoes. For some people, the judgment of value depends on their criteria for fit and comfort; for others, comfort is secondary to appearance. The purchase of the shoes will depend on that individual's comparison of the evidence against pre-established criteria. Although evaluation in this

PATIENT EDUCATION: NURSES IN PARTNERSHIP
WITH OTHER HEALTH PROFESSIONALS

example is quite subjective, formal evaluation follows the same process; the difference is that formal evaluation is carefully planned to delineate criteria, evidence, and objective methods to collect data. This is the case whether single patients or elaborate community education programs are evaluated.

WHY EVALUATE?

Evaluation of patient education must become a priority of health care educators and program planners. This is important because of the allocation of increasingly scarce resources. As competition for the health care dollar increases, health care professionals must justify patient education to agency, institutional, and organizational decision-makers; and, patient education coordinators must demonstrate that they are accountable for their activities. This requires documentation of effectiveness. Furthermore, evaluation is necessary as program developers revise programs so that they will be more effective, and as bedside nurses attempt more effective interventions with patients, families, or communities. Evaluation will assist them in using these scarce resources in the best possible way.

Another important reason for evaluation, although not as compelling as the allocation of resources, is the need to add to the existing knowledge base. Documentation of the effectiveness of patient education is needed to guide others in selecting teaching interventions and in designing programs. Techniques that patient educators have found to be helpful in achieving instructional goals in their own programs might also assist other patient educators in teaching individual patients or in designing teaching methdology for programs. For example, if a goal-setting exercise was an effective technique in a weight-loss program or with a specific client, it might also have merit in other programs, like smoking cessation, hypertension, and diabetes education. Unless results are documented, patient educators won't have scientific rationale on which to base their actions.

It should also be noted that evaluation is not necessarily research, even though evaluation designed and conducted in a rigorous manner will have equally valid results. While both research and evaluation involve objective, systematic collection of data, evaluation is conducted to make decisions in a given setting. Research is designed so that it can be generalized to other settings and replicated in other settings. Furthermore, research seeks new knowledge, examines cause and effect relationships, tests hypotheses, whereas evaluation determines mission achievement, examines means-end processes, and assesses attainment of objectives (Isaac and Michael, 1981).

BARRIERS TO CONDUCTING EVALUATION

Unfortunately, evaluation is a process often neglected by patient educators. If attempted, it is usually an afterthought, rather than an important, planned element of program development. The probable reasons for this are many and varied. For some people, evaluation is a word that carries tremendous negative connotations—perhaps associated with anxiety-provoking evaluations as a school child or uncomfortable performance evaluations as an adult. Some perceive evaluation as too complicated and technical, too reminiscent of research and statistics to be realistic for the average health care professional. Other people find the very act of evaluating anticlimactic after they've finally got a program up and going; they have no energy left to evaluate it, or perhaps, they are wary of discovering that the intended results were not achieved. Still others go about collecting volumes of data for which they have no plan—data that will remain totally unmanageable and useless when they try to sort it all out. All of these circumstances give evaluation an ill-deserved reputation and serve to make it a rather formidable, emotion-laden subject. They can be dealt with if evaluation is built into the program development process, however, so that it isn't an afterthought and collected data will be helpful. Evaluation doesn't have to be formidable if a few common sense steps outlined in this chapter are followed, and if patient education coordinators do not make the process more difficult than it need be (Ruzicki, 1985).

THE MANY FACES OF EVALUATION

Even though evaluation involves a straightforward judgment based on a comparison, there are a number of ways the process can be used. An evaluation can be targeted at individuals or programs. Evaluation can also be initiated for a variety of purposes such as needs assessment, or for what is called formative or summative evaluation. And, evaluation can examine the processes and/or the outcomes of an educational activity. A discussion of these various kinds of evaluation will provide some clarity and should assist the neophyte evaluator in planning an appropriate evaluation.

Who: Targets of Evaluation

Evaluation efforts can be directed at either individual progress or program function. Descriptions and illustrations of individual and program evaluation follow.

Individual evaluation is conducted to determine the progress of an individual patient in achieving established objectives. This type of evaluation might be a physical therapist's observation that a patient used crutches properly or a community health nurse's observation that a patient selected the correct items for a low-fat diet from a restaurant menu. Individual evaluation, important for ascertaining a person's progress toward a goal, is also important in evaluating a total program, if data from an entire group of patients are examined.

Program evaluation is conducted to determine if a program is functioning effectively and if the overall group of participants achieved established objectives. Assessing the effectiveness of an outpatient diabetes program in increasing confidence or ability of participants to monitor blood glucose is one aspect of program evaluation. It might also include an examination of the use and distribution of program materials, the costs involved, the amount of teaching time.

Why: Purpose of Evaluation

Evaluation is undertaken for differing purposes. Determining the purpose will help identify the evaluation techniques to be used. Several purposes of evaluation are discussed below.

Needs assessment is an analysis of a current situation or set of circumstances to determine necessity and feasibility of installing a program. For example, a needs assessment would probably be conducted before a decision was made to start an arthritis program in a community where another such program already existed. Needs assessments of individual patients can also be undertaken. A needs assessment of a single patient occurs during the assessment phase of the nursing process. Assessment is evaluation of the individual's need for teaching and readiness to learn before the teaching plan can be developed. For example, if a hospitalized patient denied the need for a low-salt, low-cholesterol diet, the dietitian's plan for teaching would probably be different from one developed for a patient who called a nutritionist for information about low-salt, low cholesterol diets.

Formative evaluation is implemented in order to make decisions about program revision as the program is being developed. In this way, resulting data can be used to "form" or change the program. It would be wise to use formative evaluation with any new program to determine if changes should be made in the teaching plan before it is implemented institution-wide.

Summative evaluation is a summary evaluation. It judges effectiveness of a program already in place for some time. Summative evaluation involves "looking back" at an existing program. For example, a cardiac teaching program in place for several years should be evaluated, particularly as decision-makers seek evidence of worth in order to allocate scarce resources.

What: Subject of Evaluation

What should be examined in the evaluation? Outcomes, the effects of the teaching strategies on patients' knowledge, attitudes and psychomotor skills (based on the established behavioral objectives), or process, the teaching interaction itself, can be examined. A comprehensive evaluation will examine elements of both process and outcome.

Outcome evaluation examines the results or the effects of an intervention or program; it seeks evidence of what has been accomplished. Written objectives usually delineate outcomes. Evaluation of an individual patient's progress toward goals set for that particular person would be an outcome evaluation, e.g., whether or not a hemodialysis patient could draw up and inject heparin correctly. Outcome evaluation for an entire program might determine how many self-care hemodialysis patients could draw up and inject heparin correctly after completing the program. Outcomes are most often evaluated in summative evaluations but can be covered in formative evaluations as well.

Process evaluation is used to judge the procedural or structural elements essential to program functioning. Procedural and structural elements include such concerns as if and how materials such as pamphlets are distributed, how learning resources are used, numbers of families involved in a program, methods by which content is taught, how patients are referred, documentation of teaching outcomes, numbers and qualifications of staff, and so on. Processes are less frequently specified by objectives than are outcomes, but nevertheless are necessary for smooth program implementation.

Process evaluation is usually emphasized in formative evaluation when procedural matters are critical to successful implementation. However, program processes can also be evaluated in a comprehensive summative evaluation of a long-standing program, particularly if the program is having implementation problems. Process evaluation is usually conducted in program evaluation rather than individual evaluation; however, the process by which an individual patient is taught can also be examined, particularly if the methods for teaching the client are not adequate, for example, if the client had sensory deficits or low literacy skills and was being asked to read some handout material.

A Word about Evaluation Models

Numerous evaluation models can be found in a variety of books and publications (Brinkerhoff, Brethower, Hluchyj, and Nowakowski, 1983; Morris and Fitz-Gibbon, 1978; Patton, 1982; Zapka, Schwartz, and Giloth, 1982). While many of these models provide excellent information, they can also be confusing to a new evaluator and should not be used as cookbooks. They tend to be written in evaluation jargon for professional evaluators. Patient educators with limited evaluation experience would be wise to follow the basic suggestions for planning an evaluation that are presented here, and as experience is gained, draw from some of the other approaches and models. That way, one can construct a personal, flexible, and composite model applicable to one's own situation. Several basic publications are available that can assist inexperienced evaluators throughout the process. These include the *Program Evaluation* sourcebook (Brinkerhoff, Brethower, Hluchj, and Nowakowski. 1983) and the *Program Evaluation Kit* (Morris and Fitz-Gibbon, 1978).

The Issue of Cost

With increasing emphasis on efficiency in health care and the need to carefully allocate resources, cost analysis is an important element in the total patient education evaluation picture. Awareness of cost issues is essential for coordinators who must attempt to provide the highest quality of patient education for the least expenditure.

Patient education, delivered in institutional settings, is not generally reimbursed by third-party payers; it is considered to be covered under the amount allowed for general patient care. Therefore, as hospital revenues shrink, and competition increases for those revenues, patient education coordinators must become very aware of all program costs as well as all program benefits. Program benefits, reported along with costs involved, will assist decision-makers in planning for future use of resources.

Costs to be identified in patient education programs include personnel costs (salaries of personnel who implement programs), equipment costs (audiovisual equipment acquisition and depreciation), printed material costs and facility costs (Crabtree, 1981). Other costs that should not be overlooked are program development costs like meetings, administrative costs such as secretarial assistance and managerial time, marketing costs, and inservice costs.

Methods of Evaluating Cost

Two different methods, cost-benefit and cost-effectiveness analysis, should not be confused nor should the terms be used interchangeably. Although these two techniques can be quite complex and may not be practical for every practicing nurse given the limitations of their settings, patient education coordinators should become familiar with how they work.

In cost-benefit analysis, a technique to determine if a program is worth the money invested in it, benefits as well as costs are quantified and expressed as a ratio (Crabtree, 1981; DeFriese and Beery, 1982). The resulting ratio can then be used to compare programs. For example, if two programs teaching patients how to give themselves intravenous antibiotics at home were compared, benefit might be translated into cost savings resulting from decreased length of hospital stay. Costs would include all of the costs involved in implementing each educational program (Table 8-1). The program with the

Table 8-1

Cost-benefit Comparison of Two Programs

	Benefits	Costs	Ratio
Program X	$150,000	$1600	93.8:1
Program Y	$150,000	$2000	75:1

Table 8-2

Cost-effectiveness Comparison of Two Programs

	Number of participants	Program cost	Cost/Client	Average number of visits	Cost/Visit
Program X	10	$1600	$160	5	$32.00
Program Y	10	$2000	$200	4	$50.00

higher ratio of benefit to cost would be considered optimal. The difficulty in using cost-benefit analysis is that benefits resulting from patient education are not easily quantified, because they include intangibles like enhancing quality of life, preventing complications, and minimizing suffering (DeFriese and Beery, 1982).

More useful in a practical sense is cost-effectiveness analysis, whereby outcomes are not assigned quantitative values as in cost-benefit analysis (Levin, 1985). Instead, outcomes are specified, and then costs are compared. If the program goal was that patients would give themselves intravenous antibiotics at home, program costs to achieve that goal for the same number of patients could be compared. Suppose program X entailed the services of a registered nurse for all teaching, while program Y relied on audiovisual assistance in addition to a registered nurse and took less professional contact time overall (DeFriese and Beery, 1982). Which program would be more cost-effective? Using cost-effectiveness analysis, data can be compared in different ways, such as cost per client, cost per visit, and so on (Table 8-2). The program with the lower cost would most likely be considered optimal.

Although rigorous research on cost may be beyond the scope of nurse teachers, an important source of data is the reporting of research in current journals like *Patient Education and Counseling* and *Nursing Research*. These reports can be used to justify patient education programs to decision-makers. For example, Devine and Cook (1983) using meta-analysis, demonstrated that preoperative teaching could reduce length of hospital stay by an average of 1.25 days. Keeping abreast of the literature will allow nurses to cite such results.

Planning a Program Evaluation

There are many things in any program that can be evaluated. However, in order to isolate what is meaningful and to be certain that essential data are collected and that necessary resources are available, evaluation must be carefully planned. If undertaken as an afterthought, evaluation will rarely yield useable data.

Planning involves focusing and designing the evaluation. The most important first step is to focus it by determining the audience, purpose and scope, delineating specific questions and assessing the resources available to conduct the evaluation. After the evaluation is focused, the design can be developed, which includes determining criteria and evidence and selecting methods and techniques. Designing the evaluation might also involve constructing instruments for data gathering.

Focusing the Evaluation

Because so much can be attempted in an evaluation, focusing is an essential, initial step. By focusing, the evaluator can zero in on the specifics to be examined. This step will clarify for whom the evaluation is being done, why it is being done and exactly what is to be evaluated. Focusing makes the job much easier and more manageable by sorting out important elements from all the things that could be evaluated (Brinkerhoff, Brethower, Hluchyj, and Nowakowski, 1983). Also, it is at this early stage that the evaluator can assess resources available to assist in the evaluation; if resources are limited, the evaluation design will, of necessity, be scaled down.

Audience.   The first step in focusing includes identifying the audience, or person(s) or group(s) for whom the evaluation is being done. Because responsible patient educators undertake evaluation as an aspect of program development, they are rarely requested to evaluate programs by outside parties; therefore, evaluation audience and purpose are more obscure than if professional evaluators were retained to conduct the evaluation. Considering who might want the information and who might benefit from it will be helpful in determining the audience.

Sometimes, there are several audiences. For example, administrators might want data demonstrating that a particular series of maternity education classes heightened awareness of their institution's maternity services, or they might want data about the cost of the series. Clinicians might want to know how those same classes assisted consumers in coping with the birth experience. The planning committee might be interested in knowing how the program was working and how many couples attended.

Purpose.   It is also necessary to determine why the evaluation is being conducted. Was the program just started, and does it need to be monitored so that it can be improved, if needed? Frequently, planners pilot programs before implementing them on a broader scale in order to identify and resolve problems, such as supply and distribution of materials, use of teaching aids, teaching strategy feasibility (does it work), time (is it sufficient), and so on. These types of evaluations would be formative in nature with an emphasis on process. Resulting data would assist planners in revising the program during its implementation. Or, is an established program to be evaluated to determine if it's doing what it was intended to do and if it should be continued as is? Then, the evaluation would probably be summative with an emphasis on outcome.

Scope.   Should the evaluation cover both process and outcome? Probably one of the great deterrants to evaluation is the conviction that everything should be evaluated in one overall, comprehensive design. Because overambitious evaluation designs can end up not being implemented, it is important that patient educators determine the scope of their evaluation in a realistic manner. Availability of assistance and resources will affect

Table 8-3
Planning a Summative Evaluation That Emphasizes Outcome Evaluation

Question	Evidence	Criteria	Technique
Does the program meet the stated patient objectives?	Knowledge related to objective Demonstration of skills	(Stated in objectives)	Pre/Posttest Return demonstration
Were techniques seen as helpful by patients?	Patient opinions	Teaching techniques will be helpful to all patients	Patient questionnaire
Are MDs satisfied with the program and do they observe differences in their patients' risk factor behavior following their discharge from the hospital?	MD opinions and perceptions	90% of surveyed MDs will express satisfaction and will observe at least one change	MD questionnaire

how comprehensive the design can be; a more limited design might be more practical, and ultimately, more useful.

Questions. Identifying the questions the evaluation will answer further defines the task at hand. Delineating these questions will be a crucial step before the design can be planned. Often, the questions become obvious as audience, purpose, and scope are discussed. It is best to brainstorm the questions with the audience, if accessible. Other-

Table 8-4
Planning a Formative Evaluation That Emphasizes Process Evaluation

Question	Evidence	Criteria	Technique
Does the program protocol "work"?	Existence of problems	Protocol guidelines will be followed	Log of occurrences; staff interviews; chart audits;
Are the staff using the content outlines?	Staff perception	50% of the staff will refer to the outlines	staff interviews
Are the assessment tools used?	Use of tools and staff perception	Assessment forms will be marked on and present in the chart	Chart audit; staff interviews
How frequently are the teaching booklets used?	Number of booklets	Each patient will receive a booklet	Booklet count; chart audit for documentation

wise, the evaluator and program planning committee can do so. Delineated questions should be realistic about what can and cannot be answered, given the setting and available resources. Examples of evaluation questions can be found in Tables 8-3 and 8-4.

Resources.   The type and quantity of questions that the evaluation can answer will be limited by available resources. These include such considerations as time or presence of assistants to help evaluate, postage to mail evaluation surveys, availability of experts to help design valid and reliable data collection tools and to assist in analysis, people and/or equipment to tabulate, describe, and store data. It will not be feasible to attempt to determine if a cardiac teaching program decreased incidence of heart attacks if a controlled and extensive research study is not possible. However, it might be possible to gather self-report data on diet and exercise following such classes. Limited resources will affect the number of clients interviewed, but it's still possible to acquire useful data.

Although limited resources can compromise accuracy and objectivity, the evaluation is not necessarily invalid. It is important, however, that the evaluator be aware of such limitations, acknowledge them and not intimate that it has qualities it does not have.

Designing the Evaluation

Once the overall parameters for the evaluation are determined through focusing, the evaluator is ready to begin on the design construction. The design provides the structure or framework that enables the evaluation questions to be answered. It includes deciding on appropriate evidence, establishing criteria, and selecting methods and techniques to collect the evidence. If needed, instruments are developed to assist with data collection.

Evidence.   Evidence is something that shows what the existing situation looks like. According to Boyle (1981), evidence consists of acts, words, numbers, or things that provides proof of the extent which the quality we are examining is present. When accumulated into a pattern, evidence provides a picture adequate for judging the extent to which criteria have been met.

Determining appropriate evidence begins with the evaluation question to be answered. What evidence can be collected that will answer the question? For example, if the question asks what patients learned during the class, evidence might include their response on a paper and pencil test, demonstrations of a procedure and so on, depending upon what activity would show what the patients had learned. If the evaluation question refers to use of handouts, evidence might include the number of materials distributed or a report on how often they were used by the patients. Examples of evidence for specific questions can be found in Tables 8-3 and 8-4.

Criteria.   Criteria are the standards set that depict the ideal situation. While evidence is the evaluator's indication of what is actually happening, criteria are the "what should be," the goals that have been set. Criteria describe an ideal situation, against which evaluators can compare evidence gathered from the actual situation. Program criteria, particularly for outcome evaluations, are often found in the program objectives. If the evaluation question is directed at what the patient learned from the class, the written objectives should specify the overall learning outcomes, e.g., participants will demonstrate the postural drainage technique correctly (this objective assumes participants will demonstrate all of the procedure correctly).

If the objectives do not specify criteria for all of the evaluation questions, the evaluator, together with the planning committee and/or audience, will need to do so. For example, a committee might wish to know about physician support of the program. They will need, then, to determine in advance what an acceptable level of physician support would be. Will it be sufficient if 50 percent of the physicians indicate satisfaction with the educational program in an interview or on a questionnaire? For which portions of the program will their support be most crucial? To establish criteria for process evaluations where no process objectives exist, evaluators can refer to the teaching plan or description of program procedures and structures.

It can be very helpful to organize these initial stages of evaluation design by making a chart similar to the ones in Tables 8-3 and 8-4, listing the evaluation questions, the evidence, and the criteria. The fourth column, technique, can be added once method(s) and technique(s) are selected.

Methods and techniques.   Used here, method refers to the overall evaluation plan, while technique denotes the specific data gathering procedure used within that method. For example, if the method of study is descriptive/survey, the technique used might be either interview or questionnaire.

There are a variety of methods available to evaluators that can be used alone or combined in a single evaluation. Although they may be categorized differently by various writers on research and evaluation, methods usually include the following types: experimental and quasiexperimental research designs; and, descriptive methods such as surveys, correlational studies, patient assessment, expert judgment, clinical or case studies and informal observations (Anderson and Ball, 1983). Quasiexperimental and experimental studies are seldom conducted by patient education evaluators outside more rigorous evaluation research, but should not be totally ruled out when it's possible for an evaluator to manipulate variables and randomly assign subjects or treatments. Descriptive methods are most frequently used for evaluating patient education programs, particularly when resources like time and expertise are not readily available.

Techniques for gathering data include many possibilities. Both quantitative and qualitative techniques can be used. Quantitative data are numbers, amounts that can be counted and manipulated, while qualitative data include characteristics or attributes that are described. Qualitative data are more difficult to summarize and compare than are quantitative data. Qualitative techniques might include chart audits describing use of program documentation tools, descriptions of experiences kept in a log, interviews with staff nurses about problems they've had or portions of the program they've found to be especially workable.

Quantitative techniques should produce numbers that can be tabulated and manipulated; these data are generally obtained from instruments that count frequencies or assign numbers to variables, as in scaled responses. Quantitative techniques might include the following: scoped rating tools, as when a patient demonstrates a skill and is given a numerical rating for the performance, such as 5 on a scale of 1 to 5, with 5 being able to perform without assistance and 1 being unable to perform; knowledge tests that result in scores as when a test is given to determine if a patient on anticoagulants understands the side effects of the medication; usage counts as when patient handouts that are stored on a particular unit are counted to determine amount used; attitude surveys where numbers are assigned possible responses as when "strongly disagree" equals one point and "strongly agree" equals five points.

Techniques can be identified for each evaluation question after evidence, criteria and method are determined, as in Tables 8-3 and 8-4. It is important to note that one instrument can often answer more than one evaluation question (Brinkerhoff, Brethower, Hluchyj, and Nowakowski, 1983).

Developing Measurement Instruments

Because descriptive methods are so frequently used in evaluation, development of valid (measures what it is supposed to measure) and reliable (consistent) instruments is critical to accurate evaluation results. Unless the patient education evaluator has had advanced coursework in this area, however, development of such measurement tools is easier said than done. Furthermore, anything more than a cursory overview is beyond the scope of this chapter. Help can be obtained from a knowledgeable person locally such as quality assurance personnel or experts from a nearby college, or the evaluator can refer to several good references. Particularly helpful for surveys are Dillman's *Mail and Telephone Surveys* (1978) and Sudman and Bradburn's *Asking Questions* (1983). If tests are to be constructed, standard educational measurement texts such as *Principles of Educational and Psychological Measurement and Evaluation* by Sax (1980) should be consulted. An excellent reference for constructing attitude measures is Anderson's *Assessing Affective Characteristics in the Schools* (1981).

It is best to use an instrument that is already developed if it meets the evaluator's purposes and specifications. This ensures that validity and reliability have been reported. However, it is infrequent that ready-made instruments can be used because program evaluations usually seek data very specific to the program under investigation.

Questionnaires

Questionnaires, especially those intended for physicians, hospital staff, and patients, should be clear and brief, only including those items absolutely essential to the evaluation. It is important that extra items for which no use has been planned are not added. Directions should always be included in simple, straightforward language.

Questionnaires can use either open or closed response formats. Open-ended questions allow respondents freedom to express themselves but are also very difficult to tabulate and analyze. Neophyte evaluators. when confronted with 100 questionnaires containing 15 to 30 questions with narrative responses, will wish that they had determined some of the possible responses in advance. Furthermore, respondents will be more inclined to answer questionnaires where they don't have to spend a lot of time thinking about their answers. Closed-ended questions can use scaled, ranked, yes/no, multiple choice, fill-in-the-blank, and checklist responses (Table 8-5).

All questionnaires should be piloted prior to use with actual respondents (Windsor, Baranowski, Clark, and Cutter, 1984). This way, ambiguous questions, unclear instructions and errors can be corrected before the questionnaire is distributed. The evaluator should always be wary of questions that seek socially desirable responses. Even though anonymous, respondents generally will not describe themselves in a negative way, and may answer with a socially acceptable response.

Interviews

Another often used technique for collecting descriptive data is the interview. Feedback is immediate, and there is less chance of sample bias due to nonresponse. An interview can be as structured as a questionnaire or unstructured, allowing the interviewer to explore topics with the respondent. An unstructured interview might begin

Table 8-5
Examples of Question Formats

1. Open-ended
   What problems have you had in controlling your diabetes?
   Scaled

	Strongly Disagree	Disagree	Neither Agree nor Disagree	Agree	Strongly Agree
I felt very prepared for my surgery	1	2	3	4	5

2. Ranked
   Please rank the following activities from "1" to "5," with *1* representing what you believe is *most* important for you to learn now and *5* representing what is *least* important for you to learn now:
   Diet
   Exercise
   Medications
   Signs and symptoms of problems
   Disease process

3. Yes/no
   Do you wear or carry some kind of diabetes identification?
   1. Yes
   2. No

4. Multiple choice
   You should call your doctor if you notice which of the following symptoms (circle all that apply):
   a. your temperature goes above 100°F.
   b. you have a severe headache
   c. you notice redness, swelling, drainage at the operation site
   d. you get tired easily

5. Fill-in-the-blank
   One food I should avoid on a low-cholesterol diet is _____ .

6. Checklist
   Which of the following programs did you watch on the closed-circuit television? (Please check all that apply.)
   Bathing your baby
   Breastfeeding your baby
   Infant CPR for parents
   Newborn jaundice: what now?
   Parenting
   Postpartum exercises

with open-ended phrases such as "what do you think of the nurse's instructions," "please describe how your family participated in the classes," "please explain what you'd do if your community stopped the health discussion groups." In an unstructured interview, each response might then lead to other questions to clarify, expand, elucidate. In the structured interview, the interviewer would follow a very specific outline and not deviate into other topics suggested by the respondent.

With either unstructured or structured formats, the interviewers can clarify questions and probe to motivate or obtain additional information. Well-trained interviewers are needed so that responses will be recorded accurately without bias. Major drawbacks to interviewing include lack of time and personnel and difficulty in summarizing and analyzing data.

CONDUCTING THE EVALUATION

The difficulty of completing the implementation phase of the evaluation is frequently underestimated and can be particularly problematic for people with many other responsibilities. Although unforeseen during the design phase, time and money concerns can suddenly surface. Implementation requires consistent and persistent attention.

An action plan listing all activities, person(s) accountable and deadlines for initiation and completion of all steps is necessary and will be of tremendous assistance in keeping the evaluation on schedule. Table 8-6 shows an example of an implementation action plan.

A simple method for developing the plan is to first brainstorm all possible steps or activities that will need to be accomplished during the evaluation. Many of the activities will occur simultaneously and will frequently cover more than one evaluation question. After brainstorming, the steps can be listed in sequential order. A person should be designated accountable for each step, and projected initiation and completion dates should be listed, as in Table 8-6.

Table 8-6
Implementation Action Plan

Action step	Accountable person	Start date	End date	Completed
Physicians				
Mail questionnaires.	M.B.	1–4–88	1–20–88	✓
Tabulate questionnaires.	K.L.	2–10–88	2–25–88	
Patients				
Select sample for knowledge tests/interviews	J.S. in consultation with patient education coordinator	1–4–88	1–18–88	✓
Administer knowledge tests before surgery. Administer knowledge tests after surgery,	J.S.	1–4–88	1–18–88	✓
Score tests	K.L.	1–18–88	1–30–88	
Conduct interviews	K.L.	1–9–88	2–10–88	

ANALYZING AND REPORTING THE EVALUATION

Ultimately, analysis and subsequent interpretation should provide answers to the initial evaluation questions. Methods of analysis will be determined by the type of design and data collection procedures. If a quasiexperimental or descriptive method with appropriate sampling was used, it may be possible to look for hypothesized differences or relationships among variables, employing inferential statistical procedures. More frequently, however, patient education evaluators will be interested in describing what they've found; in this case, basic descriptive statistical techniques will be appropriate and certainly easier for the less experienced evaluator.

The kinds of data collected will dictate analysis. For example, open-ended, narrative responses on questionnaires can be summarized. Similar responses can be grouped together in categories and counted; these categories can then be tabulated and graphed according to frequencies and percentages (Table 8-7). If quantitative data from scaled responses on questionnaires or scores on written tests or demonstrations are available, frequency tables, frequency distributions, histograms can be assembled, and statistics like mean, median, mode, standard deviation, variance, skewness can be used to describe results.

For inexperienced evaluators, basic statistical texts can be helpful, or better yet, a research-oriented colleague can be consulted. Generally, people who have masters degrees have had at least one course in statistics. Local colleges and universities are also a potential resource.

Of extreme importance, regardless of statistical ability, is the evaluator's objectivity. If the evaluator believes that the results might be due to factors outside the program being examined, those factors should be acknowledged. For example, patient success in self care might be due to community health nurse home visits, rather than a hospital program that covered the skills. Also, because evaluations are conducted for decision-making purposes within specific settings, evaluators should be cautious about generalizing their results to other programs and settings.

Most audiences tend to prefer that the results be interpreted by the evaluator and that some conclusions be drawn. Therefore, an evaluator's objectivity will influence credibility with audiences when reporting findings.

Table 8-7
Summarizing Narrative Data for O.B.

Type	Number	Percent (approximate)
Difficult	10	21
Moderate	30	62
Easy	8	17
Total	48	100

Frequencies and percentages of types of labor experiences, reported by class participants on their labor description forms.

Reporting Evaluation Data

Reporting format will vary with audience and evaluation purpose. If the evaluation was formative, most reports will probably be informal. They can take the form of oral, interim progress reports to planning committees and administrators. These oral reports can be enhanced by summaries of data in graphs, tables, and figures. Important points should be stressed, and results should be discussed along with conclusions and recommendations. These should be summarized in memos or minutes.

Reports of summative evaluations, by nature, tend to be more formal, written summary reports. However, brevity and clarity are important. These written reports can be organized like the evaluation itself. There should be an introduction, describing the background, purpose and audience for the evaluation. The body of the report should include evaluation questions, a brief description of the plan, listing evidence, criteria and techniques, and a section on results. The concluding portion should discuss the evaluator's conclusions and recommendations.

Whether accomplished informally for an individual patient as part of the nursing process or conducted to formally examine a patient education program based in a hospital or community agency, evaluation should not be excluded or overlooked because of discomfort with analytic methods. By following the steps described in this chapter, especially by isolating the parameters to be measured and by following through with a plan once the evaluation is designed, it is possible to make objective comparisons and derive judgments upon which decisions can be made.

Summary of Evaluation Steps

I. Focus the evaluation
    A. Determine the audience
    B. Determine the purpose and scope
    C. Identify the evaluation questions
    D. Identify potential resources
II. Design the evaluation
    A. Determine the evidence
    B. Identify the criteria
    C. Determine methods and techniques
    D. Develop chart listing evaluation questions, evidence, criteria, and techniques
        E. Develop measurement instruments, if needed
III. Conduct the evaluation
    A. Develop implementation plan. (Look for ways to combine activities so data can be collected simultaneously.)
        B. Collect data
        IV. Analyze results
        A. Tabulate data
        B. Describe data
        C. Interpret data and draw conclusions
V. Report results

REFERENCES

Anderson, L. W. *Assessing affective characteristics in the schools.* Boston: Allyn and Bacon, Inc., 1981.

Anderson, S. B., and Ball, S. *The profession and practice of program evaluation.* San Francisco: Jossey-Bass Publishers, 1983.

Boyle, P. G. *Planning better programs.* New York: McGraw-Hill Book Co., 1981.

Brinkerhoff, R. O., Brethower, D. M., Hluchyj, T., and Nowakowski, J. R. *Program evaluation. A practitioners guide for trainers and educators (sourcebook).* Boston: Kluwer-Nijhoff Publishing, 1983.

Crabtree, M. Cost-benefit and cost-effectiveness analysis of patient education programs. In D. A. Bille (Ed.), *Practical approaches to patient teaching.* Boston: Little Brown and Company, 1981.

DeFriese, G. H. and Beery, W. L. (Eds.) Cost-benefit and cost-effectiveness analysis for health promotion programs. *Baseline,* A newsletter of information about the evaluation of health promotion programs, 1982, *1*(2), 1–5.

Devine, E. C., and Cook, T. D. A meta-analytic analysis of effects of psychoeducational interventions on length of postsurgical stay. *Nursing Research,* 1983, *32,* 267–274.

Dillman, D. *Mail and telephone surveys.* New York: John Wiley & Sons, 1978.

Isaac, S., and Michael, W. G. *Handbook in research and evaluation.* San Diego: EdITS Publishers, 1981.

Levin, H. M. *Cost-effectiveness, a primer.* Beverly Hills, CA: Sage Publications, 1983.

Patton, M. Q. *Practical Evaluation.* Beverly Hills, CA: Sage Publications, 1982.

Morris, L., and Fitz-Gibbon, C. *Evaluator's Handbook,* Beverly Hills, CA: Sage Publication: 1978.

Ruzicki, D. A. Evaluation: it's what you do with what you've got that counts. *Promoting Health,* 1985, 6(5), 6–9.

Sax, G. *Principles of educational and psychological measurement and evaluation.* Belmont, CA: Wadsworth Publishing Co., 1980.

Sudman, S., and Bradburn, N. *Asking questions.* San Francisco: Jossey-Bass Publishers, 1983.

Windsor, R. A., Baranowski, T., Clark, N., and Cutter, G. *Evaluation of health promotion and education programs.* Palo Alto: Mayfield Publishing, Co., 1984.

Zapka, J. G., Schwartz, R., and Giloth, B. *Locating resources for evaluation.* Chicago: American Hospital Association, 1982.

The difference is that for professional workers, the creation, processing and distribution of information IS the job.

9

Role of the Patient Education Coordinator

Barbara Schroeder

OBJECTIVES

1. Define the role of the patient education coordinator (PEC).
2. Describe areas of expertise or competencies which are necessary for the PEC to be effective in his/her role.
3. Determine methods to gain support for the PEC position within the agency.
4. Develop methods to facilitate patient education activities throughout the agency.
5. Develop a patient teaching plan illustrating the role of the PEC.

There is a wide gamut of professional workers in health care today. These include nurses, social workers, dietitians, physicians, chaplains, pharmacists, and health educators, to name a few. Patients, families, and community groups will seek information from each of these professionals. Creating, processing, and distributing this information in formats that facilitate learning is the goal of patient teaching. The person whose role it is to meet this goal is the patient education coordinator (PEC).

Many agencies are discovering a need for the coordination and management of patient education. A systematic approach to patient education can more likely be achieved when a designated person has been given the responsibility and accountability to coordinate and manage patient education. This person may have various titles but most often is referred to as a patient education coordinator.

A patient education coordinator is basically an individual who is aware of and guides the effective use of an agencies teaching resources. These coordinators may be nurses, health educators, or people with public health backgrounds. PECs may be employed by a variety of agencies including hospitals, public health departments, physician's clinics, be in private practice, or even have their own radio or television show. Whatever their title or employment position, there are competencies established for those in the role of patient education coordinator.

PATIENT EDUCATION: NURSES IN PARTNERSHIP
WITH OTHER HEALTH PROFESSIONALS

© 1987 by Grune & Stratton, Inc.
ISBN 0-8089-1833-8 All rights reserved.

COMPETENCIES OF A PEC

Young and Johnson (1984) described several competencies or areas of expertise needed by the person in this coordination position. These competencies will be discussed and expanded to illustrate the skills and challenges found in these positions.

Program Development Competency

The most time-consuming but important aspect of the PEC's role is facilitating patient education activities wherever possible in the agency. The PEC needs to develop an overall plan on how to facilitate patient education activities within the agency. The development of this over-all plan may be time-consuming but is ultimately time well spent. One way to organize such a plan is to utilize the steps of the teaching process.

Assessment

Initially when starting in the role of PEC it will be beneficial to document the current status of patient education activities within the agency. Based on the assessment of patient education needs and current resources, decisions can be made about future program developments. The assessment phase should be carefully conducted in order for the process to be efficient and the outcomes useful for the agency.

The PEC should determine what are appropriate sources for collecting information about current programs and the human and material resources being utilized. It can be helpful to meet with the Admissions Department to get statistics on the number of patients admitted to the agency and the specific illnesses or surgeries most often seen. The PEC can use this data as she or he meets with the various agency department heads and staff.

The PEC needs to make a list of all the people they will be interviewing and determine a timetable for completing these interviews. It is beneficial to have an interview tool, so that similar data can be collected at each interview. Questions that could be included in the interview are presented below.

Interview Guides for Assessing Needs

1. Identify the current patient education programs in your department.
2. Identify teaching your department does for patients with specific diseases.
3. Review written and audiovisual materials currently being used in your department.
   - Determine when they were written or purchased.
   - Determine who approves the materials.
   - Determine who paid for the materials and their cost.
   - Determine who is responsible for keeping the information current.
4. Identify what strengths and/or weaknesses your department has in the area of patient education.
5. What are the priority patient education projects for your department?
6. What are the current skills of your staff in providing patient education?
7. What areas do your staff need assistance with?
8. How do you see the PEC position being of assistance to you and your staff?

Some of the key people necessary to interview during the assessment phase are listed below. A form that enables the staff to request the development of certain patient education programs can be used.

Individuals to Interview During the Assessment Phase

1. Nursing
   Directors of Nursing
   Assistant Directors of Nursing
   Head Nurse
   Clinical Specialist
   Education Specialist (i.e., diabetes, cardiac, ostomy, discharge planning)
   Persons Teaching Classes to Clients in the Community
2. Physicians
   Chairpersons of Departments
   Physicians who coordinate specific programs (i.e., Cardiac Rehabilitation, Home Enteral Nutrition, Bone Marrow Transplant)
   Chief of the Medical Staff
3. Pharmacy
   Director of the Department
   Individual Pharmacists Who Teach Specific Education Programs
4. Dietetics
   Director of the Department
   Clinical Dietitians Who Teach Specific Education Programs
5. Physical/Occupational Therapy
   Director of the Department
   Staff Who Teach Specific Education Programs
6. X-Ray/Laboratory Department
   Director of the Department
   Physicians/Technicians Who Perform Specific Procedures

Planning

After the completion of the data collection phase the PEC will then need to plan the priorities for patient education activities. A priority list can be made of the educational programs that need development. The opinions of administration as well as those of the Patient Education Committee should be sought in determining the priority listing.

Typically, the coordinator will set up a planning committee for developing each program after the priorities have been set. Table 9-1 lists the program that a PEC in a community hospital developed last year. The table lists the priority topics of programs to be developed, describes members of the planning committees, and outlines the type of program to be developed.

In facilitating the planning the PEC will be involved in a variety of activities.

Generally, when planning it helps to review the nursing literature about the specific content. It is also helpful to review materials from similar patient education programs, each of these give direction to the project. The logical start in developing a program or materials is to determine who is the patient population, what are their learning needs, and then put this information into objectives. If a stroke educational program was a

Table 9-1
Program Developed for a Community Hospital

Priority listing of program topics	Planning committee members	Type of program
Written cataract surgery discharge instruction	• Discharge planning nurse, • Staff registered nurse • Community health nurse	Written materials for patients
Materials for families on the isolation procedure	• Head nurse on a medical unit • nurse epidemologist	Written materials providing a demonstration of the correct procedure.
Pre-op teaching materials for same-day surgery patients.	• Physician/surgeons, • operating room nurse, • admitting clerk	Written materials and videotape to be mailed home
Cardiac Exercise Program	• Local YMCA representative • cardiologists, • cardiac patients	Program for middle-aged adults demonstrated at YMCA
Diabetic cooking and diet	• Dietitian • Diabetic patient • Diabetic nurse specialist	Outpatient program for newly diagnosed diabetics and spouse

priority, the PEC thus would start by having the librarian review the literature for current educational materials, and audiovisual programs. He or she would also ask the respective physical therapy, occupational therapy, and speech pathology department staff for their input. Once the objectives are written, it is easier to start writing the content that will be taught to the patients, families, and community. Interviewing patients and staff can often give some direction to determining the content.

The committee or task force developing the program needs to write objectives from the three domains of learning. Many times this requires direction from the PEC as the committee members may not be familiar with these concepts.

The evaluation methods to be used should also be determined in the program planning phase. The evaluation component should not only judge the patient's behavior or learning but the teacher's effectiveness. The expectations of the agency regarding documentation of patient education must also be outlined during the planning phase. Plans must also be made to train staff who will implement the program.

Implementation

Those involved in planning of the program can be used to implement the program or orient staff who will teach in the program. At a minimum, the staff must understand the program objectives, content, and how and when to implement the program with the designated patient population. The third column in Table 9-1 illustrates that implementation of patient teaching can vary from simply using written materials to demonstration exercises or meal preparation, depending on the type of education program planned.

The PEC can use principles of adult learning as she or he informs the staff about the educational program. The PEC is a role model in these classes. During the implementation phase it is beneficial to inform the medical staff of when they can expect to see the new program, and how they can refer their patients to it. Many physicians like to be involved in the review of the program content and written materials.

Evaluation

A system for evaluation and feedback from each educational program must be developed by the PEC. If the program is new, the PEC may want to closely assess its implementation by having a system for evaluation done on a routine schedule. This evaluation should assess the patient's satisfaction with the program, the patient's ability to achieve the desired behaviors, and determine the staff's effectiveness as teachers. As the program is evaluated, this may help to determine if revisions in the program are necessary.

Costs and time expenditures by staff should be monitored. Table 9-2 lists the patient outcomes, costs and sources of budget for three of the community hospital programs described in Table 9-1.

The PEC needs to keep administration, as well as the patient education committee informed of the evaluation of the program. Feedback from the evaluation should be reported to the planning committee, staff, and even written up for publication.

The development of patient education programs is possibly the most challenging competency for the PEC. To competently develop programs the PEC must have skills in all steps of the teaching process. In addition competencies in coordination, communication, staff development and other activities are required of the person in this role.

Table 9-2
Evaluation of Patient Education Outcomes and Costs

Program	Outcomes	Costs	Budget sources
Cataract surgery, written discharge instructions	Less emergency room admissions. Patients following the discharge plan.	$1.00 per patient including printing	Surgery unit budget
Pre-op education for 1 day surgery	Less time spent by doctors preparing patients for surgery, also less time spent in unit for patient due to cooperation with turning, coughing, and deep breathing	$3.50 for printed materials sent to patient's home. Purchase premade videotape for $350.00.	Physicians's office budget, as well as same day surgery budget.
Diabetic diet and cooking	Increase patient's understanding of the diet, and regulate blood glucose to within acceptable limits.	Instructor time for six, one hour classes at $10.00/hr. plus $15.00 for handouts, and diabetic refreshments.	Outpatient Clinic budget (Patient Fees)

Coordination Competency

Coordination is a process that ensures harmonious functioning of patient education activities within an agency. Coordination often means eliminating duplication of efforts among departments. Also inherent in any coordination is the necessity to keep people informed, about patient education materials, program evaluation or current state of the art. The process of keeping people informed is a substantial time commitment for any PEC.

Communication Competency

The PEC should demonstrate effective communication skills both verbally and in writing. Memos, policies and national statements or grants may need to be produced to get a program underway.

The challenge for accounting cost to boards of directors, to speak at national conferences about patient eduation, or give presentations to public groups or organizations regarding patient education requires that the PEC be knowledgeable in the theory and practice of public speaking. The PEC must also be able to listen critically to issues related to patient education activities. For example ethical issues must be articulated to the appropriate persons in the agency.

The PEC is also needed to facilitate group meetings in order to coordinate patient education projects. As a group facilitator the PEC must be able to conduct and run meetings efficiently, where all members are given an opportunity to voice their opinions, but in which a consensus is obtained.

The current trend is toward more outpatient education; thus the PEC is also responsible for marketing, and public relations and communicating with the appropriate community organizations' or services.

Initially the PEC should determine which community services would enhance programs within his or her own agency or improve the quality of patient care or followup. Next the PEC could become a member of that service organization or be placed on their mailing list to keep informed of their programs. These organizations could provide individuals to serve on the planning committees, actually teach in the programs or provide learning resource materials.

As a liason to these organizations the PEC could negotiate for funds in the form of grants, donations, or partial budget assistance for programs from which outside agencies would benefit. Local organizations certainly could be referral sources for recruiting patients or families into the education programs themselves.

On a national level the PEC must develop networks with other institutions and organizations across the country regarding patient education activities. These networks can be both formal or informal. Membership in national organizations and attendance at local, state, and national patient education meetings can be excellent vehicles for keeping current and abreast of issues and trends. The information obtained from these liaison activities will be helpful in determining policies for patient education that are in line with national research and philosophy on patient teaching.

Policy Development Competency

Policies provide direction and regulations to patient education development. The PEC is instrumental in making policies regarding patient education in the agency. This includes developing goals and philosophy statements related to patient teaching. The

PEC should be up to date on the policies and discuss these in terms of standards of care with the agency staff. Policy for cost containment, required evaluation mechanisms, approval processes and use of learning resources may be spelled out in a book or set of guidelines available to planning committees. Any legal and/or ethical concerns may also be addressed in policy statements.

Consultation Competency

Consultation means a person provides professional or expert advice concerning patient education activities. The PEC consults both in his/her own agency and in the larger community if not nationally. Consultation with departments on their patient education needs and reviewing the status of programs within the agency is a larger part of the PEC's function. The PEC must develop consultation skills to become effective in meeting the needs of the agency. Visibility is a key element to achieve a good consultation arrangement between departments.

Staff Development Competency

The key to the success of any patient education program is a comprehensive plan for staff development. Staff development is basically providing staff with the skills and information on how to do patient teaching. The staff development should provide information about the patient's learning needs. Staff teaching cardiac patients must be taught not only this information but also what to do if, for example, the patient is in a stage of denial and refuses patient education.

Not only should the staff be educated about the content in the new program or the learning resource materials, but the PEC must also take the opportunity to instruct the staff on how to be patient educators. Cardiac patients, for example, require information about risk factors, diagnostic tests, exercises, and medications. This can be done by role-playing of bedside patient teaching in the clinical area. Another method is to provide workshops for the hospital staff on how to be educators. Topics for these staff workshops are presented and information about each topic can be found throughout this text.

Topics for Staff Workshops on How to be Patient Educators

- How to create a learning environment
- Assessing patient's learning needs
- Determining a patient's readiness to learn
- Prioritizing the patient's learning needs
- Developing a teaching plan
- Advantages and Disadvantages of various teaching strategies
- Evaluating the patient's learning
- Evaluating the teacher's effectiveness
- How to troubleshoot with audio-visual hardware

Evaluation/Quality Assurance Competency

Evaluation is a process by which the value of something is judged. Most commonly in patient education that 'something' is teaching and learning with a particular patient or group of patients. Evaluation involves measuring behavior and interpreting the results in terms of desired behavior change. Chapter 8 describes in detail the evaluation activities a PEC must undertake.

Quality assurance is a system in which problems related to patient care are identified. Evaluation and quality assurance are instrumental in providing patients with the skills and knowledge they need to change behavior. The PEC will often find himself or herself conducting evaluation or quality assurance studies. Quality assurance studies often reveal patient education needs. For example, in an acute care hospital the staff on a general-surgical unit did a quality assurance study on wound care. The PEC was involved in this project by helping the staff develop standards for wound care, and then assisted in developing written materials for patients on how to continue wound care at home.

Marketing Competency

Marketing is the process of "selling" or increasing the use of patient education resources and programs. Marketing starts within the agency and expands to local and regional areas. First the PEC needs to determine how to gain support from administration, physicians, and other agency staff for utilizing patient education resources. The PEC also routinely promotes use of patient education materials and programs to the appropriate outside agencies. If staff do not utilize teaching pamphlets or physicians do not refer patients to available classes, it is the PEC's job to determine why not and to ensure the programs become well attended.

The PEC must be aware of competitive programs and how these influence the development of new programs for the agency. For example if the agency has obstetrics as part of their patient care, the PEC must be aware of what maternity education programs other agencies within a short distance offer. The PEC can then determine what programs should be retained and how these may be used to increase revenue or the number of potential patients coming to the agency.

These competencies are areas of expertise that each PEC will develop as they spend time in their positions. Although not always listed formally the above mentioned competencies are often reflected in the job description of the PEC.

A PEC Job Description

Table 9-3 describes a variety of the PEC's major responsibilities and the behaviors used to evaluate whether the performance is acceptable. The scope of the responsibilities will vary from agency to agency depending on the philosophy stressed by each employer. Qualifications of a PEC are listed. Certainly an expectation of every employer. however, is that the PEC motivate and educate staff so that they provide patients and families with expert patient teaching.

Qualifications for a PEC
1. Master's Degree in Nursing or Public Health Education
2. Current nursing license
3. Demonstrates effective communication techniques

Specific Qualifications and Job Knowledge
1. Demonstrates ability to perform leadership skill
2. Minimum of one year's experience with an education focus
3. Able to accomplish goals through coordination and direction of others
4. Demonstrates skills in education methods and learning principles

Table 9-3
Major Job Responsibilities of a PEC

Major performance responsibilities	Performance evaluation
1. Promotes the hospital philosophy of patient education.	Establishing objectives reflecting the agency's philosophy.
2. Assists the head nurse in identifying the learning needs of a specific patient population.	Head nurse is informed of what resources are available within the agency for specific patient population.
3. Assists the head nurse in providing staff development opportunities for selected registered nurses	Staff are assisted in learning knowledge and skills to develop and implement specific patient education programs.
4. Assists nursing staff in knowing how to document patient education activities	Examples of documented patient education.
5. Collaborates with agency department to publicize and market patient education within and external to the agency.	Publicity and marketing creates an audience and economic support for programs
6. Works closely with the Learning Resources Department in the development of patient education resources.	Works with learning resources department and director of nursing education to develop a budget for each project
7. Counsels and serves as a resource for problem-solving with conflicts that may stem from patient education activities.	Feedback indicates that counseling and assistance are effective and problems resolved within adequate time frame.
8. Writes the annual report for the patient education committee activities	Submits annual report to patient education committee review

GAINING STAFF SUPPORT FOR PATIENT TEACHING

The PEC will have to demonstrate to many health care professionals that patient education activities are important to the agency. Because nurses, physicians, administrators, and other staff have many demands on their time their efforts to conduct patient teaching activities or participate in the development of a program may be minimal. The PEC will need to determine the most effective and realistic method to gain staff cooperation and support.

Staff will support activities they value. Thus the PEC needs to understand the reasons certain activities are valued or considered worthwhile. Examples from a multitude of reasons people value activities are listed in Table 9-4.

It is critical that the PEC be aware of the importance that various staff members place on patient education activities. A clear understanding may make it easier to gain their support and cooperation.

It is important for this person to be perceived as one that uses coordinated effort to benefit all the agency departments. The following sections will review possible methods of gaining support and cooperation of the various health care professionals working within the agency.

Table 9-4
Reasons Staff Value Patient Education

Stated reasons for patient education	Possible motivation for patient education
1. Accreditation desired	1. Outside regulations
2. Cooperative, educated patients desired	2. Increase positive outcomes of early discharge
3. Patient education is a current trend in the health care field.	3. Want to be competitive in the health care market with other agencies within the same community
4. Desire added challenges and responsibilities of patient education	4. Provides staff with a sense of accomplishment and decreases staff turnover

Gaining Administrative Support

The PEC will need to determine the best method within the agency to keep abreast of patient education activities that are priorities for administration. This information can be gleaned from memos, policies or goals, and discussions. The PEC also needs to keep the administration current with what's happening in the patient education arena across the country. This can be through presentations at meetings, sharing of articles, or personal discussions with the administrators.

Rather than being reactive in terms of communication the PEC can be proactive and provide administration with information and trends that will affect the health care field. Administration should be presented with innovative and cost-effective methods for underwriting the patient education activities. Planning ahead for future patient education activities is also necessary. Many times the administrative staff can provide the PEC with insights about the agency's long-term goals. This is also true of the department directors in the agency.

It is also beneficial to attend administrative meetings in various departments. This can increase the PEC's visibility and also establish credibility with the staff. The attendance at staff meetings can also be a good method to get first hand information regarding patient education activities. Health care personnel will perceive that their input is valued if the PEC comes to their meetings.

Gaining Support of Other Health Professionals

Patient education activities are carried out by personnel in all agency departments. Dietitians may work with nursing staff for diet teaching, respiratory therapist and nurses may work together to do an inservice class about respirators, or sanitation workers may work with public health nurses to teach well water contamination control. The PEC needs to develop credibility and visibility in these other departments or it may be perceived that the PEC's main role is with the nursing department. The PEC should meet each department director in person to discuss their current patient education activities as well as to determine priorities for education activities.

If the agency has a patient education committee it is advisable to have administrators as well as other department directors as members. This gives these people the opportunity to keep informed and share their own patient education activities. Minutes from the patient education committee meetings can also be sent to each administrator or department director as a method of communication.

Gaining Physician Support

There are several methods the PEC can use to involve physicians in patient education activities. Physicians can have memberships on the agency's patient education committee. This opens an official avenue for exchange of ideas between medicine and the other departments represented on the committee. It can be beneficial to have a physician as a medical advisor on the program planning committees. The physician can review the written materials for medical accuracy, and also present the project when it is reviewed by other physicians.

Physicians may participate in staff development activities by providing educational classes for the staff on specific topics related to the patients' learning needs.

The PEC may find it valuable to include physicians in a needs assessment session for patient education activities. By providing the physicians with the opportunity to determine what information should be taught they will be likely to refer patients to the education programs. Physicians may act as consultants for activities such as evaluation of the results of teaching, cost accounting program expenses, or determining ways to increase physician referrals to teaching programs.

Involvement of the physicians in the assessment, planning implementation, and evaluation of patient education activities will assist them in carrying out their medical responsibilities. This involvement may also assist in getting them to "sell" or market teaching programs to their colleagues.

Gaining Nursing Staff Support

It cannot be emphasized enough that whenever feasible, nursing staff and other department staff should be included in making decisions about patient education activities for programs which they will later be responsible to teach. By involving the staff in the development of the programs or materials they are more likely to view the program as their own rather than the PEC's.

The first opportunity in which the PEC can involve the nurses in patient education is during their initial employment orientation to the agency.

At this time the PEC can review the following information:

1. Philosophy of the agency toward patient education.
2. Purposes of conducting patient education activities.
3. Barriers to providing patient education.
4. Identifying teachable moments while providing nursing care.
5. Describing basic patient teaching principles.
6. Describing the documentation system for patient education.
7. Reviewing available patient education resources.

This initial interaction with the new nurses provides the PEC with the opportunity to motivate the new employee to incorporate patient teaching into their daily activities.

After the nursing staff has worked with a specific patient group for several years many start looking for new challenges. One way to keep nurses challenged is to get them involved in developing patient education materials. Staff can be taught how to sequence information, do readability testing, critique audiovisual resources, and develop the final teaching program.

If the staff nurse is involved in the development of the materials they then become the best person to promote this product to others as they have an investment in the program.

Those involved in the development of the program/materials should present their patient teaching program in an inservice to their own peers. This helps the staff to gain skills in how to present or teach to groups.

Gaining Support of Nursing Managers

The PEC also needs to market patient education and gain the support of the staff in middle management positions. These staff are generally responsible for the day to day activities in the patient care areas.

At most hospitals, clinics, nursing homes, public health departments and physicians' offices a significant amount of patient education activities are carried out by nurses in various departments. For this reason the PEC needs to gain the support and cooperation of the head nurse or manager of the nursing area and the next level of authority within this same department.

One way of gaining support is to ask the manager of each nursing area to complete an assessment of needs for their own patient care areas and asking if the PEC can facilitate meeting these needs. The first line manager needs to see that the PEC is interested in improving the quality of patient care, as well as improving the patient education skills of the staff nurses.

ADDITIONAL ACTIVITIES OF THE PEC

The PEC will find several additional activities related to their role and to their responsibilities for patient teaching. Many such activities are self-initiated by the creative, committed individuals in the PEC role.

Liason to Academic Programs

If the agency where the PEC is employed has any students in training, the PEC should meet with them to discuss the agency's philosophy of patient education. The PEC can also review available resources that relate to each student's clinical rotation.

Students from a variety of training programs (e.g., medicine, physical therapy, nursing) should be brought together in such an orientation so they can begin to see the multidisciplinary aspects of patient education.

On a more individual basis the PEC may want to function in the role of a preceptor for certain students. Generally this type of commitment is with baccalaureate or graduate programs. This interaction can be beneficial for both the agency and the student, as well as showing the PEC's support for continuing life-long education.

The PEC can help bridge the gap between academics and the real world. This can help the students see the PEC as a resource person and a role model for patient teaching.

Patient Education Open House

A patient education open house is a gathering in which staff can drop by and view available patient education materials/programs developed by the agency staff. The staff who developed the patient education materials should display these materials at a patient education open house. These staff members will portray their enthusiasm to others, as they discuss the materials and programs they have worked so hard to develop.

Patient Education Newsletter

A newsletter is a method of informing and complimenting the staff about patient education activities. The patient education newsletter can describe new programs, materials or other learning resources. The newsletter can also include teaching tips for certain patient groups or can discuss current programs being developed or evaluated in the agency. Staff should also be encouraged to write about their experiences with patient education for a newsletter article or professional journal.

Patient Education Directory/Patient Education Pamphlet Rack

Having patient education materials readily available for the staff on a pamphlet rack or listed in a directory helps centralize them for review. A directory listing all of the patient education programs and materials available and where they are located within the agency can save the staff a significant amount of time.

Article Review or Reference Finding

The PEC can assist in keeping the staff current on patient education issues by routing articles from appropriate journals to the various departments. The PEC saves the staff time by finding the articles, summarizing the content, and underlining areas for the staff to read. By routing articles to the staff, the role of the PEC as a resource person is displayed. These activities also provide visibility of the PEC to the staff who may feel more comfortable approaching the person in this role.

Staff Meetings

Attending staff meetings for the various departments can be an effective method of gaining support and cooperation of the staff. It provides the PEC with a means to keep the staff informed of new services or programs and to get feedback from the staff on their reactions to certain patient education activities.

The PEC can also get a formal or informal assessment of needs for specific patient groups at the meetings, as staff are the one's most familiar with the educational needs of their patients and families. This is the place for the PEC to applaud the staff for their endeavors and share evaluation results from various teaching programs.

Patient Education Representatives

Another method that rewards staff who have shown a commitment to patient education, is to have these staff serve as Patient Education Representatives. These representatives can be responsible for facilitating information about patient education activities to their peers. The PEC needs to meet with these representatives on a routine basis to discuss their roles and responsibilities, as well as provide them with direction on how and what to communicate to their colleagues.

Each of the additional activities described, as well as the responsibilities and competencies cited earlier must be carried out so that the patient teaching undertaken reflects the agencies' goals and philosophy.

PECs will work with persons in many departments who have varied backgrounds, education, training, and job expectations. The effective PEC creates a situation in which these staff members perceive a need to include the PEC in their assessment, planning, implementation, and evaluation of patient education activities. The PEC must also create a milieu in which all of the staff are working toward the common patient education goals of the agency.

The vital aspect of the PEC's role, is advocating patient education to the agency's administration, various departments, and health care professionals. As this chapter illustrates, the PEC is at the center of an exciting, challenging and ever-changing position.

TEACHING PLAN FOR A PATIENT WITH A MYOCARDIAL INFARCTION

The following teaching plan describes the education of a patient who has had a myocardial infarction (MI) and is used to illustrate the many aspects of the PEC's role. The topic of exercise was selected to show the many contacts the PEC must make to facilitate the development of such a component in a patient teaching program.

Assessment

Initially, the PEC reviewed literature on exercise programs for MI patients. Several articles were shared with the staff in the cardiac care unit, physical therapy department, and cardiology physician clinic, who then gave their input as to what should be taught in this program. The PEC also attended a session of the outpatient cardiac support group to elicit directly from patients and their spouses the types of information they felt was needed to be taught about exercise after their MI. The PEC also made contact with the legal staff of the agency to ascertain the institution's liability for patients participating in such a program. The PEC then developed an assessment form for patients who enter the exercise program to complete (see assessment column on cognitive care plan.)

Planning

The PEC asked an exercise physiologist from the local clinic, a cardiologst, staff nurses from the cardiac care unit, and a patient who had recovered from an MI to sit on the program planning committee. The patient was very useful in planning ways to motivate participants to put exercise into their daily routine (see planning column on the affective care plan.) The planning committee had acted on the PEC's advice in developing learning objectives that focus on modifying the patient's lifestyle.

Implementing

The planning committee decided that the local YMCA could be a place for the exercise program to take place, so the PEC contacted the manager to ascertain interest and availability of space. The committee stated that audiovisual aids could be used to introduce, motivate, and demonstrate exercise to the patients. Thus the PEC worked with the Learning Resources Specialist and the librarian to locate and critically review available videotapes on this topic. In addition the committee selected to use a section of the text the PEC had published on cardiac rehabilitation to teach patients how to check their pulse rates relative to exercise (Schroeder, 1982).

Evaluation

The PEC established an action plan for evaluating the cost-benefits of the MI exercise program. This encompassed evaluation of development costs, teaching effectiveness, patient satisfaction and alignment of outcomes with the agency goals.

In addition, evaluation for specific behavioral change from the program was undertaken by the PEC. One of the evaluation mechanisms utilized with patients was the graph depicted in Figure 9-1. This graph was given to patients initially and then periodically throughout the exercise program. The PEC called upon the services of a nurse researcher to statistically analyse this data and to write reports on the results. These reports and other evaluation results will be shared with the planning committee, staff involved in teaching, the agency's administration and will then be used as a basis for a publication. In this way the PEC allows others to benefit from the research data, the essence of which is following the steps of the teaching process as outlined in the following teaching plan chart (Tables 9-5, 9-6, and 9-7).

Resting	Warm-Up	Conditioning	Cool-Down	Recovery
	5-10 minutes	20-30 minutes	5-10 minutes	as needed so BP/HR back to normal limits
		Target HR		
		__ beats/min		
Normal HR __				Normal HR __

Figure 9-1. Stages of an exercise program. The educator can use this graph to teach the MI patient about the stages of an exercise program. The educator should identify the patient's target heart rate.

Table 9-5
Teaching Plan for MI Patient—Exercise

Assessment	Plan/Learning objectives	Interventions	Evaluation
		Affective	
Ask the patient to identify the importance of incorporating cardiovascular exercise into lifestyle	Patient will identify the physical benefits for incorporating exercise into lifestyle	Give the patient the information on the benefits of participating in an exercise program	Patient lists the physical benefits of an exercise program. • decreased heart rate • regain strength/endurance after a MI • reduce high blood pressure • decrease obesity • improve the chance of survival if patient has another heart attack
	Patient will identify the psychological benefits for including a routine exercise program into lifestyle	Have the patient/family view a videotape on closed-circuit television on the benefits of an exercise program	Patient identifies the psychological benefits of participating in an exercise program: • improve self image • decrease feelings of tension and anxiety • enhance well-being
		PEC serves as a facilitator of a cardiac patient/spouse support group to ventilate fears, and set realistic goals post-MI for participation in an exercise program	

Table 9-6
Teaching Plan for MI Patient—Exercise

Assessment	Plan/Learning objectives	Interventions	Evaluation
		Cognitive	
Ask the patient if he or she has participated in an exercise program before the MI, and then determine the following: • type of exercise • frequency of exercise • intensity of exercise • duration of exercise PEC gives registered nurse listing of available materials and asks learning resource experts to critique these for use with patients and/or families.	Patient will identify appropriate types of aerobic exercise for an MI patient. Patient will describe how to determine appropriate intensity of exercise. Patient will describe the appropriate frequency of exercise. Patient will describe the appropriate duration of an exercise program.	Give patient information on appropriate types and review why these types are selected. Instruct patient on target heart rate limits. Obtain heart rate limits from patient's doctor Inform patient of frequency of exercise to 3–5 times per week, with a day's rest between each session. Have the patient review chart on the stages of an exercise program. • warm-up • conditioning • cool-down • resting Have the patient review section in Steps to Heart Health (Schroeder et al. 1982) on an Exercise Program.	Ask patient to list the appropriate types of conditioning exercise for an MI patient. • swimming • stationary bicycling • walking • aerobic dancing • jogging Patient will identify the pulse rate limits given by patient's doctor and/or physical therapist. Patient identifies 3–5 times per week as adequate for cardiovascular fitness on nonconsecutive days. Patient describes each stage of an exercise program and identifies time limits. • warm-up 5–10 minutes • conditioning 20–30 minutes • cool-down 5–10 minutes • resting Enough time for heart rate and blood pressure to return to normal.

Table 9-7
Teaching Plan for MI Patient—Exercise

Assessment	Plan/Learning objectives	Interventions	Evaluation
		Psychomotor	
Review chart to determine if registered nurse has assessed learning needs in area of exercise e.g., checking radial pulse	Patient/family will identify the steps involved in taking a radial pulse Patient/spouse will demonstrate use of appropriate equipment in the exercise laboratory	Have the patient review the chapter in *Steps to Heart Health*, written by the PEC on how to take a radial pulse Demonstrate technique of taking a radial pulse using checklist in "Steps to Heart Health" Have patient return demonstration of taking radial pulse and obtain an accurate heart rate	Have the patient return demonstration on taking a radial pulse, as identified in the chapter pulse rate obtained should be within 6 beats of the heart rate obtained by instructor

REFERENCES

Schroeder, B. J., Zarling, K. K., Harrison, C. E., and Maxon, M. L. *Steps to heart health*, Rochester, MN: Mayo Foundation, 1982.

Young, B., and Johnson, L. The development of hospitalwide patient-education director competencies. *Patient Education and Counseling*, 1984, 6(1), 19–24.

BIBLIOGRAPHY

American Hospital Association. *Strategies to promote self-management of chronic disease*, American Hospital Association, 1982.

American Hospital Association. *Implementing patient education in the hospital.* American Hospital Association, 1979.

American Hospital Association, *Managing cardiac patient education*, American Hopsital Association, Chicago, IL.

Bille, D. *Practical Approaches to Patient Teaching*, 1981.

Crosson, Cathy. Consultation Corner, *Patient Education Newsletter*, October, 1984, 7(5), 5–7.

Corkadel, L. & McGlashan, R. A practical approach to patient teaching, *The Journal of Continuing Education in Nursing*, 1983, 14(1), 9–15.

Czerwinski, B. S. *Manual of patient education for cardiopulmonary dysfunction*, St. Louis. C. V. Mosby Company, 1980.

DuBrey, R. J. *Promoting wellness in nursing practice*, St. Louis: C. V. Mosby Company, 1982.

Hinthorne, R., and Jones, R. Coordinating patient education in the hospital, *Hospitals*, June 1, 1978, 85–88.

Kernaghen, S., and Giloth, B. *Working with physicians in health promotion: A key to successful programs.* American Hospital Association, 1983.

Rankin, S., and Karen, D. 15 Problems in patient education and their solutions, *Nursing*, April, 1984, 67–81.

Ruzicki, D. Motivating patient care staff to teach: A plan for action, *Promoting Health*, July–August, 1984, 6–8.

Zonca, B. M. The role of the patient education coordinator, *The Journal of Nursing Leadership and Management*, December, 1980, 21–27.

10

Teaching Patients, Families, and Communities About Their Medications

James W. Kleoppel, David W. Henry

OBJECTIVES

1. Discuss why it is important to educate patients on their drug therapy.
2. Formulate a basic plan for pharmacist involvement in patient education about proper drug usage.
3. Describe assessment of the patient's attitude toward drug therapy.
4. List the various types of educational tools available to help teach patients about their drugs.

Traditionally, pharmacists have been perceived as providers of prescription drugs and over-the-counter remedies. Their role was to prepare a drug product in accordance with a physician's written recipe. Due to increases in the number of drugs available and their potential for side effects, present day pharmacists also may function as a potential gold-mine for drug information and education for other health care professionals and, more importantly, for the lay public.

The 1980s may be remembered as a time for increased consumer awareness in health. Numerous books and magazines are directed toward the lay public on all types of health issues, i.e., diet, exercise, and prescription drug usage. In fact, a consumer-based survey reported that the lay public actively seeks out drug information on their own, the most used source being the *Physician's Desk Reference (PDR)* (Ruffner, 1984). This being true, why is there still a compliance problem with drug therapy? A complete discussion of noncompliance will be provided later in this chapter but the two following reasons illustrate why pharmacists and nurses should be involved in educating patients about their medication.

One reason may be that patients do not have enough information to make a decision. A recent survey of 210 hypertensive outpatients and 50 clinicians found that 41 percent of the patients preferred more information about hypertension. Clinicians under-estimated this need by 29 percent and overestimated the patient's desire to participate in decision making by 11 percent (Strull, Lo, and Charles, 1984). The authors further concluded that clinicians should ask a series of questions to assess the patient's preference

PATIENT EDUCATION: NURSES IN PARTNERSHIP
WITH OTHER HEALTH PROFESSIONALS

for information, discussion, and decision making and to individualize the care accordingly.

Another reason for noncompliance may be that the consumers rely too heavily on their own interpretation of medical information. This encourages self medication with left-over or borrowed prescription drugs without seeking the advice of a health professional. Some might try to treat their condition with an over-the-counter (OTC) product. Additionally, patients frequently do not understand the potential benefits versus risks of their therapy, or how to properly take their drugs, based on what they have read. This provides initially a nurse and subsequently a pharmacist, who usually is the last member of the health care team seen, with an enormous opportunity and responsibility to educate the patient.

Noncompliance with drug therapy can result in potential problems. First, the patient's condition may not improve. Second, the physician may increase the dose, so that if the patient then takes the prescribed amount, he or she has side effects. Third, the physician may start a new drug regimen thinking the first was not effective. The second choice of drugs may be less effective, or a more potent drug might be prescribed that could adversely affect the patient's health, i.e., an increased number of side effects, potential drug interactions, or a toxic effect. Finally, increased cost to the consumer, both in terms of drug expense and physician followup may occur (Hill and Goeden, 1976).

Professional liability concerns are also a reason for pharmacists to become more involved in patient teaching. Historically, a pharmacist's liability for negligence was related to the mechanical functions of drug provision such as misfilling a prescription or typing the wrong directions on a prescription label. Currently, pharmacists are also being held liable for failure to inform patients of potential hazards from their therapy. This is due in part to the emergence of patient-oriented clinical services (Brushwood, 1984, Part 1). This is a gray area because the standard of practice is not uniform among all pharmacists. Less than 50 percent of the states have laws that address the duty of the pharmacist to counsel patients.

A portion of this liability is the result of the numerous advances in pharmaceutical research, which have supplied us with an arsenal of new drugs. Because of these advances, physicians and nurses find it increasingly more difficult to be familiar with drugs outside their own specialties. This is where the pharmacist can be utilized as an authority on drug information (Brushwood, 1984, Part 2). As a result, many pharmacists are now initiating the process of counseling their patients as to proper drug use, storage, and potential problems with long-term use. The rest of this chapter will explain how this is accomplished and provide ideas for all health professionals to consider when educating the lay public about their medications.

ASSESSMENT

To improve patient compliance with prescription drug use, a health professional must first obtain some background information on the patient using the product or family member responsible for administering it. This requires communication skills by both parties. The pharmacist may have to learn techniques to improve his or her own skills as well as those of the patient.

The pharmacist must be able to elicit the patient's background knowledge about the disease and familiarity with the drug therapy. For example, a newly diagnosed patient with glaucoma may be familiar with administration of eye drops either from a family member or because of some prior training. In both cases, the level of questioning and the information needed will be extremely different from that of someone not familiar with glaucoma.

The most effective way to obtain this type of information is by a medication history (Fig. 10-1). This is best accomplished by reviewing the patient's medical record. The pharmacist should become familiarized with the patient's diagnosis, special diet, age, social history, past medical history and lab test results. This is where a hospital pharmacist has an advantage over the community pharmacist.

Assessment of the patient should include evaluating the patient's medication to avoid duplication or a potential adverse reaction between drugs. An example of this involved an elderly woman who received a prescription for salsalate (Disalcid, Riker Labs Inc., St. Paul, MN) and 2 weeks later another prescription by a different doctor for salsalate. Both products are identical, but the patient was not informed of this and later developed salicylate toxicity. This factor is more important than ever due to the increased use of generic drugs and the lack of communication between patients and their doctors regarding drug therapy ordered by other physicians. Therefore, the pharmacist should make a point of obtaining the drug profile of the patient before each new prescription.

There are several factors that can affect the outcome of the medication history, two of which are verbal and nonverbal communication. Verbal communication is the easiest to explain and understand. It involves a systematic approach to questions in a language comprehensible by the patient. Nonverbal communication is more difficult and usually is developed with experience. It includes components like pitch and tone of voice, facial expression, gestures, and body posture. This is true for both the interviewer as well as interviewee. Nonverbal communication allows interpretation of the patient's attitude and can be a signal for the interviewer to modify the approach either to gain the confidence of the patient or to explain the information in a different manner.

Other factors that can affect the medication history include (a) the patient's need for social acceptance, which may cause them to omit or distort facts to gain approval, e.g., a patient may not tell the interviewer he or she is on a phenothiazine because that would reflect on his or her mental status; (b) hospitalized patients may have fears about being in a hospital or about the nature of their illness which can affect their communication exchanges; (c) educational differences and the ability of the patient to understand the interviewer; and (d) the number of medications the patient is taking and his or her familiarity with these drugs. These points must be considered when interpreting the information from the medication history.

A major reason for counseling patients is to educate them about their drugs to promote compliance. To aim the educational effort at a specific individual, one must assess the potential causes of noncompliance in that patient. A medication history may provide the pharmacist with information on noncompliance to which patients sometimes admit in the interview. There are many factors that can affect patient compliance (a) the patient's understanding of the directions for use; (b) the complexity of the drug regimen and its conflict with the patient's lifestyle; (c) the patient's realization that they need treatment; (d) tolerance of side effects caused by the therapy; (e) different cultural beliefs existing among the various ethnic groups about medicine; and (f) the cost of drug therapy.

Some patients will not or can not pay the cost of drug therapy. High drug costs could

The University of Kansas Medical Center
College of Health Sciences and Hospital
3900 Rainbow Boulevard
Kansas City, Kansas 66103

DEPARTMENT OF PHARMACY
MEDICATION HISTORY

Informant: Patient_____ Spouse_____   Diagnosis: _____
            Family_____ Other_____   _____

Admission Date:_____
History Date:_____

MEDICATION TAKEN PRIOR TO ADMISSION: (Up to 1 year)
     NAME   DOSE   ROUTE   SCHEDULE   HOW LONG TAKEN   WHY TAKEN

MEDICATION AT BEDSIDE: (Assure Proper Use)

PRESENT MEDICATIONS: (From Chart)

KNOWN ALLERGIES AND HYPERSENSITIVITY:
A. Drugs (Note type and severity of reactions)

B. Foods or Pets

ADVERSE DRUG REACTIONS: (Note dose limiting side effects, etc.)

NONPRESCRIPTION MEDICATIONS: (Name, Dose, Route, Schedule, Reason and Extent
of Use)
     a. Laxatives/Antidiarrheals_____

274

  b. Antacids/Antinauseants_____
   _____
  c. Vitamins_____
  d. Aspirin/Pain Relievers_____
  e. Sleep_____
  f. Cough/Cold Products_____
  g. Allergy/Asthma Products_____
  h. Menstrual Products_____
  i. Eye Products_____
  j. Topicals_____
  k. Misc._____
Caffeine products: Coffee, Tea, Cola_____
Alcoholic beverages:_____
Tobacco:_____
Illegal Drug Use:_____

COMMENTS:

_____
(Signature)

Figure 10-1. University of Kansas medication history form. (Courtesy of Sara J. White, Mary Ann Toll, Patrick Parker, David W. Henry, and James W. Kleoppel. Reprinted with permission.)

deter compliance in one or more ways, failure to have a prescription filled, failure to obtain needed refills, failure to take the medication as frequently as instructed, and premature discontinuance of the medication to "save" for a future episode of illness (Smith, 1976). If a physician writes a prescription for a trade product when a generic or different dosage form is available at a significant price reduction, that difference could affect whether the patient fills the prescription or not.

Another potential area for noncompliance that is sometimes overlooked includes a patient's physical handicaps. Special procedures will be essential for deaf or blind patients especially if they are self reliant. Other physical handicaps which need to be addressed are the use of non-childproof caps for arthritics, the use of liquid preparations in patients who have dysphagia, or the use of calendars or medication-reminder dispensers for complex regimens.

Patients often comment that their physician is too busy for them to take time asking questions about their illness. Other patients are so overwhelmed with the health care system that they can not listen attentively to their doctor's recommendations. The pharmacist thus should assess their knowledge about their condition and complement the remarks made by the doctor.

Plan

There are several different ways to educate the patient as to the appropriate use of prescription drugs. The most common way is to use the prescription label on the bottle (Ivy, Tso, and Stamm, 1975). From this, the pharmacist and nurse can inform the patient about drug name (both trade name and generic); route, dosage form, and schedule, e.g., take the drug with meals or on an empty stomach; refills available and quantity in the bottle; and the appearance of the drug (identity of tablet, etc.). The remainder of the information that is verbally presented includes: intended use, special directions for storage, special directions prior to administration (shaking the bottle prior to use), side effects of the drug and what to do if they occur, how to avoid potential drug–drug, drug–food, drug–laboratory interactions, actions to take for a missed dose, and techniques for self monitoring. One can see that well over half of all information is presented verbally. The next question would be: how well is it remembered?

The patient's ability to recall information about his or her drug therapy has been examined and most authors agree that the recall after verbal counseling alone is poor. The average level of knowledge of 109 patients on prescription drugs was 26.6 percent of the total knowledge of which they should have been aware (Crichton, Smith, and Demenuele, 1978). These authors further stated that the average could be increased to 89.2 percent after the patient received both verbal and written information. Other studies have shown comparable results (Morris and Halperin, 1979; McKercher and Rucker, 1977). Most counseling methods utilized to date include a mixture of verbal and written information. Studies show that patients were best informed when given verbal counseling and written information (Baker, 1984).

For this reason, other ways to educate patients should be used. Items like patient package inserts (PPI) and auxiliary labels emphasize certain points on proper administration. The Food and Drug Administration (FDA) required mandatory PPIs up to 1982. They were designed to provide consumers with information on certain prescription drugs. The most commonly available PPI deals with oral contraceptives. A survey of 50 women, in childbearing age, found that 84 percent had taken or were currently taking oral contraceptives. Of these women, 90 percent received a PPI, but only 61 percent read all of it (Sands, Robinson, and Orlando, 1984). This is apparently not the best source of patient information. Since 1982, various private groups have published books and pamphlets to educate the consumer on prescription drugs (Table 10-1).

Recently, additional aids have become available like *USPDI* (*United States Pharmacopeia on Drug Information Advice for the Patient*) (Table 10-2), a consumer-oriented book containing written information on numerous drugs in lay terminology. This service is also available on computer discs so that a pharmacist can print out the information requested by the patient. Disadvantages with the computer system are the initial costs and the expense to update. Another method is the use of computer-generated prescription labels (Table 10-3), which allow space on the receipt for additional written information similar to auxiliary labels.

Videocassette recorders (VCRs) are being utilized to teach patients about drug therapy. Tapes are available to provide instruction on drugs, especially oral antidiabetic agents and insulin. The American Society of Hospital Pharmacists (ASHP) also has

Table 10-1
Sources for Prescription Drug Information [*]

Sources for prescription drug information

Following are detailed descriptions of some available patient information programs—and how to contact them—excerpted from a compilation prepared by the National Council on Patient Information & Education.

Patient leaflets

Medication Information Leaflets for Seniors (MILS)

Written in cooperation with the Food & Drug Administration by the Pharmacy Service of the American Association of Retired Persons. These leaflets are geared to the elderly. Organizations can request permission to reprint MILS from AARP Pharmacy Service.
Contact: Nancy Otins
    AARP Pharmacy Service
    National Headquarters
    510 King St., Suite 420
    Alexandria, Va. 22314
    (703) 664-0244

Patient Advisory Leaflets (PAL)

Pharmex produces patient advisory leaflets on 250 brand-name drugs for doctors and pharmacists to give to their patients. Cost: $3.49 per box of 200. Subject to quantity discounts.
Contact: David Bardsley
    Pharmex
    Division of Automatic Business
        Products Co. Inc.
    P.O. Box 57
    Willimantic, Conn. 06226
    1-(800) 243-8192

USP Patient Drug Education Leaflets

Abstracted from *Advice for the Patient* (1983 *USP DI* Volume II; see also "Books"), the U.S. Pharmacopeial Convention's one-page patient drug education leaflets are available for all of the most commonly used medicines, both prescription and over-the-counter. Leaflets are 5½ by 8½ in. and are available in English and Spanish. Space is available for printing the name, address, and telephone number of the health professional who provides the leaflet. Cost: $1.50 per 50 leaflets, with quantity discounts.
Contact: Alice E. Kimball
    USP Convention Inc.
    12801 Twinbrook Parkway

(continued)

277

Table 10-1 (*Continued*)

    Rockville, Md. 20852
    (301) 881-0666

Patient Medication Instructions (PMI)

The American Medical Association has prepared one-page patient medication instruction sheets on 60 most commonly prescribed medicines. Space is provided to write in the dosage and any individualized instructions for the patient. PMIs are available to all health professionals. Cost: minimum order of 10 pads (100 sheets per pad) at 50 cents per pad.

To order PMIs write:
    PMI Order Department
    American Medical Association
    P.O. Box 52
    Rolling Meadows, Ill. 60006

Patient Information Leaflets

Offered to members of the National Association of Retail Druggists. PILs are abstracted from *USP Dispensing Information*. Program currently covers 32 drugs and drug classes. Cost is $1.50 per pad of 50 leaflets or $45 for entire set.

Contact: NARD
    205 Daingerfield Rd.
    Alexandria, Va. 22314

Positive signs

The American Pharmaceutical Association (APhA) has produced six stand-up signs urging consumers to ask questions about products, directions for use, cigarettes, immunizations, and child-resistant enclosures. The signs are intended to be used in pharmacies as patient education resources. Cost: $3 per sign, set of six for $15. (A prepayment is required with each order.)

To order, contact:
    APhA Order Desk
    2215 Constitution Ave., N.W.
    Washington, D.C. 20037

National Medication Awareness Test, Health Check Test, and Self-Medication Awareness Test

These three slide tape programs are designed for pharmacists to use as a presentation to community groups. They can be ordered by health professionals other than pharmacists, however. Cost: $50 rental for one slide/tape program, the purchase price is $225. These prices include enough written material to hand out to 50 people.

To rent or purchase, contact:
    Transit Media Inc.
    779 Susquehanna Ave.

Franklin Lakes, N.J. 07417
(201) 891-8240

Digoxin, warfarin, theophylline, and tricyclic antidepressant patient education programs

This slide/cassette tape program helps teach patients about their disease and drug therapy. These 15- to 20-minute programs consist of 35mm slides and an accompanying cassette tape. A printed script is also provided. Cost, $25 each.

Contact: Francis Ahern
American Society of Hospital
    Pharmacists
4630 Montgomery Ave.
Bethesda, Md. 20614
(301) 657-3000

Books

Consumer Drug Digest, American Society of Hospital Pharmacists, 1982 (also available in bookstores, published by Facts on File Inc., 1982). An authoritative reference book for patients, with entries on more than 200 of the most frequently prescribed prescription medicines. The medications included in the book comprise more than 1,000 brand-name products. Cost: $9.95.

Contact: Francis Ahern
American Society of Hospital
    Pharmacists
4630 Montgomery Ave.
Bethesda, Md. 20614
(301) 657-3000

Advice for the Patient (1983 *USP DI,* Volume II). United States Pharmacopeial Convention Inc., 794 pp., 1982. Drug information written in lay language, covering almost all drugs, both Rx and OTC. Cost: $17.95.

Contact: Alice E. Kimball
USP Convention Inc.
12601 Twinbrook Parkway
Rockville, Md. 20852
(301) 881-0666

About Your Medicines, United States Pharmacopeial Convention Inc., 400 pp., 1982. Cost: *About Your Medicines* display case of 12 copies, $36; single copies, $5.95.

Contact: Alice E. Kimball
USP Convention Inc.
12601 Twinbrook Parkway

(continued)

Table 10-1 (*Continued*)

Rockville, Md. 20852
(301) 881-0666

Physicians' Desk References (PDR) contains detailed drug descriptions in technical language but has become popular with consumers. Cost: $20.

Contact: Medical Economics Co.
880 Kinderkamack Rd.
Oradell, N.J. 07649
(201) 262-3030

Instructional materials

Medication Teaching Manual, A Guide for Patient Counseling, American Society of Hospital Pharmacists, 350 pp., 1983. An aid to patient educators, the material is easily adaptable for patient take-home sheets. ASHP grants permission to photocopy pages from the publication.

Contact: Francis Ahern
American Society of Hospital
Pharmacists
4630 Montgomery Ave.
Bethesda, Md. 20614
(301) 657-3000

"How to Promote Your Patient Education Program," United States Pharmacopeial Convention Inc., 1981. The promotion kit contains two "Ask About Your Medicines" posters (one in English and one in Spanish), scripts and guidelines on public speaking designed for presentations to elementary school children, high school students, and community groups; sample news release, camera-ready newspaper ad mats, and radio scripts. Each kit contains copies of the pamphlet, *General Information on the Use of Medicines* (one in English and one in Spanish), and a step-by-step guide to using all of the materials.

Contact: Alice E. Kimball
USP Convention Inc.
12601 Twinbrook Parkway
Rockville, Md. 20852
(301) 881-0666

*From Robinson, B. Patient information: Are the voluntary approaches working? *Drug Topics*, 1984, 128, 42–46. With permission.

Table 10-2
Advice for the Patient Using Sublingual Nitroglycerin Tablets˙

NITROGLYCERIN (Systemic)

Some commonly used brand or other names are:

Glyceryl	Nitrong
trinitrate	Nitrospan
Nitro-Bid	Nitrostat
Nitro-Dur	Susadrin
Nitrodisc	Transderm-
Nitroglyn	Nitro
Nitrol	

For a summary, read the bold information first. Then go back and read the other information. It is a good idea to read all of the information again later.

Nitroglycerin (nye-troe-GLI-ser-in) belongs to the group of medicines called nitrates. It is used to improve the supply of blood and oxygen to the heart. In some forms, this medicine is used to relieve the pain of angina attacks. In other forms, it is used to prevent such attacks. This medicine is available only with your doctor's prescription.

Remember:
• This medicine has been prescribed for your current medical problem only. It must not be given to other people or used for other problems unless you are otherwise directed by your doctor.
• In order for this medicine to work, it must be taken as directed.
• Keep all medicines out of the reach of children.
• If you want more information about this medicine, ask your doctor, nurse, or pharmacist.
• If any of the following information causes you special concern, do not decide against taking this medicine without first checking with your doctor.

Before Using This Medicine
In order to decide on the best treatment for your medical problem, your doctor should be told:
—if you have ever had any unusual or allergic reaction to nitroglycerin.
—if you are pregnant or if you intend to become pregnant while using this medicine. Although this medicine has not been shown to cause problems, the chance always exists.
—if you are breast-feeding an infant. Although this medicine has not been shown to cause problems, the chance always exists.
—if you have either of the following medical problems:
Anemia (severe)
Overactive thyroid
—if you have recently had a heart attack.
—if you are now taking any of the following medicines or types of medicine:
Asthma medicine
High blood pressure medicine
Sinus medicine

Proper Use of This Medicine
Use nitroglycerin exactly as directed by your doctor. It is effective only if taken correctly.
For patients using the sublingual (under-the-tongue) tablet form of this medicine:
• Testing the ability of a sublingual nitroglycerin tablet to relieve angina by the presence of a tingling or burning sensation, a feeling of warmth or flushing, or a headache, after a tablet has been dissolved under the tongue, is not completely reliable since some patients may be

---

(continued)

Table 10-2 (*Continued*)

unable to detect these effects. Newer, stabilized sublingual nitroglycerin tablets are also making such potency testing less popular, since the stabilized tablets are less likely to produce these detectable effects.

- **When you begin to feel an attack of angina starting (chest pains or a tightness or squeezing in the chest), sit down. Then place a nitroglycerin tablet under your tongue and let it dissolve there.** This medicine works best when you are standing or sitting; however, since you may become dizzy or lightheaded, or feel faint soon after taking a tablet, it is safer to sit rather than stand while the medicine is working. If you become dizzy or feel faint while sitting, take several deep breaths and bend forward with your head between your knees.
- By remaining calm you will help relieve the attack sooner.
- You should feel better in a few minutes. This medicine should not be chewed or swallowed since it works much faster when absorbed through the lining of the mouth. Do not eat, drink, or smoke while a tablet is dissolving.
- **This medicine usually gives relief in 1 to 5 minutes.** However, if the pain is not relieved dissolve a second tablet under the tongue. If the pain continues for another 5 minutes, a third tablet may be used. **If you still have the chest pains after a total of 3 tablets in a 15-minute period, contact your doctor or go to a hospital emergency room without delay.**
- You may prevent anginal chest pains for up to 1 hour by putting a tablet under the tongue 5 to 10 minutes before expected emotional stress or physical exertion that in the past seemed to bring on an attack.
- When properly stored, sublingual nitroglycerin tablets retain their strength until the expiration date printed on the original label. However, because of patient usage, changing temperature and moisture, shaking, and repeated bottle opening, the tablets may be good for only 3 to 6 months. The "stabilized" sublingual tablets may stay good for a longer period of time.
- To help keep the nitroglycerin tablets at full strength:
—keep the medicine in the original glass, screw-cap bottle.
—remove the cotton plug that comes in the bottle and *do not* put it back.
—**put the cap on the bottle quickly and tightly after each use.**
—to select a tablet for use, pour several into the bottle cap, take one, and pour the others back into the bottle. Try not to hold them in the palm of your hand because they will pick up moisture and crumble.
—do not keep other medicines in the same bottle with the nitroglycerin since they will weaken the nitroglycerin effect.
—keep the medicine handy at all times but try not to carry the bottle close to the body. Medicine may lose strength because of body warmth. Instead, carry the tightly closed bottle in your purse, jacket pocket, or other loose-fitting clothing whenever possible.
—store the bottle of nitroglycerin tablets in a cool, dry place. Average room temperature away from direct heat or direct sunlight is best. Do not store in the refrigerator or in a bathroom medicine cabinet because the moisture usually present in these areas may cause the tablets to crumble if the container is not tightly closed.

Precautions While Using This Medicine

If you have been using nitroglycerin regularly for several weeks or more, do not suddenly stop using it. Stopping suddenly may bring on attacks of angina. Check with your doctor for the best way to reduce gradually the amount you are using before stopping completely.

Dizziness, lightheadedness, or a fainting feeling may occur, especially when you get up quickly from a lying or sitting position. Getting up slowly may help. **Drinking alcohol may make these effects much worse and may cause a serious drop in blood pressure.** Check with your doctor before drinking alcoholic beverages.

After using a dose of this medicine you may get a headache that lasts for a short time. This is a common side effect, which should become less noticeable after you have used the medicine for a while. If this effect continues, or if the headaches are severe, check with your doctor.

Side Effects of This Medicine

Along with its needed effects, a medicine may cause some unwanted effects. Although not all of these side effects appear very often, when they do occur they may require medical attention. Check with your doctor if the following side effect occurs:

Rare

Skin rash

Other side effects may occur which usually do not require medical attention. These side effects may go away during treatment as your body adjusts to the medicine. However, check with your doctor if any of the following side effects continue or are bothersome:

More common

Dizziness, lightheadedness, or fainting

Flushing of face and neck

Headache (severe or prolonged)

Nausea or vomiting

Rapid heartbeat

Other side effects not listed above may also occur in some patients. If you notice any other effects, check with your doctor.

---

*Reprinted from the *USPharmacopeia Drug Information*, vol. II. *Advice for the Patient*, Sixth Edition, pp. 501–503. © 1985, the United States Pharmacopeial Convention, Inc. Permission granted.

made tapes on educating the lay public to the role of pharmacists and what to ask about prescription products. (Burns, 1986; Marshall, Rothenberger, and Bunnell; Olsen and Dube, 1985).

Besides these counseling aids, pharmacists also utilize additional items that help to improve the patient's compliance. Calendars have been used to solve a couple of different problems (see Fig. 10-2). Complex regimens can be more easily understood if presented in this form. Illiterate individuals can also understand scheduling directions if this same format is used with pictures, ie., pasting a picture of the drug at administration times corresponding to pictures of breakfast, lunch, dinner and bedtime.

Medication boxes have also been designed in several fashions. The most useful is the type that is divided into seven compartments across and four down corresponding to days of the week and schedule times respectively. These boxes are also made with braille print. Studies have shown a positive effect on compliance by both medication containers and calendars (Ascione and Shimp, 1984; Rehden, McCoy, Blackwell, Whitehead. and Robinson, 1980).

Noncompliance is a public health problem and requires a public health–oriented solution. Recently, five practical suggestions were proposed. It's important that the professions, locally, be sensitized to the critical nature of the problem. Pharmacists, nurses, physicians, and other health professionals should arrange joint meetings of their local societies to discuss the nature and scope of noncompliance and how locally organized health professionals can initiate joint solutions. The concept of interprofessional collaboration must be considered, and methods discussed for implementing it. Pharmacists should be prepared to discuss with physicians and nurses those patients whom

Table 10-3
A Graphic Illustration of a Computer-Generated Prescription Label with Counseling Information for the Patient

JIM'S PHARMACY

410 E. 50TH STREET
KANSAS CITY, MISSOURI 64110
555-5494

RX NO: 00000 DR: Jones

John Doe 6.5.86
Take one tablet daily in the
morning.
HCTZ 50mg #100
Refills 2x

PRESCRIPTION RECEIPT

JIM'S PHARMACY
410 E. 50TH STREET
KANSAS CITY, MISSOURI 64110
555-5494

RX NO: 00000
DATE: 6.5.86

COST: $3.99

PRESCRIPTION INFORMATION FOR THE PATIENT

Take the tablet at the same time each day preferably with
breakfast.

While on this medication, drink orange juice or eat bananas
daily.

If you miss a dose of this medicine, take it as soon as you
remember unless it is almost time for your next dose. Never
double the dose if you miss one dose.

*Designed by James W. Kleoppel. Reprinted with permission.

The University of Kansas Medical Center
College of Health Sciences and Hospital
3900 Rainbow Boulevard
Kansas City, Kansas 66103
MEDICATION CALENDAR

Patient Name: _____

Directions for use: The drug is listed in the far left-hand column and checks (X) made
in the time columns corresponding to the time to take the drug.

MORNING

EVENING

Drug and Dose	1	2	3	4	5	6	7	8	9	10	11	NOON	1	2	3	4	5	6	7	8	9	10	11	Midnight

Figure 10-2. University of Kansas medication calendar. (Courtesy of James W. Kleoppel. Reprinted with permission. Designed by James W. Kleoppel.)

they believe require attention so that noncompliance is avoided. Pharmacists should be prepared to discuss with physicians and nurses those patients about whom pharmacists require more information in order to assure high levels of compliance, and pharmacists should select patients for routine monitoring to assess levels of compliance (Bectel, 1984).

A few additional items have been introduced to patients that allow them to carry potentially valuable information in an emergency. Medication alert cards and bracelets are available and should be considered by individuals with special needs. These can be helpful to patients who have diabetes, epilepsy, drug allergies, or patients who wear special appliances like contact lens or ostomy products.

Advances in technology may soon make it possible for individuals to carry a small card containing the patient's medical record. This could allow the health professional to review, add, or delete information. Advantages of this type of system include availability of the complete medical record to all health care professionals providing services to the patient. Another similar idea might be the use of a clearing house that would store the information on discs, which could be accessible through an office computer.

Implementing the Plan

To effectively implement a plan to improve patient compliance, the nurse and pharmacist must possess good communication skills and provide the patient with an appropriate amount of time to express him or herself. It necessitates the pharmacist to listen when the patient is ready to talk. Interviewing the patient requires that health care professionals be empathetic. Patients need time to express concerns and fears and to be reassured that the health care system is functioning in their best interest. However, there is a need to guard against being overly sympathetic. The patient should be allowed to express his or her beliefs about drug therapy and the beneficial effect of the drug on his or her condition. This type of conversation should not be prolonged, and the patient could be redirected by a statement like, "Tell me about your past medication." The goal is to achieve proper patient education on drug therapy.

Hospital pharmacists and nurses may have an advantage in implementing a teaching plan since the patient is "in house." The pharmacist has access to the medical record and may be able to schedule several visits with the patient during the course of his or her stay. Disadvantages include that the patient may be too sick to participate or is too concerned with the process of leaving the hospital. In contrast, community pharmacists and nurses must depend on the patient's willingness to return in order to continue the counseling. Patients may be receptive to education about their drugs at this point, or they may still have distractions such as children waiting in the car or a long shopping list. Either way the patient's attentiveness must be considered.

When the patient does return, it may not be the best time for the pharmacist who might be overburdened with other patients and prescriptions. Therefore, it requires time management by nurses and pharmacists. Additionally, patients will only remember a few points from the session, therefore, pertinent points need to be made in a few minutes. There are ways to supplement this method of counseling. On each return visit, the pharmacist should continue the counseling process and review information from the first session. Drug checklists (a page of specific questions relating to their drug therapy) provide boxes which the patient can mark to act as a stimulus for later questions. Patients should be encouraged to call and talk with the pharmacist during the slow periods of the day. In some cases, pharmacists have telephoned patients to reinforce the directions and prompt any questions.

The environment where counseling is done should be private and without interruptions. Hallways and pharmacy counters are not appropriate places to conduct this personalized service. Experience with patients has shown that hospital roommates or family members curtail the conversation (Covington and Whitney, 1971). For this reason, isolating the patient with the interviewer is the ideal situation. In some instances having a family member present is important, especially if he or she is responsible for administering the medication.

Another study examined 106 outpatients' compliance with the amount of privacy provided during the interview. The results showed that the patients' questioning and comprehension was enhanced in a private setting. Some patients stated that they would not have asked as many questions in a less private setting. (Beardsley, Johnson, and Wise, 1977).

The medication history can proceed once the proper setting is determined and the interviewer is familiarized with the patient's medical record. Approaching the patient mandates an introduction and purpose of the pharmacist's interview. It is at this time the patient is deciding whether or not to participate, so it is essential that the pharmacist has good personal hygiene and a professional appearance. In the hospital, it is recommended that the interviewer sit down in a chair while in the patient's room. This relaxes the patient and prevents a feeling of intimidation. The interviewer should neither stare at the patient nor write continuously during the interview. Short notations should be taken and the form finished later.

The University of Kansas medication history form (Fig. 10-1) has a space in the upper right hand corner to stamp the patient's name and hospital numbers from the hospital identification card. There is also a section for identifying the informant and the patient's diagnosis.

The next section deals with medication taken in the last year prior to admission. In this section only prescription drug products are noted. The interviewer should use open-ended questions, e.g., "What prescription drugs have you taken in the last year?" and "How do you take it?" Appropriate questioning leads not only to a list of the drugs the patient has taken, but also to valuable information concerning the patient's level of understanding of drug therapy and the level of compliance. Typical answers to questions about dosing include statements like "I take my digoxin every morning, but if my heart feels weak that day I take two" or "I take three phenytoins per day, except when I forget. A lot of times I forget the afternoon dose." Potential compliance problems such as the above can often be corrected once they have been identified.

It is not unusual for a patient to know only the color and size of the tablet or the reason for taking the drug. If the patient can only identify the product in this way, it is recommended that the interviewer follow up with the patient or a guardian who can properly identify the product. On occasion, patients may present a list of their drugs because they are aware they do not know their drugs.

For hospitalized patients, the section on medication at the bedside is important because some patients on maintenance medication bring their personal supply or over-the-counter (OTC) products which could potentially cause an overdose or negative drug-interaction. For example, a patient who is receiving Coumadin in the hospital may be taking aspirin daily for an arthritic condition. The question, "What medications from home do you have with you?" should be asked in a manner that prevents an automatic negative response. The patient should be informed that he or she should consult the physician, pharmacist, or nurse before taking any medications from home. In a retail setting the pharmacist also needs to know about any medications the patient is taking, even if they are purchased from another pharmacy or retail outlet.

Present medications are obtained from the medical record of the hospitalized patient. However, if the patient has been using the drug in the past, asking this question will also inform the interviewer of the patient's alertness to present drug therapy.

Drug, food, and pet allergies are important and the interviewer is encouraged to ask for details of the allergic response. Patients often confuse allergic reactions with side effects. For example, a patient may state he or she is allergic to erythromycin because of an upset stomach after each dose, which is a typical side-effect.

Pharmacists and nurses can excel in taking medication histories concerning information about nonprescription drug usage. It is highly recommended that the interviewer be familiar with several trade name products as examples to cue the patient's memory. While reviewing the list of OTC therapeutic categories, patients will frequently report the use of homeopathic products, folk remedies, or even prescription drugs. For example, when the interviewer asks "What OTC product do you take for pain?" the patient may state "I don't use aspirin, but I take acetaminophen with codeine that my doctor gave me."

The concurrent use of OTC products with prescription drugs can result in significant bioavailability problems such as antacid usage with tetracycline or digoxin. Some prescription or OTC products contain sympathomimetics and/or alcohol, which could add to the patient's symptoms or disease. For example, a patient may be taking disulfiram for ethanol abuse, but at the same time be using a mouthwash with a high alcohol content.

Caffeine-containing beverages or drugs of abuse may be related to symptoms or problems the patient has. Ethanol and tobacco can also be related to the patient's problems and they can affect the metabolic clearance of other drugs. Patients should be asked if they use illegal drugs.

Asking patients about illegal drug use is controversial and involves moral, legal, and ethical issues. Policies need to be made concerning utilization of this information and its accessibility to other health professionals. It is advantageous for the interviewer to be familiar with the street names of drugs and with their method of administration, since lack of this knowledge might be equated with the interviewer's disapproval of drug-seeking behavior. Questions regarding illegal drug use must therefore be asked using the appropriate jargon and in an unbiased manner to prevent a negative response.

One approach involves asking the pateint if he or she is using, has used, or has experienced a particular drug, such as 'acid', 'crack,' or 'grass.' Never should the interviewer use the word 'abuse,' since most users do not consider their habits to be abuse of a substance. Further probing of the patient as to frequency, drug effects, and feelings about the drug might provide the health professional with insight into the truth of the statements made by the patient. The most common problem with this type of questioning is the patient's concern about the consequences.

Ending the interview should always be positive for the patient. It should allow the patient time to ask questions about his or her drugs. Questions relating to patients' illnesses should not be handled by the pharmacist, but patients should be encouraged to ask their physician. The interviewer could prompt the physician to the patient's concerns to be handled the next time the physician sees the patient.

After evaluation of the information from the medication history, the pharmacist will be able to formulate the approach needed to teach the patient and improve compliance.

The pharmacist should start by asking the patient if the intended use and dosage times were explained. In either case, the pharmacist should start by reviewing the prescription label with the patient as well as the list of other items covered in the list below on "medication counseling information." If the information was covered at the physician's office or by the discharge planning nurse, or if the patient has previously taken the drug, the pharmacist should have the patient explain the information to check the accuracy. Written information, auxiliary labels, and other counseling aids can be used at this time to highlight the points made by the pharmacist. After this counseling has been done, the pharmacist can evaluate the patient's knowledge with questions.

Medication Counseling Information

- Drug name (trade name and generic)
- Route, dosage form and schedule
- Quantity in the bottle and refills available
- Appearance of the drug (tablet identity, etc.)
- Intended use
- Special directions for storage
- Special administration directions (shake bottle)
- Side effects and what to do if they occur
- How to avoid potential interactions
- Actions to take on a missed dose
- Techniques for self monitoring

Three points require additional explanation. First, the explanation of the intended use must be simple and agree with the information provided by the physician. Second, prescription drug scheduling may conflict with the patient's lifestyle. It is therefore important to ask the patient specific questions about his or her daily activities in order to schedule the doses, and to improve understanding and compliance. One example concerns a patient who is taking ibuprofen (Motrin, Upjohn, Kalamazoo, MI) three times a day. The patient is instructed to take each dose after meals to avoid an upset stomach. If the patient does not eat three meals per day, he or she might be confused about how to take the drug. The final point relates to the amount of information given to the patient regarding potential side effects. Generally, this information is limited to the most common problems that the patient may have to deal with, e.g., drowsiness and the danger of operating machinery, upset stomach relieved by food or reporting a rash to the physician. For drugs that may cause serious side effects, the pharmacist should verify that the patient is being closely monitored by the physician.

EVALUATION

Pharmacists evaluate patient compliance in the same ways that other health professionals do. For example, an encephalopathic patient with cirrhotic liver disease receives 16 ounces of lactulose syrup with a physician's directions reading "Take 2 tablespoonfuls four times daily." The patient is seen 4 days later by the pharmacist for a refill.

Initially, the pharmacist should note an improvement in the patient's condition. He may be able to think more clearly as evidenced by his ability to handle a conversation.

With lactulose therapy, it is not the drug serum level that is being monitored as it would be with theophylline, phenytoin, or digoxin. Instead, the patient can be asked about his or her bowel movements, which should consist of two to three soft stools per day. If the patient is hospitalized, the pharmacist can note lowering of the serum ammonia level as a result of lactulose therapy. These signs would indicate an appropriate dose is being taken.

The next method for monitoring compliance is unique for pharmacists and involves the refill history. Pharmacists record refills of drugs by patients with date and quantity. From the example, this patient would be expected to need a refill by the fourth day based on dosage and the initial amount. If the patient's use does not match the directions for use, the patient can be counseled or the physician called if necessary. Poor compliance can include excessive use as well as insufficient use. Excessive use may result from the patient thinking more drug will do more good, or from sharing medications with friends or family members.

Pharmacists should also use this time to reassess two points, proper drug use, and any problems caused by the drug. The patient should be asked how the drug is administered to assess proper understanding of the dosing schedule. Assuming the patient is dosing the drug properly, but states that he is having six to eight loose stools per day, it would be the pharmacist's duty to suggest that the patient call his doctor. The therapeutic dose needs to be adjusted because the patient is experiencing the side effect of diarrhea. Pharmacists or nurses should call the physician when their patients are experiencing an apparent adverse drug effect rather than refill the prescription. Consulting with the physician may result in a dosage change and a more compliant patient.

Pharmacists can play an important role in optimizing patient drug therapy. It should be the standard of practice that pharmacists become more involved in their patients' health care. Several interventions have been discussed as methods for a pharmacist to have a definite impact on the outcome of drug therapy. Nurses and other health care professionals should utilize pharmacists for drug information and patients should be encouraged to ask questions about their drugs. By increasing consumer awareness and utilization of the vast network of professionals available to help them, one can expect to see significant improvements in patient response to drug therapy. The following plan on teaching about nitroglycerin tablets illustrates the major points made in this chapter.

TEACHING PLAN FOR THE PATIENT USING SUBLINGUAL NITROGLYCERIN TABLETS

Angina pectoris is a clinical syndrome resulting from transient myocardial ischemia. This condition is usually preceded by the development of coronary atherosclerotic heart disease. The coronary arteries have atheromatous lesions that thicken and harden the vessel walls resulting in restricted blood flow and problems with oxygen supply versus demand. There are several major risks factors which include sex (incidence being greater in males), advancing age, presence of hypertension, elevated serum lipid levels (especially low density lipoproteins and cholesterol), a family history of cardiovascular death at a young age, history of cigarette smoking, diabetes mellitus, and obesity.

Angina is usually precipitated by exertion and is relieved by rest. The most common drug used to manage this condition is sublingual nitroglycerin (NTG) tablets. The patient and family members need to be taught the proper use and storage of NTG tablets.

Assessment

The patient and family need to be evaluated as to their understanding of the condition. The risk factors should be addressed as well as the physician's recommendations modifying these risks. Patients should be encouraged to follow their physician's recommendations to attain ideal body weight, stop smoking and alter their diets and exercise plans. The patient also needs reassurance that angina does not usually mean retirement to a sedentary lifestyle, if the patient can learn to pace him or herself when performing tasks that predispose one to angina.

The pharmacist should obtain a medication history of any new patient, or review and update any history done previously. Special attention should be given to topics such as tobacco usage, diet, and potential drug interactions. Antihypertensives, nifedipine, and alcohol are especially capable of adding to hypotension and dizziness caused by nitroglycerin. The patient should be warned about the use of cough/cold preparations which have the potential to elevate blood pressure or increase the heart rate.

Plan

The patient requires instruction about the use of sublingual NTG tablets. Proper administration and potential side effects are important points the pharmacist must stress especially to the newly diagnosed patient.

In addition to verbal counseling, written information should be given to enhance the patient's retention of information about nitroglycerin. An excellent source of this information is in *U.S.P.D.I. Advice to the Patient* (Fig. 10-2).

Implementing the Plan

The patient or family member needs to know this drug is used only when the patient is experiencing or anticipating an anginal attack. He or she should be instructed that the product should be opened prior to use to remove the safety seal and cotton plug. Nitroglycerin tablets require storage in the original glass container with the lid on tight and the cotton removed.

A patient with an anginal attack should sit down and place one tablet under the tongue. There will probably be a sensation of tingling or burning followed by dizziness or light-headedness. This is one reason why it is important for the patient to be sitting down. If the angina pain does not subside in 5 minutes, an additional tablet may be taken, but no more than three tablets should be taken in a 15-minute period. Pain not relieved in this time frame necessitates calling the doctor or going to an emergency room.

Storage of the tablets is important due to the volatile nature of the drug. Patients should be warned not to carry the bottle too close to the body, store it in a refrigerator or bathroom, or to hold the tablets in the hands due to loss of tablet effectiveness. Regardless of the number of times the product is opened, the patient may need to purchase a new bottle every 3 to 6 months. Tablet efficacy can be checked when a tablet is taken by the presence of the most common drug side effects listed below. The patient needs to be warned about potential side effects. The most common rarely require medical attention, e.g., dizziness, headache, flushing of skin, nausea, and rapid heartbeat. However, patients should not ignore syncope, bradycardia (rarely occurs), skin rash (usually from topical administration), or blurred vision (especially if the patient has glaucoma).

After the patient has received verbal counseling on the use of NTG tablets, the pharmacist should ask questions that allow the patient to repeat the information. Any corrections should be made and questions from the patient answered at this time. The patient should be encouraged to read the written information when he or she gets home, prior to the need for the product. The pharmacist should be called later if the patient has additional questions.

Evaluation

Positive efficacy of the therapy involves improved ability of the patient to perform tasks without pain. In addition to an increase in exercise tolerance, the patient should have changes in diet and tobacco use and an improved mental status regarding his or her condition. Patients should be questioned on return visits as to their pattern of NTG needs and storage of the product. The patient can also be reminded when to refill the prescription. Patients should be questioned by the pharmacist to assure that they are being seen regularly by the physician. This is an excellent time for the pharmacist to have the patient express any problems he or she may be having with the drug. Teaching plan follows in Tables 10-4, 10-5, and 10-6 (pages 293–295).

REFERENCES

Ascione, F. J., and Shimp, L. A. The effectiveness of four education strategies in the elderly. *Drug Intelligence and Clinical Pharmacy*, 1984, *18*, 926–931.

Baker, D. M. A study contrasting different modalities of medication discharge counseling. *Hospital Pharmacy*, 1984, *19*, 545–554.

Beardsley, R. S., Johnson, C. A., and Wise, G. Privacy as a factor in patient counseling. *Journal of the American Pharmaceutical Association*, 1977, *17*, 366–368.

Bectel, M. Q. Improving patient compliance. *American Pharmacy*, 1984, NS24, 58–60.

Brushwood, D. B. The pharmacist's duty to warn the patient. Part I. *U S Pharmacist*, 1984, *9*, 21–29.

Brushwood, D. B. The pharmacist's duty to warn the patient. Part II. *U S Pharmacist*, 1984, *9*, 25–30.

Burns, D. How a VCR monitor helps pharmacists to counsel patients. *Pharmacy Times*, 1986, *52*, 45–46.

Covington, T. R., Whtney, H. A. K. Patient-pharmacist communication techniques. *Drug Intelligence and Clinical Pharmacy*, 1971, *5*, 370–376.

Crichton, E. F., Smith, D. L., and Demanuele F. Patient recall of medication information. *Drug Intelligence and Clinical Pharmacy*, 1978, *12*, 591–599.

Hill, R. W., and Goeden, G. R. A plan for pharmacist-conducted patient discharge interviews. *Hospital Formulary*, 1976, *11*, 651–656.

Ivey, M., Tso, Y., and Stamm, K. Communication techniques for patient instruction. *American Journal of Hospital Pharmacy*, 1975, *32*, 828–831.

Marshall, W. R., Rothenberger, L. A., and Bunnell, S. L. The efficacy of personalized audiovisual patient-education materials. *Journal of Family Practice*, 1984, *19*, 659–633.

McKercher, P. L., and Rucker, T. D. Patient knowledge and compliance with medication instructions. *Journal of the American Pharmaceutical Association*, 1977, *17*, 282–291.

Morris, L. A., and Halperin, J. A. Effects of written drug information on patient knowledge and compliance: A literature review. *American Journal of Public Health*, 1979, *69*, 47–52.

Table 10-4
Teaching Plan for Sublingual Nitroglycerin Tablets

Assessment	Plan/learning objectives	Interventions	Evaluation
		Affective	
Ask patient/family about problems they may have using nitroglycerin tablets.	Patient will discuss problems with use or storage of nitroglycerin tablets.	Patient will call nurse or pharmacist when question occurs about nitroglycerin usage.	Patient states how they are using nitroglycerin and how often it is required.
	Patient will discuss problems with side effects of nitroglycerin.	Patient will report any side effects to pharmacist and physician immediately.	Patient reports no adverse emotions about using the drug.
Ask patient/family to express fears or concerns about angina.	Patient will discuss their feelings about using nitroglycerin and angina.	Patient will make appointment with physician for follow-up and to discuss concerns about angina.	Patient is being seen by physician on a regular basis and has contacted them about any side effects.
	Patient will develop skills for coping with stress or decreased ability to exert him/herself.		

Table 10-5
Teaching Plan for Sublingual Nitroglycerin Tablets

Assessment	Plan/learning objectives	Interventions	Evaluation
		Cognitive	
Ask the patient/family what they know about angina.	Patient/family list the beneficial effect expected from nitroglycerin tablets.	Give patient/family fact sheet on proper storage and use of nitroglycerin tablets.	Ask patient/family to explain the reason they are taking the medication.
Ask the patient/family what they know about using nitroglycerin tablets.	Patient/family state how the nitroglycerin tablets are to be administered, when and how many.	Show patient/family the tablet and explain how they are given and discuss the scheduling and storage.	Ask patient/family to tell you when the patient is to use these tablets.
Ask the patient/family about the risk factors associated with the development of angina.	Patient/family describe the side effects that tell them if the nitroglycerin tablets are good.	Give patient/family information on atherosclerosis and angina.	Ask patient/family to show you how many tablets the patient can take before calling the physician.
	Patient/family describe the side effects they need to report to physician and pharmacist not related to the above.		Ask patient/family when to refill the nitroglycerin tablets and how to store them.
	Patient/family list risk factors associated with the development of angina.		Patient able to tell you about atherosclerosis and angina.

Table 10-6
Teaching Plan for Sublingual Nitroglycerin Tablets

Assessment	Plan/learning objectives	Interventions	Evaluation
		Psychomotor	
Observe/record patient's use of nitroglycerin tablets i.e., number of tablets used per day; refill history	Patient tells how many tablets are used per day.	Refer to physician for potential excessive use of nitroglycerin tablets.	Question/observe patient for: 1. Proper use of tablets 2. Proper storage of tablets 3. Increased involvement with reducing risk factors associated with angina.
Determine if patient is using prophylactically or in response to actual anginal attack.	Patient able to explain reason why tablets were taken and what precipitated anginal attack.	Refer to physician if condition not relieved by nitroglycerin.	
Observe/record patient's progress: exercise tolerance, weight reduction and ability to quit smoking.		Demonstrate appropriate storage and handling of nitroglycerin tablets, i.e., carrying in coat pocket versus shirt pocket where body heat may deteriorate.	

Olsen, K. M., and Dube, J. E. Evaluation of two methods of patient education. *American Journal of Hospital Pharmacy*, 1985, *42*, 622–624.

Rehder, T. L., McCoy, L. K., Blackwell, B., Whitehead, W., and Robinson A. Improving medication compliance by counseling and special prescription container. *American Journal of Hospital Pharmacy*, 1980, *37*, 379–385.

Ruffner, M. Consumers lack, but want, prescription help. *Drug Topics*, 1984, *128*, 12–13.

Sands, C. D., Robinson, J. D., and Orlando, J. B. The oral contraceptive PPI: Its effect on patient knowledge, feelings, and behavior. *Drug Intelligence and Clinical Pharmacy*, 1984, *18*, 730–735.

Smith, M. C. How drug cost affects patient compliance. *Drug Therapy*, 1976, *6*, 12–14.

Strull, W. M., Lo, B., and Charles, G. Do patients want to participate in medical decision making? *Journal of the American Medical Association*, 1984, *252*, 2990–2994.

11

Teaching Patients, Families, and Communities about Nutrition

Linda Snetselaar

With Teaching Plan by
Cheryl Verstraete Ratliff

OBJECTIVES

1. Discuss factors influencing adherence to diet.
2. List steps in a behavioral change plan.
3. Describe the difference between modeling and simulation.
4. Discuss two strategies for self-direction.
5. Identify potential problems in self-monitoring as an evaluation tool.
6. Develop a nutrition teaching plan to prevent malnutrition in a child diagnosed with cancer.

Nutrition education is an essential component of patient teaching. It is needed in many situations involving individuals, families, and communities. Changes in diet rarely have impact on one person without affecting others who must interact with that individual.

In all instances involving dietary change assessment, planning, intervention, and evaluation are important. In most instances measuring learning or behavior change is much more difficult than modifying it (Barlow, 1981). Before proceeding with planning, a thorough assessment of the problem is necessary in order for the patient to successfully meet goals (Cone and Hawkins, 1977). Nutrition education is the means whereby goal fulfillment is realized.

This chapter initially reviews the major studies that involve nutrition education and summarizes the results. Guidelines necessary to assess and meet the learning needs of patients are provided. Specific strategies used in nutrition education are discussed in detail. These include modeling, simulation, thought stopping, cognitive restructuring, reinforcement, extinction, tailoring, shaping, contracting, and self-directed strategies.

Research indicates that patients tend to meet dietary goals when appropriate nutrition education strategies are utilized.*

As more is learned about the benefits of nutrition education, the need for colaboration between the registered nurse and the dietitian increases. When the registered nurse sees a problem involving nutrition, referral to a registered dietitian is initiated. The nurse and dietitian should reinforce the nutrition education or counseling given to a patient, family, or community group. All health team members and significant others must work together for consistent, well-developed, and successful teaching in the area of nutrition. The dialogue between nurse and dietitian is equally as important as the dialogue between nurse and patient and dietitian and patient.

Nutrition education over the years has been a mainstay in the medical profession. Experimentation in the field has and does rely heavily upon the knowledge a health professional can impart to a patient.

A classic example of research linking diet and disease is the well-known Framingham study, in which several factors, such as overweight and physical inactivity, were found to be associated with the occurrence of coronary heart disease (CHD) in men in Framingham, Massachusetts. This research indicated that persons with serum cholesterol levels in excess of 225 mg/dl are at risk of developing CHD and that at higher levels the risk increases dramatically. The blood content of cholesterol is derived both from endogenous and exogenous sources. Americans typically ingest from 500 to 700 mg per day. It has been shown that there will be predictable elevation of serum cholesterol levels if the dietary intake of cholesterol is increased from 0 to 400 mg, but cholesterol intakes in larger amounts raise serum cholesterol levels higher in some individuals than in others (McGill and Mott, 1976).

The National Diet Heart Study of 1960 served as a prelude to two major studies, the Multiple-Risk Intervention Trial (MRFIT, 1982) and the Lipid Research Clinics Coronary Primary Prevention Trial (CPPT, 1984). To achieve even a slight decrease in serum levels, dietary cholesterol must be sharply reduced. The National Diet-Heart Study (1968) found that, after a year, men who were placed on low-cholesterol diets of 350 to 450 mg per day and who increased the ratio of polyunsaturated fat to saturated fats* (ratio of 1.5–2.0) had reduced serum cholesterol levels by an average of 11 percent, to "safe" levels slightly over 200 mg/dl. A control group put on a diet resembling the "typical" American diet (650–750 mg cholesterol, polyunsaturated fat to saturated fat ratio = 0.4), experienced a 4 percent reduction in serum cholesterol levels, suggesting that their prestudy intake had been much higher (National Diet-Heart Research Group, 1968).

Serum cholesterol levels seem to be sensitive, however, not only to cholesterol intake but to other components of lipid intake and metabolism as well. Saturated fat raises the level of plasma cholesterol; monounsaturated fat has no significant effect; and serum cholesterol is lowered by polyunsaturated fat. We do not always know whether the excess cholesterol has been excreted from the body or has shifted from the blood into tissues. There is some evidence that increasing polyunsaturated intake may have some potentially negative effects as well (Melchior, Lofland, and Jones, 1974; Reiser, Sorrels,

---

*Snetselaar, L. Unpublished data collected during workshop and nutrition counseling supported by National Heart, Lung and Blood Institute Contract # NOL-HV-02923, 1986.

*By dividing the amount of saturated fat into polyunsaturated fat the resulting number provides an indication of serum cholesterol lowering. The higher the ratio or number the greater the degree of serum cholesterol lowering.

and Williams, 1959). The mechanisms for all of these observations have not yet been fully explained and must be studied further.

The MRFIT educated patients on a three-phase diet, stressing the eventual use of the 100 mg cholesterol, P/S ratio of 1.0. The CPPT used a moderately low cholesterol diet of 400 mg cholesterol with a P/S ratio of 0.6–1.0 (MRFIT Research Group, 1982; Lipid Research Clinics' Group, 1984). Both studies relied heavily on nutrition education to maximize program intervention. Study participants learned both the hypothesized reasons and proven facts related to diet and coronary heart disease. They also became adept at learning the fat content of foods and label reading to maximize the effectiveness of diet in controlling factors related to risk in coronary heart disease.

Many other studies also use nutrition education as a major component of treatment of disease states. The Diabetes Control and Complications Trial (DCCT) was designed to determine whether very strict control of type I diabetes as compared standard treatment as is currently practiced through the country results in fewer complications such as blindness, renal malfunction, neurologic problems, or cognitive deterioration.

A second study involves nutrition education and its use in determining whether low protein diets can delay or possibly eliminate the need for dialysis. In this study nutrition education involves teaching patients how to use special low protein products in food preparation.

A third study involves use of low fat diets in those women who are at risk for breast cancer. This study uses nutrition education as a means of helping women incorporate low fat products into their diets while keeping caloric intake at a level that will not allow for weight loss.

Education in all of the above instances relies on much more than merely providing information about the disease and the effect of diet. Indeed, merely telling the patient what foods to avoid and what foods to use will not promote long-term adherence. The sections that follow provide a step-wise means of achieving client adherence to diet: assess needs; plan and mutually set goals; intervene with teaching strategies; and evaluate.

ASSESSMENT

Nutrition assessment is a crucial phase in the process of nutrition education. Several categories of assessment information should be considered in determining nutrition needs of each patient and the areas of teaching on which to concentrate. To achieve a thorough assessment the dietitian and nurse must assess in the following areas: nutrition, biology, knowledge, behavior, social support, and coping.

Nutrition Assessment

Nutrition assessment involves looking at the quality and quantity of a diet. Assessing quality can vary depending upon the disease state that one is trying to alter. For example, for the client who has diabetes the parameters of assessment would be very different from those of a person at risk for breast cancer.

In all instances, however, the diet should conform to general guidelines as recommended in the dietary prescription. In other words, when certain nutrients are prescribed or limited, the meal patterns change. In diabetes all three major nutrients, carbohydrate, protein, and fat are important. However, in the diabetic diet calorie balance with simple and complex sugars, animal protein and fat intake is essential. Fat plays a role in coronary heart disease as well where it should be limited and the type specified. In low-fat diets for women at risk for breast cancer the quantity of fat is also a focus. Of special importance then in the education of all these patients is learning to modify fat intake appropriately. This is a challenging behavioral change since the American diet is high in fat, in both a visible and invisible form.

Assessing the appropriateness of quantities of nutrients eaten is often difficult. Several factors should be considered in this assessment (Mason, Wenberg, and Walsh, 1977). First, is the variability among individuals. Never assume that all individuals eat alike. Second, a 1-day record will not provide an accurate measure of intake over time for one person. Third, is the validity and reliability of the assessment. If the questions used to interview the patient and family do not obtain accurate information then the assessment is invalid. However, taking a diet history or requesting a 3–7-day diet diary does give indepth quantitative and qualitative information that is valid.

Biological Assessment

Biological assessment includes an assessment of all areas of physiologic function relative to the total nutrition picture. The client's chart has a wealth of data that relates to biological assessment and reflects dietary intake. For example, one can determine height and weight over time, variations in laboratory tests which offer cues to general health status and nutrient levels, and a medical diagnosis or specific reason a client is seeking health care that is nutrition related.

Charting notes by medical doctors, reigstered nurses, and registered dietitions provide an excellent source for biological information. Laboratory reports also contain nutrition information such as blood or urine levels of nutrients or their byproducts. Charting notes also indicate types of drugs that may be used in altering diets. Some drugs are taken with meals and may affect the types of instruction given when the topic of diet is presented to the patient. For example the use of a lipid-lowering drug like cholestyramine, has been shown to be more effective when taken with meals.

Charting notes are invaluable in teaching diabetic persons. Ongoing values for glycosulated hemoglobin indicate diabetic control over time and thus form an indirect measure of dietary adherence. Blood glucose values indicated in averages for the week also provide a picture of control. In addition matching postprandial blood glucose values to meals may provide a clue as to which time of day a meal is most problematic. In some cases, the postprandial blood glucose values may indicate that the timing of the injection of insulin is incorrect. All of this information can be taught to the diabetic person and family who can learn to monitor many of these laboratory parameters at home.

In renal patients laboratory results are also extremely important. Declines in glomerular filtration rates may signal a need to reduce protein intake. Wasting and malnutrition is also a concern in renal patients. Falls in serum albumin and transferrin indicate potential protein wasting. Reduction in body weight or potential malnutrition is significant and should be evaluated by the dietitian who should note the patient's age, height, and sex. Any renal patient with elevated fasting serum phosphorus values on two consecutive measurements may need dietary phosphorus restriction and phosphate binders so that symptoms of renal failure do not reuslt. The patient and family will have to be taught about these potential complications and how to avoid phosphorus in the diet.

Table 11-1
Assessment of Nutrition and Biologic Factors Affecting Renal Patients

Patient Objective	Assessment Procedure
Patient will exhibit an adequate nutrition status indicated by the following parameters	Patient will be assessed for risk factors that precipitate development of malnutrition
Serum albumin, 3.5 to 5.5 g/dl Transferrin, 180 to 200 mg/dl Hemoglobin, Males=14.0 g/dl Females=12.0 g/dl Hematocrit, Males=44% Females=38%	Patient unable to achieve oral intake or unwilling to eat Patient experiencing stress from infection, surgery, and trauma from accidents Patient who has a recent weight loss of 7 to 10% body weight Patient will be provided with a computer or hand-generated diet pattern designed to meet the patient's individual needs. Foods to target are those high in protein (indicate high and low biological value), phosphorus, potassium, and sodium.

As with renal diets, working with low-fat diets in dealing with breast cancer necessitates a variety of tests such as lipoproteins and estradiol. Laboratory findings will indicate changes in blood levels of fat soluble vitamins, especially vitamin A. Alteration in these laboratory tests reflects dietary intake and can provide clues that must be stressed in instructing the patient on the low fat diet. These are only a few examples of how biological assessment contributes to the teaching plans used with each patient. Table 11-1 provides an assessment plan aligning patient objective and a specific assessment procedure.

Knowledge Assessment

Prior to any type of diet instruction it is necessary to determine the knowledge level of patients. Although assessment of knowledge varies with the diagnosis and diet prescription of each patient a general technique for determining what the patient knows is use of pretests (Klein, 1971). Such tests may actually be pencil and paper type or they may be a series of questions asked verbally. Remember to include the family members in this assessment as they often need instruction so they can assist the patient later in complex diet choices. Large groups often respond well to pretesting before a lecture or menu preparation session because this type of assessment stimulates questions relative to lack of knowledge and concerns which they share. The dietitian and nurse can collaborate on the types of questions patients with certain illnesses should be asked. For example a patient who has problems with controlling diabetes may be stimulated by a pretest to ask questions that lead to more organized changes in insulin dosages and changes in dietary intake. The nurse and dietitian are then responsible for discussing the changes step by step. A close working relationship between the dietitian and nurse is essential.

Pretests might also be used for patients with coronary heart disease. The pretest might include questions related to knowledge in the area of foods high in cholesterol and saturated fat. Additional questions might focus on foods containing no fat or small amounts of fat. Following instruction a posttest might be administered to determine the level of knowledge acquisition.

Pretests for diabetic persons might focus on a knowledge of how insulin and food interact. Since all of the major nutrients (carbohydrate, protein, and fat) are important to diabetic diets, questions about how various foods might be counted in terms of consistency in dietary intake would be of value. Additional questions might focus on use of food to avoid hypoglycemic reactions during illness when food is often forgotten. It is important to remember to drink juices as a substitute for meals. Questions on how to substitute juices for entire meals are important when determining patient knowledge in situations involving illness. Periodic assessment of postinstruction knowledge is important.

In renal disease knowledge of foods high in protein, phosphorus, and sodium is important to eventual success on the diet. Questions asking which foods are high in these substances will indicate how knowledgeable the patient is prior to instruction. Once again postinstruction knowledge assessment is very important.

If low-fat diets are used to treat women at risk for breast cancer, a knowledge of foods high in total fat is important. Asking a group of women from one community to participate in group sessions might involve giving each woman a check-off list and asking her to place a check next to foods high in fat. Following instruction in this area a posttest of knowledge gained would be appropriate.

A general rule to keep in mind when constructing a test for patients is to keep questions simple. Ask for one word or multiple-choice answers. Keep wording at a sixth grade level or lower. Use simple nonmedical terminology. Keep the number of questions between 5 and 10. Keep verbiage short and simple. Give all questions a pilot test period in which patients similar to the ones for whom the test is designed take the test and comment. Revise the test based on patients' comments following the pilot test. This type of assessment is invaluable in designing teaching plans.

Behavioral Assessment

Behavioral assessment is the act of identifying behaviors or day-to-day acts that must change in order for dietary goals to be achieved. This type of assessment provides the information to determine whether the patient will have the ability to adhere to a diet over time. Prior to diet instruction the patient might be required to keep a 3-day intake record. Instruction must be given as to the level of detail required in keeping the record. Is it necessaary to ask patients to record all foods eaten? If "yes" the Table 11-2 may be of

Table 11-2
Sample Diet Diary Chart

Kind of food	Amount	Time of day	Feeling before eating	Feeling after eating
Noodles	2 cups	8:00 am	Angry	Full
Milk, 2%	8 ounces	10:00 am	Thirsty	Satisfied
Hot Dogs	2 ounces	12:00 noon	Frustrated	Less frustrated

Table 11-3
Sample Diet Diary Chart

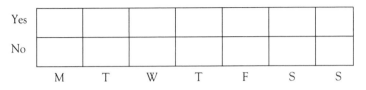

value. If this much detail is not necessary concentrate on just those areas that contribute most to lack of success in achieving a goal.

The chart used in Table 11-3 is simple and can highlight days where a problem behavior most frequently occurs.

Data from the types of records in Tables 11-2 and 11-3 show the level of precision in determining amounts of foods for diabetic diets; the care taken to use low fat, low cholesterol foods; and the creativity in selecting a diet low in protein. If the instructions indicate, a patient may provide specific labels for specialty foods and the emotional feelings at the time of eating a meal. Based on this record a sense of the patient's ability to provide details related to eating behavior is ascertained.

Questionnaires are another avenue used in assessing behavior related to diet intake. This type of instrument can delve into the frequency of use of salt, salt substitutes, sugar, sugar substitutes, low fat dairy products, low cholesterol egg substitutes, low-fat dairy products, low cholesterol egg substitutes, etc. Questionnaires can also provide information on usual food preparation habits, i.e., use of margarines, butter, oils, and spreads in frying, baking, braising, seasoning, and sandwich preparation. Additional data determined through questionnaires might include the following. When does the patient eat meals, snacks? What types of food does the patient choose if given alternatives? Does the client select seconds? Does the client avoid favorite foods for long periods of time, only to give in and eat large amounts of those favorites on a binge?

Behavioral assessment can also provide an indication of nonfood related behaviors that trigger eating habits. For example, watching TV may provide the impetus for snacking on high-fat munchies. Identifying behaviors that trigger eating may be the first step toward eliminating the unwanted eating behavior.

Social Support Assessment

Another type of behavioral assessment involves talking with those persons who have frequent contact with the patient. Studies indicate that persons who form a support system for the patient are helpful in long-term adherence to diet (Morton, Ringles, and Christakis, 1967). The spouse is a crucial factor in dietary adherence. In families where the wife does most of the meal preparation and husband is on a restricted diet her support and understanding of the dietary pattern will mean the difference between success and failure. Involving the wife by inviting her to submit recipes and provide tips on what has worked for her in terms of dietary preparation is a step toward helping the patient comply. In a situation where a patient is on a restricted diet and the spouse is not following the same diet, conflicts may arise. Assessing these problems before diet instruction can lead to the appropriate affective teaching.

A variety of questions can be posed to significant others in the patient's life to determine their involvement in dietary matters. Who plans and prepares meals? Who buys the groceries? How are parties planned, i.e., by patient, by spouse? Is money a factor in planning meals? If yes, describe the monetary concerns. Do family conflicts ever arise over meal planning? If yes, please describe. Will the patient who is on a diet eat meals prepared separately from other members in the family? How are friends and coworkers involved in eating patterns? Will friends and coworkers be supportive? Please describe how supportive or nonsupportive they might be?

Children in a family can be a supportive influence for a family member following a diet. Allowing children to get involved in meal preparation and to prompt for appropriate eating behaviors can provide a positive reinforcement for the new eating habits.

Friends can be allies in helping a patient to adhere to a specific dietary regimen. Because friends tend to be associated with social occasions (work, parties, etc.) they can give support at times when eating indiscretions are most tempting.

Coping Assessment

Assessing the ways in which people cope with problems is essential. Coping skills are a means of dealing with different situations in a systematic fashion. Without the ability to handle problems the patient is powerless in achieving goals. Coping can be assessed by giving the patient a scenario to discuss. For example, describe a situation involving mild hypoglycemia; what would the patient do to resolve the problem? During a party the patient on a low cholesterol, low fat diet is tempted to take the cheese cake. How would the patient respond? For the patient on a low protein diet how would he or she react at a barbeque where many high protein foods are being served? A coping pattern can be identified from discussing these scenerios.

Questionnaires can also provide a forum for discussion of coping skills. The questionnaires might allow multiple-choice answers to hypothetical situations. One answer might be "I'm not sure what I would do." If this answer occurs frequently it might signal the need for more thorough instruction or it might indicate the need for help in knowing how to use information in crisis or demanding situations.

Assessment in the areas of nutrition, biological, behavioral, and coping needs can influence the direction of patient education. For example, if during a behavioral and coping assessment it is discovered that the diabetic patient believes that drinking fresh fruit juices in any quantity is allowed, teaching in the cognitive domain will be necessary. If during the coping assessment, it becomes clear that the patient has problems saying "no" to friends' food offers at social events, affective teaching should be addressed. If it becomes clear through a questionnaire on meal preparation that the wife lacks the skills of food preparation skills for low-fat cookery, the psychomotor domain should be emphasized.

In summary, a thorough assessment of current nutrition status, biological data, current knowledge, behavioral skills, social support and coping skills will prepare the clinician for educating the patient. Without this assessment a major component of the total nutrition change program will be missing.

PLANNING

Planning the second step in the teaching process allows time for determining the what, where, and when of nutrition education.

An essential part of planning for nutritional teaching is goal setting and objective writing. Once assessment is complete and analysis of that data is finished, the next step involves goal setting.

Goal Setting/Objective Writing

In setting dietary goals eight steps are utilized. These steps are illustrated in Tables 11-4 and 11-5. The first step is to explain to the patient what needs to be accomplished. In Table 11-4 the explanation includes the spouse, and Table 11-5 illustrates the need to incorporate parents into this process.

Once the purpose is explained the second step is to state the dietary goals. The actual goals should be stated in behavioral terms and written as objectives. For example, "I (the patient) will be able to measure meat in 3-ounce portions for every evening meal." Once the goals are mutually identified, the advantages and risks of each objective should be discussed. The third step in Tables 11-4 and 11-5 illustrates the importance of this discussion for realizing the effort that must be put forth to change the behavior.

Following these three steps a decision must be reached. Are the goals feasible? Do advantages outweigh the disadvantages? At this point a decision must be made by the patient to either work toward the goal or not. This helps establish commitment toward the goal, motivates the patient to put forth the effort. After the decision to go forward is made the nurse and patient must further define the behavior or goal by specifying the conditions and criteria used to evaluate goal attainment. Typically this requires that subgoals be identified. Identifying subgoals are another method of providing the patient with specific details necessary for dietary compliance.

The last two steps of mutual goal setting are working toward patient commitment and discussing the patient, family or group concerns about the dietary behavior that is to be learned or changed. Are there major difficulties associated with achieving the goals that must be resolved prior to working toward success? Perhaps referral to another health professional, i.e., nurse clinical specialist, psychiatrist, psychologist, etc., is necessary before a goal can be achieved.

An indication of patient commitment should be sought following goal setting. Patient commitment is a very difficult area to assess. Frequently only subjective information is available. The following three basic behaviors may be appropriate measures indicating commitment: (a) A patient's statement indicating that the established goals are workable in their everyday lifestyle. (b) The clinician and family should carefully discuss the deterents to achieving the goal, i.e., time, money, risk, anxiety, embarrassment, etc. These barriers to dietary adherence should be discussed and solutions proposed by the patient. (c) The group or community should state clearly that they will work to make the solutions successful.

Once measures of commitment are seen, then identification of concerns is important for the eventual success in long-term dietary adherence. Some concerns may be content oriented; others may be emotionally oriented. For example, a community group

Table 11-4

Steps in Mutual Goal Setting for A Low Cholesterol, Fat-Controlled
Diet For Cardiac Patient and Spouse

General guidelines for steps	Examples for specific steps
1. Purpose of goal setting	1. "The purpose is to work together to set goals which are possible for you to reach."
2. Goal identification	2. "Limit meat intake to 3 ounces per day." "Limit whole milk to ½ cup per day." "Substitute an egg substitute for whole eggs in all breakfast meals."
3. Advantages and risks	3. "Advantages to all are lower blood cholesterol." "Disadvantages are the loss of the enjoyment of eating an 8-ounce steak and whole milk products." "Disadvantage of limited restaurant menu choices."
4. Decision	4. "Yes go on."
5. Define behavior: conditions and criteria	5. "Meat intake will occur at only one meal each day." "Whole milk intake will be limited to ½ cup per day on cereal. All other dairy products will be skim milk."
	5. "Whole eggs will not be used but egg substitutes will be used daily as a replacement food."
6. Subgoal identification	6. "Limit 4 out of 7 meals per week to only 3 ounces of meat for the first week." "Once 3 ounces of meat becomes a habit for an entire week (in approximately 1 month), limit whole milk intake to ½ cup 3 days out of 7." "Once this subgoal is achieved for an entire week (in approximately one month) begin using egg substitutes 3 out of 7 days per week as a substitute for eggs. In approximately one month only egg substitutes will be used."
7. Commitment behavior	7. Couple eats monthly with a gourmet cooking group that follows American Heart Association's low-cholesterol, low-fat recipes.
8. Identification of concerns	8. Couple joins the local "cardiac club" that has speakers and discusses problems of managing low cholesterol diets.

Table 11-5
Steps in Mutual Goal Setting for A Low-Protein Diet For Child With
Renal Failure

General guidelines for steps	Examples for specific steps
1. Purpose of goal setting	1. "The purpose is to work together to set goals."
2. Goal identification	2. "Limit meat intake to 3 ounces per day." "Limit milk intake to ½ cup per day." "Use low protein bread and cookies as a substitute for regular bread and cookies."
3. Advantages and risks	3. "Advantages are the potential of reducing the complications due to kidney failure so I can play with the other children." "Disadvantages are missing the enjoyment of what other children are eating."
4. Decision	4. "Yes go on."
5. Define behavior: conditions and criteria	5. "Meat intake will occur at two meals per day with 3 ounces divided between the two. All meat will be weighed by parents to assure accuracy." "Milk will be served at dinner and measured to assure a ½ cup serving." "All regular bread and cookies will be avoided and low protein substitutes used routinely as desired."
6. Subgoal identification	6. "A move from the current 6 ounces of meat per day, 1 cup of milk per day, and high protein bread and cookies will occur gradually." "Each reduction will occur on a weekly basis, i.e., 2 times per week meat will be dropped to 3 ounces, milk to ½ cup, and high protein bread and cookies avoided." "Eventually the goals will be followed 7 days a week."
7. Commitment behavior	7. Child states low protein cookies are good to eat. Knows to say, "This is best for my kidneys" when other children tease him about his diet.
8. Identification of concerns	8. Can't eat hot dogs and many of the fast foods other children enjoy.

who has come together to discuss nutrition for the elderly may express several content concerns such as confusion over sodium on food labels really meaning salt or the misunderstanding that coconut oil (a vegetable oil) is not a good substitute for shortening made with animal fat as they are both saturated.

On the other hand a group of parents, whose children are undergoing chemotherapy and prescribed diets high in calories and protein, may express emotional concerns such as giving in to the child's desire for candy or having to discipline the child to eat at the dinner table even when nauseated.

The dietian or nurse may feel very comfortable dealing with content but incapable of handling emotional problems. Use of a counseling psychologist or clinical nurse specialist in pediatrics may be necessary.

Behavioral Aspects of Planning

It is important to determine the circumstances surrounding the situation that concerns the patient. Under what circumstances does the poor eating behavior occur? Is eating inappropriately only a snacking problem at night? The frequency or the number of times a poor dietary behavior occurs and its duration should be determined. Duration means length of time over which a given dietary behavior occurs and how long it continues each time.

Situations that occur frequently in day to day living can trigger an inappropriate eating behavior. Very important to eventual success is identification of which reinforcers promote poor dietary behaviors and which allow that conduct to continue. If feelings of depression trigger eating, try to eliminate the depression by doing a fun nonfood activity. By listing benefits derived from continuing the inappropriate behavior, the patient can identify those cues that perpetuate a behavior.

Family and Community Involvement

Goal setting and concern definition, both discussed above, can involve a variety of people from families to the community. By initially providing suggestions for using these persons as supportive elements in dietary adherence, problems can be avoided at later points in time. Although goal setting involves the teacher and the patient, it also involves the family. The family should be present during instruction sessions. Community resources should be specified, i.e., local heart associations can provide a wealth of information to patients following a low-cholesterol, fat-controlled diet. Many communities offer group help sessions for persons making dietary changes because of their diseases. Providing support at the onset of a new diet regimen may provide the impetus for future long-term dietary adherence.

Many hospitals provide outpatient services that include special mealing planning for patients on special diets. All meals are served throughout the day and combined with classes to assist patients in learning how to apply dietary knowledge. Many hospitals have diabetic teaching units that include this feature.

Planning for dietary instruction has as its first step mutual goal setting where the purpose and identification of goals are important. Beyond these two steps advantages and risk of meetings goals should be identified, a decision should be reached, behavior should be specifically defined and subgoals should be delineated. Planning for dietary instruction and mutual goal setting also includes identifying family and community support structures. The patient who has many persons or resources to lean upon for support will more likely find following a diet much easier.

Begin a session with the patient by first identifying the responsibility of the teacher as that of listener, observer and provider of a learning environment to try out new skills and behaviors. Make it clear that the teacher is a facilitator not a dictator. Discuss the general formatting of sessions. One topic or goal will be discussed at a time. Sessions will be as focused as possible.

Whether using individual interventions with one patient or group sessions always stress that active participation is encouraged and indicate that all information will be kept confidential. Patients should be aware that there are limits to nutrition education and that referrals to nurse specialists, psychologist or psychiatrist may be arranged.

When selecting a dietary teaching intervention remember that four major elements are known to influence adherence: patient, teacher, clinic environment, and dietary regimen.

Factors That Have Impact on Adherence

Patient Characteristics

What happens in most nutrition education sessions initially is information dissemination. Research indicates that recall diminishes directly in proportion to the amount of information given (Joyce, Caple, Mason, Reynolds, and Mathews, 1969). If a patient is anxious or not attentive during a session forgetfulness tends to increase. Retention is best with moderate anxiety (Joyce, Caple, Mason, Reynolds, and Mathews, 1969). Studies have also examined fear as a factor in information retention (Holder, 1972; Leventhal, 1973). These studies indicate that high levels of fear of disease complications promote poor dietary adherence.

Living alone has also been associated with poor adherence (Archer, Seymour, and Christakis, 1967). An asymptomatic condition requiring preventive treatment also tends to be associated with lower adherence rates (Blackwell, 1973).

A patient's expectations of the ease of following a diet can affect adherence if incongruent with his or her actual experience (Dunbar, 1977). It seems that when the family expects the patient to adhere well, performance is better (Dunbar, 1977). In selecting intervention strategies these factors should be carefully considered.

Nutrition Teacher

Studies show that the patient's satisfaction with the caregiver and care increases adherence (Hagen, Foreyt, and Durham, 1976; Hulka, Zyzanski, Cassel, and Thompson, 1971; Hurtado, Greenlick, and Columbo, 1973; Kaim-Caudle and Marsh, 1975; Kincey, Bradshaw, Ley, and Ratoff, 1975). Adherence also increases if the patient sees the same caregiver at each visit (Alpert, 1964; Becker, Drachman, and Kirscut, 1972; Becker and Maiman, 1975; Sackett and Haynes, 1976). The diabetic person who is having variations or swings in blood glucose levels will feel more comfortable contacting a caregiver with whom he or she is familiar. Knowing that one person is familiar with past and is ready to help; imparts a feeling of confidence in the patient.

In summary, patient characteristics associated with higher levels of adherence to a medical regimen include: patients who are moderately anxious without being fearful, patients who do not live alone, patients who are symptomatic, and patients whose expectations are equal to the actual experience of following a regimen. Interactions with the caregiver are very important. Patients who are satisfied with and able to see the same caregiver at each visit also tend to exhibit higher degrees of adherence to a medical regimen.

Clinic Environment and Dietary Regimen

Clinic atmosphere influences adherence but frequently receives little attention. A bright, well-lit room would seem to be more inviting then a dark, dingy one. A minimum of waiting time would also seem to be effective in enhancing learning.

In addition to the clinic environment the complications and difficulties of the medical and dietary regimen effect adherence. When many life changes occur at one time it may be difficult to ensure adherence (Davis and Eichhorn, 1963; Johannsen, Hellmuth, and Sorauf, 1966). The following factors involving medical regimens have been shown to affect adherence: difficulty in combining dietary restrictions with current life style; irregularity of the routine required by the dietary regimen; difficulty with the complicated dietary regimen itself; carrying out the regimen at work or in a restaurant (Dunbar, 1977).

It is possible to overcome these negative factors by carefully reviewing existing habits and incorporating some of them into the patient's new dietary pattern. Cultural traditions can frequently be incorporated into the diet to make it more acceptable. For example, planning for religious holidays and rearranging the dietary pattern to accommodate such meals can be accomplished without changing the dietary prescription.

Cooking demonstrations to show how to prepare a low-protein bread for a renal patient will provide practical advice in a concrete fashion. A similar demonstration for the low cholesterol diet to illustrate how to prepare a patient's favorite casserole with low cholesterol, low fat foods can be a great asset to dietary adherence.

When restaurant eating is a frequent problem, assisting the patient in making menu selections can be helpful. Keep a large selection of restaurant menus on hand. Ask the patient to act out a typical restaurant situation. Provide assistance in making selections when the patient needs help. Praise those efforts that allow the dietary prescription to be followed.

Adherence Predictors

Up to this point factors to maximize adherence have been described. In some cases the dietitian or nurse may wish to screen for those patients who will have difficulty in following a regimen. Those who can be predicted to have difficulties might be placed on a modified regimen until they work into the more stringent regimen.

Researchers have looked at these potential predictors of good adherence: attitudes of the patient, judgment of the dietitian, and patient prediction of eventual adherence (Dunbar, 1980). Negative aspects associated with these factors, i.e., poor patient attitudes, the dietitian's predictions of low adherence, dietitian's preconceived negative judgments of patients, and patient's statements indicating lack of confidence in being able to meet the goals set, have been linked with future problems. It is important to note here that these factors do not identify who will fail to follow any specific regimen. To date, no single factor has been pinpointed as an absolutely accurate predictor of adherence.

Research indicates that changes in patient beliefs about a medical regimen are not related to changes in long-standing diet patterns (Dunbar, 1980). For example, just because the patient believes diet is helpful does not mean that he or she will follow it. The performance of a given dietary pattern can predict subsequent adherence more clearly than can client attitudes or beliefs.

Numerous researchers have looked at self-prediction of adherence to medical regimens. In some cases clients were asked how well they could follow a regimen over time. One study showed that while 77 percent of 154 new patients expressed a willingness to comply with a clinician's advice, only 63 percent actually exhibited compliant behavior over time (Davis, 1968). A second study reported that of subjects who agreed to participate in a blood pressure study, 38 of 230 did poorly in following a regimen and needed added counseling (Haynes, Gibson, Hackett, Sackett, Taylor, Roberts, and Johnson, 1976).

With these adherence predictors in mind (attitudes, judgment of the dietitian and patient prediction of adherence) adequate interventions can be developed to maximize adherence to diet.

IMPLEMENTING NUTRITION EDUCATION

Once preliminary planning has taken place intervention begins. Intervention is the act of working with a patient to solve a problem. This process may be aimed at maintaining recommended dietary behaviors, preventing indiscretions, and dealing with existing problems. The major purpose of intervention is to provide the patient with problem-solving skills to be used in applying dietary information.

Remediation Interventions

Frequently remediation or reteaching is needed when dietary lapses occur. Six steps are used in implementing a remediation strategy (Table 11-6).

First, divide nutrition teaching related to the inappropriate behavior into manageable steps arranged in sequence. Second, arrange steps so that the first step can be managed with little effort. Third, sequence the section of information so that the patient is capable of attaining each one. Fourth, make each step within the nutrition instruction small enough to achieve but not too easy or trivial that the patient will consider it worthless. Fifth, make the planning of steps a mutual situation involving the clinician and the patient. Finally, discuss specifically what is expected in the successful completion of steps. Intervention to remediate inappropriate dietary behaviors is illustrated in Table 11-6). Many intervention strategies may be directed at helping the patient learn new responses, others are designed to achieve a change in a specific habitual behavior that remained unchanged over time, and still others seek to promote behaviors that are self directed. These are discussed below.

Simulation

Two interventions that promote new learning responses are simulation and modeling. Simulation is the act of going through a mock experience (Stewart, Winborn, Burks, Johnson, and Engelkes, 1978). Examples of simulation are role playing, group decision-making practice, menu planning and meal preparation practice, grocery expeditions, and restaurant menu selections. In role playing the teacher takes the role of a friend offering the patient food not on the diet. The patient responds as he or she would to the friend. He then expresses his feelings about the way he "role modeled" appropriate behavior (refusing the restricted food). By discussing feelings he also learns how emotionally uncomfortable this may be. After several role plays the patient feels less distress emotionally and more confidence in turning down the restricted food.

Table 11-6
Remediation Intervention Using a Low-Cholesterol, Fat-Modified Diet

A	B	C	D
			Step 6: Criteria for successful completion of a goal
		Steps 3–5: Sequence information	1. Patient associates low cholesterol, low-fat snacks with a decrease in serum cholesterol.
	Step 2: Easily Managed Information Patient will:	Keep tasks small Mutually agree on the goal toward which the task is aimed for example: Patient substitutes low cholesterol, low-fat snacks for high-cholesterol, high-fat snacks.	2. Tests show a decrease in serum cholesterol.
Step 1: Divide nutrition information 1. Need for reduction in cholesterol and fat (decrease serum cholesterol). 2. Need for increasing low cholesterol, low fat foods (decrease serum cholesterol).	1. Identify high cholesterol, high fat snacks. 2. Identify low cholesterol, low fat snacks.		3. Diet record shows that patient is eating low-cholesterol, low-fat snacks.

In group decision-making one member of the group describes a difficult situation such as eating at a party. Other members of the group respond in constructive ways to deal appropriately with the real life situation. This simulation allows a patient to work on a problem by providing a variety of options for responding.

Menu planning, meal preparation, grocery shopping, and restaurant menu selection provide a way of simulating what happens in the real world. Simulation provides a safe environment for experiencing new responses. It is preferred to an actual situation for several reasons. It allows the patient to succeed. It allows for compression of time. It makes it possible to focus on one or two variables at a time. It provides for control of circumstances so that learning is managed more easily than in real life encounters.

Planning for a simulation is very important. Begin by identifying and describing the environment in which the inappropriate eating behaviors occur. Carefully work as a patient-counselor team to develop the situation and roles. Discuss with the patient the roles, situational elements, and the purposes of the simulation. Act out the simulation. Ask the patient to recall experiences and emotions. Discuss relevant aspects of the patient's performance. Do another role play concentrating on the behavior options learned in the first trial. Vary the simulation to promote the generalization of learning to other situations. For example, if a simulation has concentrated upon eating at a friend's home do a further role play to illustrate selecting foods in a favorite expensive restaurant. Continue role playing until the objective of the simulation has been reached.

Modeling

Another teaching intervention that promotes learning of new responses that can be used in dietary instructions is modeling. Modeling allows the patient to learn by mimicking and observing others (Bandura, 1976 and Stewart et al., 1978). Modeling a new response can increase the patient's awareness of performance and behavioral outcome. A second use of modeling is to demonstrate a behavior in a situation that in real life may be associated with fear, failure, anxiety, and pain.

Dieticians or nurses can model a behavior in order to help the patients learn to solve a problem with eating behaviors. It may be valuable for clinicians to point out environmental models, asking what persons in the patient's estimation have excellent eating behaviors. These then can be used as models.

Symbolic models may also be valuable. With this type of model, presentation is through written materials, audiotapes or videotapes, films, or slide-tape exercises. An example of a symbolic model might be an actor on videotape performing an appropriate response to a relative who offers a high-fat snack on a special holiday such as Thanksgiving or a religious feast.

In preparing a symbolic model, carefully consider patients and their make-up. Assess those who might be viewing, reading, or listening to the model. What is the average age, sex, ethnic origin, cultural practices, coping behaviors, mastery of the model portrayed? A second step is to identify goal behaviors and provide instructions for the modeling. The script should include instructions, modeled dialogue, practice, written feedback, written summarization of what has been modeled, and why it is important to change behavior. It is most important that the script be field tested on a sample of patients and modified on the basis of their comments and responses.

Modeling may not be suited to all nutrition problems. Some patients who must restrict salt intake may cook with spices that are not obtainable. In this case a model is not sufficient for behavior change. Modeling will work best in situations where the patient is unaware of the response necessary to achieve an ultimate goal, is unfamiliar with the conditions that cue a proper behavior, is unsure of the reward potential of a proper response, and connects the appropriate eating behavior with a bad experience, making it unlikely that the performance will be attempted again. Many obese patients are working toward a goal without knowing the appropriate response needed to achieve that goal. For example, fasting is frequently used to attain weight loss. Although this may be an appropriate response to an overweight condition in a very few cases, it is not appropriate for the majority.

Many diabetic persons who are not in good control will become so familiar with feeling badly that they lose the desire to strive for a proper response—feeling good.

In families where the spouse or children are unsupportive of appropriate eating behaviors, following a diet may be connected with a bad experience. Each of these examples illustrates a situation where modeling may be beneficial.

Many persons faced with difficult eating situations may be unaware of how to cue appropriate eating behaviors. If television watching tends to initiate snacking, change this cue to aerobics instead, thus avoiding snacking.

Before the modeling or simulation, a typed sheet of questions for discussion can be handed to the group observing the model or role play. These questions will form the basis of discusssion following the teaching intervention used.

1. What precipitated the model's response?
2. What were the situational conditions and social stimuli?

3. What was said? What emotions were experienced?
4. What was the manner of speech?
5. What did the model do? What did the patient do?
6. What were the consequences of the role play response?
7. How did others react?
8. How did the model seem to feel about the experience?

In summary, modeling allows patients to observe and learn behaviors. Both simulation and modeling are interventions to promote new learning responses. The next interventions discussed are designed to motivate behavior change through cognitive therapy, reinforcement, extinction, tailoring or shaping, and contracting.

Cognitive Therapy

Cognitive therapy involves change in thought patterns. Thought stopping and cognitive restructuring are two types of cognitive therapy. Thought stopping involves controlling unproductive thoughts by suppressing or eliminating them. In cognitive restructuring positive coping thoughts replace negative or self-defeating ones. Thought stopping is a two-step sequence: The patient allows all thoughts related to eating behavior to come to mind. When the patient identifies a self-defeating thought, he or she stops it by covertly saying, "Stop!"

This process continues until the patient is able to eliminate the negative thoughts with only the covert interruption. Once thought stopping is accomplished cognitive restructuring can proceed. At this point a positive coping statement including positive or reinforcing self-statements can proceed. An example of these two strategies follows.

"If it weren't for my busy schedule, I could follow this low-cholesterol diet." Patient inwardly says "Stop!". (This covert response is called thought stopping). Next cognitive restructuring uses the appropriate monologue to substitute such as:

"My schedule isn't any more hectic than anyone else's. I will be more creative in ways I try to improve my eating habits. I'm a creative person; I can handle this."

Reinforcement

Reinforcment is another intervention for motivating change in eating behaviors. Reinforcement may involve verbally praising, giving privileges, monetary reward, token rewards, etc. Reinforced desirable behaviors will be more likely to recur than unreinforced ones. Reinforcement can be used effectively in nutrition education by identifying the response to be reinforced, selecting appropriate reinforcers, monitoring and affixing these at the proper time. The following steps are necessary in setting a reinforcing structure.

1. Identify the behaviors that will be reinforced.
2. Describe both the behavior and the circumstances under which the behaviors are to be performed.
3. Describe the reinforcement (praise, privileges, money).
4. Affix a quantity to the reinforcement, i.e., for every seven high fat snacks which you avoid in a week you can reward yourself with a trip to your favorite clothing store and you are allowed to spend $10.00.
5. Decide which will be reinforced: each occurrence of the behavior or the persistence with which patients perform a response for a period of time.

Several factors are important to consider when reinforcing dietary behaviors. A system should be set up whereby appropriate eating behaviors are reinforced immediately. In cases where this is impossible, reward the end product of a series of such behaviors. Reinforcement can take many forms. Social reinforcement can be given through verbal or nonverbal signs by a person, group, spouse, family, and/or peers. In some instances it is possible to use tangible reinforcement such as money, clothes, or a valueless token that can be exchanged for some object or privilege related to eating behavior. Physical activities such as swimming, hiking, and skiing are meaningful reinforcers. They not only act as reward systems but also help increase caloric expenditure, firm muscles, and decrease appetite (if exercise is strenuous).

All of these types of reinforcers are affected by scarcity (deprivation) or overuse (satiation). If the reinforcer has been enjoyed before its administration, its influence will be increased. Rewards that are readily available are poor reinforcers, however.

Timing is very important in reforcement of eating behaviors. While the patient is learning new eating behaviors frequent rewards are most effective. Reward each occurrence or step toward a new behavior. Dispense rewards often and regularly in order to help the clients learn to associate the appropriate eating behavior with the compensation. As the appropriate eating behavior becomes habitual, reinforcement should be administered less frequently and on a variable schedule.

The following three conditions should exist before using the reinforcement strategy.

1. The eating behavior to be learned requires a great deal of practice before becoming habitual. A low-protein diet may be extremely complicated, requiring major changes. Practice is necessary for it to become habitual.
2. The initial learning attempts are painful. Weight loss can be a very painful experience as some see it as constant denial.
3. The actual outcomes of the new eating behavior are far in the future. Losing a large number of pounds may seem to be distant goal while lowered cholesterol blood levels may be quickly accomplished.

Extinction

Extinction is an intervention used to stop unwanted eating behaviors. Basically extinction works by eliminating a behavior associated with a reward. Begin by identifying the associated reward. Record when and under what circumstances the inappropriate eating behavior occurs, including conditions that make it more intense or more frequent. Factors that appear to reduce the inappropriate eating behavior should be listed. Patients should identify when they are eating inappropriately, how others react, and what feelings are at the time.

An example of extinction follows:

Patient: "I have most problems following my low protein diet when I am depressed. I will immediately head for the kitchen."
Nutrition Educator: "Many people have the same problem. It sounds as though you use food as a positive experience to eliminate feelings of worthlessness or despair. Is that a fair thing to say?"
Patient: "Yes, eating is my crutch."
Nutrition Educator: "Are there other things that make you feel good when you are depressed?" (Not eating is the response to be reinforced.)
Patient: "I feel good after I have my hair done, or when I go shopping for new clothes, or just reading a good mystery."

Nutrition Educator: "Good, let's make a list of those things that are rewarding for you. (Describe behaviors and circumstances under which behaviors are performed.)

Patient: "I can replace eating with an equivalent substitute that's rewarding" (A noneating behavior will be substituted for an eating behavior.)

This is an example of extinction of an inappropriate eating behavior with another more positive rewarding behavior.

Tailoring or Shaping

Another intervention designed to achieve change in eating behaviors, requires fitting the behavior into the patient's daily lifestyle. Crucial to the success of this strategy is a careful scrutiny of the patient's dietary intake (what, where, and when food is eaten). This data forms the basis for setting up the dietary pattern necessary to meet the dietary prescription. The tailoring intervention assumes that there is no standard dietary pattern for a standard patient but that each has unique circumstances to which the therapy must be adapted. For example, instead of asking the patient to fit into a low protein diet pattern, fit the pattern to the patient. Use a preplanned list of foods placed in categories such meat, vegetables, fruits, milk, etc., as a basic planning guide. Ask the patient to star the items used and discard those items that are not used. This allows for a new listing uncomplicated by foods which the patient never eats.

Once the diet has been tailored to the patient each component of the diet instruction should be approached gradually in a process called shaping.

Shaping is a behavior change intervention involving a gradual building of skills. Patients proceed in steps to achieve subgoals and gradually reach the food objective. For example, if the patient currently eats 400 mg of cholesterol, the patient might gradually drop down to 300 mg, then 200 mg, and at last to the goal of 100 mg.

Contracting

Another intervention utilizes a written agreement between the clinician and the client. The contract clearly indicates the responsibilities of all parties. The agreement is signed by both parties and includes agreement to carry out certain eating behaviors with rewards contingent upon performance. Reinforcers may be money or other valuables. Patients play a large role in designing their own treatment. Clinicians provide advice and support while encouraging the patients to plan and implement a self-managed treatment. A prerequisite to self-managed treatment is a well-informed, well-taught patient. In educating patients for nutrition health a contract can be used to specify the learning goals or objectives and the actions necessary to achieve them. Contracts can also contain the actual information to be learned. For example, if the diet prescription for protein intake is 0.6 gms. of protein per kilogram of body weight, determine which meats the patient currently eats and include those in an individual listing of meats high in protein and those low in protein. Concentrate on the foods frequently used by the patient and place secondary emphasis in educating on a standardized list. In this way the contract lists the foods the patient will have to learn that are appropriate protein sources. Also with mutual negotiation the meats currently eaten are listed so that the contract is realistic for the patient. Other characteristics of a well-written contract are outlined.

1. Instructions are written, specific, positive, realistic, and mutually arrived at.
2. Goals can be measured, recorded, and evaluated at specified dates.

Table 11-7
Contract (An Example)

"In the next week I agree to limit my meat intake to 3 ounces at the evening meal for the next month ending on December 21st, 1985. I have chosen three reinforcers. Each evening, I will allow myself to watch TV, call my girlfriend, or go out for the evening only if I have been successful in eating the weighed 3 ounces allowed for meat. If I fail to achieve the goal I will not allow myself to engage in any of the above behaviors."

Signed _____(Patient)
        _____(Spouse/Parent/Friend)
        _____(Dietitian)
        _____(Nurse)
        _____(M.D.)
        _____(Physical Therapist)

---

3. If goals are not achieved then instructions for alternative actions are provided.
4. Space is indicated for signatures by patients and significant others who will be involved in the process of behavior change.
5. Space also is provided for signatures by the health care team, including all persons involved in achieving the goal, i.e., nurse, dietitian, medical doctor, physical therapist, etc.

Contracting has several advantages. Because the contract is a written document, there is an outline of behaviors to be accomplished. Since the patient has control over treatment; discussion of potential problems as well as solutions is possible. The contract provides formal commitment to the treatment. It gives incentive value by establishing rewards from self or others for attaining goals. See Table 11-7 for an example of a contract.

Once the contract is in use, periodically the health care team should assess the patient's progress in achieving goals. The patient may need added advice from the dietitian on how to follow a diet more closely. Other members of the health care team, i.e., nurse, medical doctor, psychologist, physician's assistant, etc., should reinforce the dietitian's teaching. The spouse should be the primary reinforcer providing the patient with encouragement in complying with the contract at home.

Self-Directed Interventions

Eventually at the end of every nutrition education session the teacher strives for patients who are self-directed. The next two interventions, decision making and self-management, help in promoting self-direction. It is crucial to eventual success with a diet that patients feel in control when their nutrition education sessions end.

Decision Making

Decision making is an information-processing operation. The teacher's task is to assist patients in achieving accurate self-information and feedback. Decisions begin with problem solving by asking the following questions:

1. What is the inappropriate eating behavior?
2. What interferes with a solution?
3. When does the inappropriate eating behavior occur?

4. With whom does the eating behavior occur?
5. Under what circumstances does the eating behavior occur?
6. Under what conditions is the eating behavior most or least in variance from the recommended dietary pattern?
7. When must a decision be made or the problem eating behavior resolved?
8. How much effort is necessary to find a solution?
9. What behaviors contribute to the problem or interfere with its solution?
10. What evidence will indicate that the inappropriate eating behavior has been extinguished? (Snetselaar, 1983; Stewart et al., 1978)

Once these questions are answered, both actions and goals must be re-evaluated. The patients might then generate a list of possible or alternative courses of action. Each alternative should be examined in terms of time, money, effort, and advantages and disadvantages. Then the patient can choose some tentative course of action.

Decision making is the nutrition education intervention of choice when patients are concerned about choices to be made and are unsure of alternatives. When information is lacking or a method of systematically examining options and making decisions is not apparent decision making can be valuable.

Self-Management

Self-management goes beyond decision making in that the patient becomes totally self directed.

Interventions for self-management include self-monitoring, stimulus control, alternate responses, and altering response consequences.

Self-Monitoring

Self-monitoring requires use of food diaries and intake graphs or charts. Through these means patients can learn more about their existing eating behaviors. Role playing may also be a way of reviewing eating patterns. Self-monitoring allows the patient to identify the environmental factors affecting intake.

Stimulus Control

After the patient has monitored eating habits he or she must control the environmental factors that are associated with the inappropriate eating behavior. To assist the patient or family with this begin by looking at eating behaviors as a chain of events. Identify elements in the eating behavior chain and alter conditions at one of the points that is early in the sequence. These steps comprise the intervention of stimulus control.

Cueing may be one way of interrupting a normal chain of events that leads to an inappropriate eating behavior. Environmental cues are used to effect long-term changes in eating behaviors. For the patient following a cholesterol-modified eating pattern, notes on the refrigerator emphasizing the use of vegetables as snack foods may serve as cues. This strategy works best with habitual eating behaviors. For eating behaviors that are excessive or inappropriate the environmental conditions under which the behavior is allowed to occur must be gradually reduced. For example, where bingeing is a problem, the environmental conditions such as stress or depression should be gradually reduced to eliminate this behavior.

Alternate Responses

In self-management the patient must identify the situation in which the inappropriate eating behavior occurs and develop an alternate response or behavior. If snacking at night while watching TV is a problem, replace the snack with a new nonfood behavior, i.e., needle-work cued by watching TV.

Alternating Response Consequences

A final component in the process of becoming self directed is altering response consequences. Patients will use self-rewards to modify their eating behavior by monitoring their own responses and rewarding goal directed actions. Patients begin by identifying desirable self-statements, monitoring positive self-thoughts, using a cue to elicit the desired ones, and finally reinforce the positive ones.

Ultimately all nutrition education interventions should lead to successful self-directed diet management by the patient themselves. However, health care personnel must evaluate whether the interventions are successful or not.

EVALUATION

Evaluation of the strategies discussed above is the final step in nutrition education. Do the strategies work? Focus on the patient's behavior. Were the goals originally set achieved? Begin an evaluation by comparing initial and current dietary intake. How far has the patient come? Success should be measured on an individual basis. There are several techniques that can be used in evaluating the outcome of nutrition education.

Techniques for Evaluation

The patient's dietary performance can be measured by doing an initial and final 7-day food record. Other options are two 2-week food records or weighed food records 1 day a week. Questionnaires and interviews can also be used to collect this data. (Coplin, Hines, and Gormican, 1976; Research Committee, 1965; Shorey, Sewell, and O'Brien, 1976). The validity of interviews depends upon the patient's memory and willingness to report dietary adherence behaviors honestly. Research indicates that nonadherence is underreported (Stewart et al., 1978). Reliability of an evaluation tends to be better when patients are aware that their behavior is being assessed (Stewart et al., 1978). Specific nutrient's in the diet may also be misreported (Madden, Goodman, and Guthrie, 1976).

Biological or laboratory assessment provides a more direct means of measuring adherence but it is not adequate over time (Dunbar, 1980). Biochemical methods at best provide little information on the current degree of adherence, and individual variations may give misleading values (Soutter and Kennedy, 1974).

Vital to the improvement of each nutrition education session is dietition performance evaluation. Determine if the teacher has helped the patient achieve goals as efficiently as possible. Assess if other strategies would have been more effective. Sometimes a referral to a counseling psychologist would have made the sessions more productive. Evaluate whether or not patient needs were met. Were techniques used suited to this individual patient?

Nutrition education is a process that involves assessment and planning as well as a

variety of interventions, and evaluation. The process is ongoing and constantly changing. It does not involve one health professional but rather a team of interacting, open
individuals who respond to patient needs in a group effort. Throughout this process aimed
at long-term diet adherence, the patient is central to all efforts.

The following teaching plan illustrates the use of some of the nutrition education
interventions discussed in this chapter. The dietitian, nurse, physician, parents and child
described in the plan are all involved in teaching to prevent nutritional deficits from
occurring.

TEACHING PLAN FOR THE CHILD WITH POTENTIAL NUTRITIONAL DEFICITS RELATED TO CANCER AND ITS TREATMENT

Cheryl Verstraete Ratliff

No parent is prepared to hear the words: Your child has cancer. Feelings of confusion, fear, denial, and helplessness, and a desire to protect the child surge as the diagnosis
is revealed. News of the cancer diagnosis is soon followed by a discussion of the pathophysiology, recommended therapy, and the aspired outcomes of therapy. Abruptly,
out of necessity, the child and parent are faced with a myriad of physiological and
psychological effects of cancer diagnosis and treatment.

Problems Related to Potential Nutritional Deficits in the Child with Cancer

One of the major challenges encountered in the management of children with
cancer is that of preventing nutritional problems. Veninga (1985) reported that while the
survival rate for those children with cancer is increasing, there exists a significant risk of
developing malnutrition.

Risk of malnutrition is high because the nutrients available for growth in the person
with cancer are utilized by the normal and the cancerous cells. Depending on the type
and stage of the disease, there are three potential systemic effects: anorexia, hyper-
metabolism, and negative nitrogen balance. Anorexia may contribute to the insufficient
intake of nutrients. In addition, the rapidly dividing abnormal cells have increased the
metabolic requirements and established a competition for nutrients between the normal
and cancerous cells. Thus normal food intake fails to keep pace with nutrient requirements. Ultimately, unable to meet the energy requirements by food ingestion, the body
utilizes protein stores to feed the cancerous host.

There are other factors contributing to the risk of malnutrition. The emotional components of the diagnosis, which may include painful or frightening procedures and separation from family, decidedly influence the child's nutritional status (Neumann, Jelliffe, Zerfas, & Jelliffe, 1982).

Malnutrition can also be related to the treatment of disease. Each of the major forms of cancer treatment has impact on the nutritional status of the child and requires nutritional support. Anorexia, nausea, vomiting, weight loss, diarrhea, constipation, and mucosities are common side effects of cancer treatment.

Assessment

The nutritional assessment is essential to the development of a comprehensive nutritional plan. Assessment of the nutritional status consists of a medical history, psychocultural history, dietary assessment, clinical examination, anthropometric measurements, and biochemical and hematological assessment (Neumann, Jelliffe, Zerfas, & Jelliffe, 1982).

Assessment of the learning needs of clients and families is the cornerstone for developing a nutrition therapy education program. It is important that the data base include a family profile and a nutritional assessment of the child.

The family profile describes the child in the context of his or her family and developmental level. The purpose of the profile is to identify ways in which the family members interact, as a means of determining potential coping skills and available support (Coping with cancer: A resource for the health professional N.I.H. 80-2080, 1980; Scipien, Barnard, Chard, Howe, and Phillips, 1986).

In addition to obtaining a profile, the nurse has an active role to play in the collection of data for the psychocultural history, dietary assessment, and anthropometric measurements. The psychocultural history compliments the family profile data. Information is obtained pertaining to the family's lifestyle and food habits, which may be affected by cultural or religious beliefs. The dietary assessment includes a diet history and inventory. The anthropometric measures include stature or height, weight, and head circumference.

The child's level of development, which affects self feeding and food intake patterns, is also assessed. This information may be obtained by interview and by observation of the client and family particularly during mealtime. Assessment should also revolve around the potential problems resulting from cancer therapies.

The child who undergoes surgical intervention for a malignancy experiences pain in the area of the incision. Surgery itself alters the child's nutritional status and needs. Wound healing further increases the caloric and nutrient requirements.

Radiation therapy has various local and general side effects. In the areas irradiated, the client may experience varying degrees of radiodermatitis. Gastrointestinal reactions that should be assessed include mucosities, nausea, vomiting, and diarrhea. Radiation therapy to the oral cavity may cause a dry mouth and difficult swallowing. Bone marrow suppression induced by irradiation increases the client's risk of developing anemia and infection.

The chemotherapeutic agents administered to combat malignant cell proliferation do not act selectively on the cancer cells. Any rapidly dividing cells such as bone marrow, skin, gastrointestinal mucosa, and hair follicles are subject to the drug's effects. Consequently, bone marrow depression, gastrointestinal side effects, skin, and hair damage are the common side effects of antineoplastic agents. Bone marrow depression causes anemia and increases the client's susceptibility to a life threatening infection or spontaneous bleeding. The troublesome and uncomfortable gastrointestinal side effects are nausea, vomiting, and anorexia. Painful mouth ulcers, altered food tastes, and feelings of malaise or fatigue compound the problem of meeting the child's nutritional and fluid requirements.

The child recieving treatment for a malignancy experiences psychological, as well as physiological effects from the cancer diagnosis and treatment. Suddenly, the child is in unfamiliar surroundings where daily he or she may encounter painful or frightening procedures, separation from family, and alterations in sleeping, eating, and playing routines. Withdrawal, regression, aggression, separation anxiety, sleeping, and eating problems are potential effects of the illness and hospitalization experiences.

The entire family of the child with cancer experiences many tensions and stresses. Some of the problems are marital stresses, siblings' feelings of being abandoned by their parents, increased medical expenses, misunderstandings with teachers and classmates when the child returns to school, and living with the possibility that a son or a daughter, a brother or a sister may die (University of Kansas Medical Center Bulletin, October, 1978). It is important to assess the potential impact of these stresses on the child and family. Planning to address the common learning needs related to nutritional support of the child with cancer is discussed below.

Planning

During the diagnosis and initial treatment phase, the family is asked to begin to grasp information about the malignancy and its management. Upon the child's discharge from the hospital, the family must administer medications and observe for possible complications. The family must also encourage the child's usual activities while resuming the customary routines and activities in the family's life. The nurse must, therefore, design a teaching plan aligned with the family's lifestyle, concerns, and course of therapy.

Common learning needs of the child and family coping with a potential nutritional deficit brought on by the cancer or its treatment are (a) measures to cope with a lack of appetite and weight loss, (b) ways to deal with diarrhea or constipation, (c) foods to provide when oral lesions exist, (d) approaches to discipline revolving around eating, (e) sources and types of nutrition supplements, and (f) psychomotor skills necessary for providing nutritional supplements such as intravenous feedings. These learning needs address the nutrition topics related to caring and coping with cancer. Strategies which focus on providing optimum nutritional support and preventing complications are discussed below.

Implementation

Numerous activities can be used to implement teaching to both the child and significant others. In the case study and teaching plan presented in the following chart, psychomotor activities are of less importance because the focus is on preventing any potential nutritional deficits. Should definitive nutritional therapy be required to combat a malnutrition state or nutritional complication, learning strategies pertaining to the administration of tube feedings, preparation of blended food mixtures, and management of intravenous nutritional feeding would be utilized.

The affective learning goals deal with the child's and parents' feelings, attitudes, and perceptions about the nutritional management. Many of the counseling techniques described in this and earlier chapters would be implemented to address such problems. The nurse must remember that the initial treatment phase is stressful for the entire family. Behavioral strategies such as written contracts, cognitive therapy, stimulus control, and modeling often help to reduce anxiety as well as to reinforce the teaching.

Evaluation

Periodic evaluation checks the progress of the patient and family in meeting the learning objectives. Data by which to evaluate the results of certain teaching interventions may be obtained by observing or questioning the child and/or family. For example, the nurse may note that the parents utilize certain behaviors modeled by the staff to avoid conflict at meals. Should oral lesions occur and nutritional interventions be initiated early by the family, one has evidence that the teaching strategies were effective. More objective measures of the effects of teaching aimed at preventing malnutrition are the anthropometric measures and other laboratory data.

Teaching Plan

The case study cited deals with a newly diagnosed pediatric cancer patient beginning chemotherapy. The teaching plan focuses on the promotion of nutritional health and the prevention of nutritional complications.

Damon is a 6-year–old male diagnosed with a childhood malignancy called rhabdomyosarcoma. Three weeks prior to surgery at a local hospital, Damon's mother noted scrotal swelling while bathing him. There had been no pain or tenderness. Damon had been feeling well.

Surgery was performed for testicular removal and a partial right-sided scrotectomy. Seven days after surgery, Damon was admitted to the medical center 75 miles from home to undergo tests to rule out metastasis and to initiate chemotherapy.

On the day of admission to the pediatric oncology unit, the nurse learned that Damon is the oldest child in the family. He lives with his mother, stepfather, and 3-year–old brother. Damon's mother works in the home and his stepfather is employed by a small home improvement company. Damon's maternal grandparents live in the same rural community. Assessing the family's understanding of the purpose of hospitalization, Damon's mother related to the nurse that he had "a cancer of the testicles." Both parents anticipated "more tests" and the initiation of the "cancer medicines." Damon's mother indicated that she had never known anyone with cancer. Damon's stepfather recalled his grandfather who died of cancer. He named several chemotherapeutic drugs which he received. He spoke of caring for him at home and visiting him in the nursing home.

Damon's mother states that she has told her son he will need more tests and then some medicine before he can return home. Damon appears comfortable in the room with his parents. He intently watches the nurse and glances from time to time at his mother during the initial interaction.

Teaching plan follows in Tables 11-8, 11-9, and 11-10.

Table 11-8
Teaching Plan for Child with Potential Nutritional Deficits

Assessment	Plan/learning objectives	Interventions	Evaluation
		Affective	
Assess parent(s) openness with the health care team: —comfort in sharing feelings, concerns —desire to participate in decision-making —ability to raise questions	Parent(s) will comfortably share concerns about the child's nutrition with the health care team.	Encourage parent(s) to make a list of questions and concerns. Tell family to discuss nutritional topics at subsequent clinic visits. Introduce family to nutritions and dietitian.	Parent(s) asks questions or volunteers information regarding the child's nutritional status.
	Parent(s) will express confidence in ability to implement home nutritional management.	Use "what would you do if" exercises to explore options in dealing with home nutrition problems (*simulation*). Use the decision-making strategy to begin problem solving, identified concerns, potential interferences in employing nutrition recommendations.	Parent(s) convey confidence in making decisions pertaining to nutrition, i.e., selection of food, institution of mouth care, use of positive reinforcement techniques.

Determine child's developmental level, especially assess language skills.	Child will feel at ease in interactions with the nurse and nutritionist.	Utilize therapeutic play to establish rapport and teach the child.	Child engages in conversation and play with the nurse or nutritionist.
	Child will experience satisfaction and reward for efforts to comply with nutritional interventions.	Teach parents to focus on and reward "positive" rather than "negative" behaviors associated with eating (*reinforcement*). Use stickers as reinforcers for meeting nutrient requirements.	Child displays his "chart of stickers." Expressed pride in attempts to meet nutritional requirements.
Determine usual atmosphere at mealtime at home. Ask parents what approaches are used when the child does not eat or refuses to eat.	For child and parent mealtime will be a pleasant relaxed experience.	Avoid discussing disturbing topics at mealtimes (*extinction*). Show parents how to make meals pleasurable in the hospital by adding adventure, surprise or novelty (*modeling*).	Observe the child at meal time: Relaxed? Socializing? Nagging and bargaining are not observed.

Table 11-9
Teaching Plan for Child with Potential Nutritional Deficits

Assessment	Plan/learning objectives	Interventions	Evaluation
		Cognitive	
Ascertain parent(s) knowledge of basic functions of nutrients.	Parent(s) will describe the basic functions of the nutrients.	Give parents pamphlets on nutrition facts and food groups.	Ask parent(s) the role of the basic nutrients. Ask parent(s) to name examples of foods containing concentrated sources of each nutrient.
Obtain a diet history and inventory which may include 24 hour recall 3–7 day intake record or list of food intake by food groups.	Parent(s) will indicate awareness of the child's food consumption patterns.	Identify nutritional requirements by food groups. Record in pamphlet. Review pamphlets with parents after they have had the opportunity to read them and record foods.	Ask parent(s) to state the daily nutritional requirements by food group.
	Parent(s) will identify interventions for coping with the potential side effects resulting from the cancer and cancer treatment.	Review, using printed materials, interventions to cope with anorexia oral lesions diarrhea/constipation weight loss	During problem-solving exercises parents are able to discuss interventions to use.

	Parent(s) will self report use of at least one recommended nutritional interventions at each meal or snack.	Parent will keep a diary of interventions employed and their effectiveness. (contract to review this)	Observe parents for use of nutrition interventions at meals/snacks. Review shopping list
		Prior to discharge, parents/child make a shopping list of nutritious foods.	
	Parent(s) will select a minimum of two foods which fortify the diet with proteins or calories on a daily basis.	Have parent(s) complete daily menus. Determine nutritional adequacy by comparing against recommendations according to food groups.	Review menu selections made by parents.
Determine child's favorite nutritious foods.	Child will name favorite foods from each of the four food groups.	Play a game of naming favorite "energy" foods using pictures. Include child's selection of foods from menu. (*stimulus control*)	Ask the child to name favorite "energy" foods.
	Child will keep a food chart which shows food consumed from each food group at each meal or snack.	Establish a chart in patient's room. At each meal use stickers to record the intake of food by food groups (*reinforcement*).	Note effectiveness of reinforcement techniques in encouraging food intake.

Table 11-10
Teaching Plan for Child with Potential Nutritional Deficits

Assessment	Plan/learning objectives	Interventions	Evaluation
		Psychomotor	
Assess home for best location to carry out sterile procedure.	Parents will administer parental nutrition through Hickman catheter.	Demonstrate to parents care of Hickman catheter on a model.	Child remains free of sepsis. Child's blood laboratory and body measurements indicate stable nutritional status and positive nitrogen balance.
	Maintains sterility during procedure.	Parents demonstrate procedure with their child several times before discharge.	
Assess parents emotional reactions to carrying out invasive procedures on their own child.	Parents state they feel confident to provide parental nutrition.		Child and parents practice with doll that has tube connected to chest.
			Observe the child for cooperation during procedure.

REFERENCES

Alpert, J. J. Broken appointments. *Pediatrics,* 1964, *53,* 127–132.

Archer, M., Seymour, R., and Christakis, G. Social factors affecting participation in a study of diet and coronary heart disease. *Journal of Health and Social Behavior,* 1967, *8,* 22–31.

Bandura, A. Effecting change through participant modeling. In J. D. Krumboltz and C. E. Thoresen (Eds.), *Counseling methods.* New York: Holt, Rinehart and Winston, 1976.

Barlow, D. (Ed.). *Behavioral assessment of adult disorders.* New York: The Guilford Press, 1981.

Becker, M. H., and Maiman, L. A. Sociobehavioral determinants of compliance with health and medical care recommendations. *Medical Care,* 1975, *13,* 10–24.

Becker, M. H., Drachman, R. H., and Kirscht, J. R. Predicting mother's compliance with pediatric medical regimens. *Journal of Pediatrics,* 1972, *81,* 843–845.

Blackwell, B. Drug therapy: Patient compliance. *New England Journal of Medicine,* 1973, *289,* 249–252.

Charney, E. Patient-doctor communication: Implications for the clinician. *Pediatric Clinics of North America,* 1972, *19,* 263–279.

Cone, J. D., and Hawkins, R. P. (Eds.). *Behavioral assessment: New directions in clinical psychology.* New York: Brunner/Mazel, 1977.

Coplin, S. S., Hines, J., and Gormican, A. Outpatient dietary management of the Prader-Willi Syndrome. *Journal of the American Dietetic Association,* 1976, *68,* 330–334.

Davis, M. S. Physiologic, psychological and demographic factors in patient compliance with doctors' orders. *Medical Care,* 1968, *6,* 115–122.

Davis, M. S., and Eichorn, R. L. Compliance with medical regimens: A panel study. *Journal of Health and Social Behavior,* 1963, *4,* 240–249.

Dunbar, J. M. Adherence to medical regimen. In Foods and Nutrition Resource Center (Eds.). *Nutrition counseling manual for lipid research clinic nutritionists.* Iowa City, IA: University of Iowa, 1980.

Dunbar, J. M. *Adherence to Medication Regimen: An Intervention Study with Poor Adherers.* Unpublished doctoral dissertation, Stanford University, 1977.

Hagen, R. L., Foreyt, J. P., and Durham, T. W. The dropout problem: Reducing attrition in obesity research. *Behavior Therapy,* 1976, *7,* 463–471.

Haynes, R. B., Gibson, E. S., Hackett, B. C., Sackett, D. L., Taylor, D. W., Roberts, R. S., and Johnson, A. L. Improvement of medical compliance in uncontrolled hypertension. *Lancet,* 1976, *1,* 1265–1268.

Holder, L. Effects of source, message, audience characteristics on health behavior compliance. *Health Service Representative,* 1972, *87,* 843–850.

Hulka, B. S., Zyzanski, S. J., Cassel, J. C., and Thompson, S. J. Satisfaction with medical care in a low income population. *Journal of Chronic Disease,* 1971, *24,* 661–673.

Hurtado, A. V., Greenlick, N. R., and Colombo, T. J. Determinants of medical care utilization: Failure to keep appointments. *Medical Care,* 1973, *11,* 189–198.

Johannsen, W. J., Hellmuth, G. A., and Sorauf, T. On accepting medical recommendations: Experiences with patients in a cardiac work classification unit. *Archives of Environmental Health,* 1966, *12,* 63–69.

Joyce, C. R. B., Caple, G., Mason, M., Reynolds, E., and Mathews, J. A. Quantitative study of doctor-patient communication. *Quarterly Journal of Medicine,* 1969, *38,* 183–194.

Kaim-Caudle, P. R., and Marsh, G. N. Patient-satisfaction survey in general practice. *British Medical Journal,* 1975, *1,* 262–264.

Kincey, J. A., Bradshaw, P. W., Ley, P., Ratoff, L. Patient satisfaction in general practice. *British Medical Journal,* 1975, *3,* 97–98.

Klein, S. P. Choosing needs for needs assessment. *Procedures for needs assessment education: A symposium.* CSE Report No. 69. Los Angeles: Center for the Study of Evaluation, 1971.

Leventhal, H. Changing attitudes and habits to reduce risk factors in chronic disease. *American Journal of Cardiology*, 1973, *31*, 571–580.

Lipid Research Clinics Group: The Lipid Research Clinics Coronary Primary Prevention Trial Results I. Reduction in incidence of coronary heart disease. *Journal of the American Medical Association*, 1984, *251*, 351–364.

Madden, J. B., Goodman, S. J., and Guthrie, H. A. Validity of the 24-hour recall. *American Journal of Clinical Nutrition*, 1976, *68*, 143–147.

Mason, M., Wenberg, B. G., and Welsch, P. K. *The dynamics of clinical dietetics*. New York: John Wiley and Sons, 1977.

McGill, H. C., and Mott, G. E. Diet and coronary heart disease. In D. M. Hegsted (Ed.), *Present knowledge in nutrition* (4th ed.). Washington, D.C.: Nutrition Foundation, Inc., 1976.

Melchior, G. W., Lofland, H. B., and Jones, D. C. Influence of dietary fat on cholelithiasis in squirrel monkeys. *Federal Proceedings*, 1974, *33*, 626.

Morton, A., Ringles, S., and Christakis, G. Social factors affecting participation in a study diet and coronary heart disease. *Journal of Health and Social Behavior*, 1967, *8*, 22–31.

Multiple Risk Factor Intervention Trial Research Group. Multiple Risk Factor Intervention Trial: Risk factor changes and mortality results. *Journal of the American Medical Association*, 1982, *248*, 1465–1477.

National Diet-Heart Study Research Group. National diet-heart study final report. *Circulation*, 1968, *37*(Supplement 1), 1–419.

National Institutes of Health. *Coping with cancer: A resource for the health professional*. (NIH Publication No. 80-2080). Washington, DC: U.S. Government Printing Office, 1980. Source: Office of Cancer Communications, National Cancer Institute.

Neumann, C. G., Jelliffe, D. B., Zerfas, A. J., and Jelliffe, E. F. *Nutritional Assessment of the Child with Cancer*, 1982, *42*(Supplement), 699–712s.

Reiser, R., Sorrels, M. F., and Williams, M. C. Influence of high levels of dietary fats and cholesterol on atherosclerosis and lipid distribution in swine. *Circulation Research*, 1959, *7*, 833.

Research Committee. Low-fat diet in myocardial infarction: A controlled trial. *Lancet*, 1965, *2*, 501–504.

Rockart, J. F., and Hofmann, P. B. Physician and patient behavior under different scheduling systems in a hospital outpatient department. *Medical Care*, 1969, *7*, 463–470.

Sackett, D. L. Priorities and methods for future research. In D. L. Sackett and R. B. Haynes (Eds.), *Compliance with therapeutic regimens*. Baltimore, MD: The Johns Hopkins University Press, 1976, 169–189.

Scipien, G. M., Barnard, M. U., Chard, M. A., Howe, J., and Phillips, P. J. *Comprehensive pediatric nursing*. New York: McGraw-Hill, 1986.

Shorey, R. A. L., Sewell, B., and O'Brien, M. Efficacy of diet and exercises in the reduction of serum cholesterol and triglycerides in free-living adult males. *American Journal of Clinical Nutrition*, 1976, *29*, 512–521.

Snetselaar, L. *Nutrition counseling skills*. Rockville, MD: Aspens Systems Corporation, 1983.

Stewart, N. R., Winborn, B. B., Burks, H. M., Johnson, R. R., and Engelkes, J. R. et al. *Systematic Counseling*. Englewood Cliffs, NJ: Prentice-Hall, 1978.

Soutter, B. R., and Kennedy, M. C. Patient compliance assessment in drug trials: Usage and methods. *Australian and New Zealand Journal of Medicine*, 1974, *4*, 360–364.

University of Kansas Medical Bulletin, October, 1978.

Veninga, K. S. Improving nutrition in children with cancer. *Pediatric Nursing*, 1985, *11*, 18–20, 73.

12

Teaching Patients, Families, and Communities About Their Medical Problems

John H. Renner

With Teaching Plan by
Carol E. Smith

OBJECTIVES

1. Discuss the rational for teaching patients about their medical problems.
2. Assess patients and families for learning needs related to their medical problems.
3. Plan appropriate use of personnel, time, facilities and community resources in patient teaching.
4. Utilize educational materials to teach patients about their medical problem.
5. Evaluate one to one communication skills used in teaching patients, families and communities.

This chapter follows the steps of the teaching process to illustrate the partnership of the physician, patient, nurse, and other health care professionals in educating individuals, families, and communities about their medical problems.

RATIONALE FOR TEACHING PATIENTS ABOUT THEIR MEDICAL PROBLEMS

Patient education is a vital component of quality clinical care. The physician may make an astute diagnosis and may prescribe a sound treatment plan, but if the patient is not informed or not motivated to carry out the plan, the quality of care will not be high caliber.

Most physicians routinely practice informal patient education in their clinical work as they provide explanations, recommend treatment plans, offer reassurance, and suggest behavior changes for improving health. Physicians typically carry out these educational efforts on an intuitive and impromptu basis.

PATIENT EDUCATION: NURSES IN PARTNERSHIP
WITH OTHER HEALTH PROFESSIONALS

© 1987 by Grune & Stratton, Inc.
ISBN 0-8089-1833-8 All rights reserved.

The number of medical practices implementing systematic programs of patient education, however, is on the rise as more physicians recognize the value of education in patient care. Among the factors behind this growth is the convincing evidence that has been produced to document the positive effects of patient education on compliance, health outcomes, savings to the health care system, and patient satisfaction.

Patient compliance or adherence is a critical issue in health care (Evans and Haynes, 1984). Although it can be affected by numerous factors, several studies have shown that the physician's attention to patient education is one of the most important variables and that it affects the end results substantially.

The value of patient education in health outcomes has been particularly notable with chronic conditions and with surgery. For example, a study of an outpatient group with congestive heart failure found that about 30 percent of the patients in an organized education program improved their functional status as compared with only 1.1 percent of the control group (Rosenberg, 1971). The educated patients also had significantly fewer hospital readmissions and shorter hospital stays when compared with the control group and with their own previous experiences. Similar findings have been reported with asthmatic patients and with patients expecting to undergo surgery. Additionally, in the Maryland High Blood Pressure Control Program, individuals with high blood pressure who reported that their physician told them their exact blood pressure measurement and what it meant were more likely to have achieved blood pressure control and to have visited their doctor about their high blood pressure in the last six months. (Levine, Bone, and Steinwachs, 1983). Patient education also has been found to be effective in enhancing patient responsibility and in encouraging self care.

A substantial dollar savings to the health care system was reported in a 2-year study of a large group of diabetic patients who were educated about their health problems and given access to a "hot-line" for consultation. The savings of approximately $1.8 million resulted from reductions by half or more in the number of diabetic comas, emergency room admissions, and hospital admission. (Miller and Goldstein, 1972) In addition, a recent analysis of studies found considerable evidence that preoperative patient education shortens the postoperative length of stay (Mumford, Schlesinger, and Glass, 1982).

Patient education also has been shown to be effective in increasing patient satisfaction, which in turn, is correlated with retention of patients, appointment keeping and the prevention of malpractice suits. Satisfaction generally is related to the extent to which the physician meets the patient's expectations for information and to the patient's perception that the physician volunteers information.

Another factor contributing to the rise in the number of formal patient education programs is the right of the patient to full information about his or her health status. This right is well established and has won acceptance from major health care organizations such as the American Medical Association, the American Hospital Association, the American Academy of Family Physicians and the American Nurses Association.

Also acting as a significant impetus to patient education is the doctrine of informed consent, which imposes a legal obligation on the physician to assure that patients agree to treatment with full knowledge and understanding (see Chapter 2). The information which must be conveyed includes the diagnosis, treatment alternatives, and the benefits and risks of various options.

Certainly, one of the most compelling factors behind the increase in formal patient education programs is the public's strong interest in health topics and in greater control over individual health care. In a 1982 nationwide poll undertaken by a presidential commission studying ethical problems in medicine, 92 percent of Americans indicated that they want to participate with their physicians in making decisions about their health care. At the same time, the percentage of the public reporting that their physicians discussed case and treatment information with them was 12–25 percent lower than the percentage of physicians who reported discussing these matters. In a period of increasing competition for patients, some physicians recognize patient education as an effective marketing tool.

For the purposes of this chapter, patient education is defined as planned learning experiences in the clinical setting that encourage and enable the patient to take better care of him or herself. Such learning encompasses experiences that enhance patient, family and community's information, skills and attitudes.

ASSESSMENT PRIOR TO INITIATING
A PATIENT EDUCATION PROGRAM

Several considerations should be kept uppermost in starting a program of patient education. To be effective, the program must be tailored to the individual practice. It should be started on a small scale, and its components should be evaluated before expansion is undertaken.

Prior to embarking on a new or expanded program of patient education, it is critical that the physician and his or her associates in practice examine their own thinking about the field (Griffith, Attarian, and Harrison, 1983). A philosophy of patient education should be developed from a vague concept into a guide for practical application. Some of the questions that may prove helpful in developing a philosophy are presented below:

1. To what extent should the practice be person oriented rather than illness oriented?
2. To what degree should patients be accepted as partners in health care?
3. What roles will the physician and associated take in providing patients, families, and communities with health education?
4. What level of commitment exists to the development of attitudes and skills that are necessary to conduct patient education?
5. What goals will the physician and associates set for the patient education program?

In initiating a systematic approach to patient education, the physician is confronted with a multitude of opportunities for action. A prudent way to begin is to select three to five areas for concentration of effort. Among the most potentially productive areas are medication information, prenatal education, management of hypertension or other chronic condition, treatment of upper respiratory infections or other acute illness, and physical examinations.

The major determinant of priorities is patient needs, and the first step in establishing a patient education program will be assessing those needs. The physician may rely on the results of surveys that indicate the most common diagnoses in family practice, such as the National Ambulatory Medical Care Survey. Other sources of input for assessing patient needs include surveys of patients, suggestions offered by patients, questions asked by patients, and observations of patient behavior.

However, most physicians will find it more effective to develop priorities based on data from their own practice. Figure 12-1 illustrates a sample survey done to determine priority areas for patient education. First, this requires listing all the problems for which

PROBLEM	Column 1 FREQUENCY ENCOUNTERED IN YOUR PRACTICE Rare 1 2 3 4 5 Freq.	Column 2 SEVERITY Minor 1 2 3 4 5 Severe	Column 3 LIKELIHOOD OF IMPROVEMENT BY EDUCATION INTERVENTION OR PREVENTION OF COMPLICATIONS OR RECURRENCE Unlikely to Help 1 2 3 4 5 Treatment of Choice	SCORE Col. 1 × Col. 2 × Col. 3
UPPER RESPIRATORY ILLNESS	3	2	3	18
BIRTH CONTROL ADVICE	4	2	4	32
DEPRESSION	3	3	3	27
URINARY TRACT INFECTION	4	3	4	48

Figure 12-1. Sample practice survey to determine priority areas for planning patient education packages. From Patient Education: A Handbook for Teachers, Society of Teachers of Family Medicine, 1979, p. 59. Used with permission of the Society for Teachers of Family Medicine Kansas City, Missouri.

patients are treated in the practice. Then, relative weights are assigned to each problem according to factors considered important, and finally a total score for each problem is calculated by multiplying the figures. A scale of 1 thorugh 5 can be used for such factors as the frequency of the diagnosis, the severity of the problem, and the likelihood of improvement by patient education.

In establishing priorities, it is wise to consider the special interests or expertise of the physician and staff. A physician's personal concern for physical fitness and a nurse's interest in prenatal development, for example, suggest these areas as natural starting points and high priorities for patient education.

PLANNING FOR APPROPRIATE USE OF RESOURCES

Much of the responsibility for patient education falls on the physician, who educates primarily on a one to one basis. Many Americans consider their own doctor to be the most useful and reliable source of information about health and medical care. Moreover, by the nature of the medical encounter, the physician is in the best position to educate patients. In some settings, a physician and nurse work together to direct the patient education effort in a practice, and the nurse assumes responsibility for a large portion of the program.

Transforming the educational efforts of a medical practice into a formal program of patient education requires the development of plans and the collection of materials. The essentials of a basic program comprise a "physician's starter kit" for patient education as listed.

1. Leaflet or booklet for patients expressing the practice philosophy of patient education.
2. Patient questionnaire to assess educational needs and interests.
3. Written plans for each patient education priority area, including standard content and methods of delivery.
4. List of patient education responsibilities and tasks for each employee.
5. List of available community health resources with names of contact persons.
6. Office floor plan indicating areas designated for patient education (posted in waiting room).
7. Patient education handouts on major problems treated in the practice.
8. Collection of health education materials, including books, pamphlets, posters, models, and audiovisual aids.
9. Patient education prescription forms.
10. Forms for evaluating the patient education program.

To carry out patient education endeavors as listed it is necessary to have across the board support and enthusiasm from all staff. To achieve this support, all personnel should be recognized for their educational contributions as well as their clinical or office work. Staff members should be invited to develop their own ideas for contributing to the patient education program, and a system of rewards for the most effective suggestions should be implemented. In addition, staff who are interested in developing their patient education skill should be afforded opportunities to attend conferences or workshops.

Involving all staff as providers of patient education is a practical approach for several reasons. Time, of course, is a paramount consideration. Patient education is an involved, sometimes repetitious activity which cannot be handled by the physician alone. More patient education can be delivered when other staff assume responsibilities. Patients often are reluctant to take the time of the physician or to ask questions that might appear foolish or uninformed but they may be more at ease with other staff. The content of patient education can be quite complex or detailed in some areas, for example, in explaining laboratory procedures, and the expertise of others is useful. Another reason for involving staff is to take advantage of a strong patient orientation which some have because of background or training.

Nurses, in particular, are especially well-suited for the role of patient educators for several reasons. Their education includes the methodology of learning and emphasizes the care of patients; moreover, their experiences in patient education often are more extensive than that of medical students (see Chapter 1).

The job description of each staff member should include a paragraph about patient education, and the contribution of each staff member to patient education should be monitored and modified as necessary. Responsibilities must be clearly defined for the different types of patient education to be delivered. In addition to individual responsibilities, everyone should have periodic opportunities to play a role in the overall program, which might involve reporting feedback, evaluating materials or promoting patient education.

Specific individual responsibilities for a variety of positions might include the following:

1. Office manager. Send a welcome letter and practice information guidebook to new patients; insert timely health announcements on statements; analyze information from patient data bases to determine needs for group health education.

2. Receptionist. Familiarize new patients with opportunities for patient education; encourage all patients to read or view current patient education materials in the office; ask patients to complete the first part of their reminder form for the office visit, as shown in Figure 12-2.

3. Head nurse. Educate patients on phone and in person, helping them to deal with routine health care problems; check patient's reasons for office appointment and select helpful material for patients to read or view prior to the examination; carry out the physician's patient education prescription, offering additional explanation and reinforcing instructions.

4. Nurse educator, physician assistant, or health educator. Provide one-to-one skills instruction, e.g., breast self-exam or glucose monitoring; teach classes on health topics such as self care, weight reduction, parenting, or self management of chronic illness; coordinate reviews of educational materials and create materials as needed. (See Chapter 9)

5. Laboratory technician. Explain laboratory procedures to patients and furnish with written instructions; monitor indicators of compliance.

6. X-ray technician. Provide written instructions and oral explanation concerning x-ray procedures; inform patient about radiation safety devices. Medical records clerk: Audit records for patient education in the treatment plan; compile a practice problem list that can serve as a baseline for patient education.

7. Billing/insurance clerk. Educate patients about the insurance process; create a hotline for inquiries on health insurance.

8. Dietician, pharmacist, physical therapist, and other health care professionals: Can

---

Figure 12-2.   Reminder list for visit to doctor.

BEFORE THE VISIT (complete this yourself):
1. What is main reason for coming to the doctor today?_____
   _____
2. Is there anything else that worries me about my health? ____Yes ____No. List:____
3. What do I expect the doctor to do for me today? (In ten words or less):_____
DURING THE VISIT (complete with help of doctor):
1. What is the diagnosis or problem?_____
2. Why did I get it and how can I prevent it next time?_____
   _____
3. Are there any helpful patient education materials available for the condition?
   ____Yes ____No Describe:_____
   _____
4. Are there any medicines for me to take? ____Yes ____No
   Describe:_____
5. If a prescription drug:
   Name of drug:_____
   Purpose of drug:_____
   How and when to take drug:_____
   When to stop taking drug:_____
   Foods, drinks, other drugs to avoid while taking drug:_____
   _____
   What side effects may result (serious, short-term, long-term, etc.)_____
6. Will I need a refill? ____Yes ____No
AFTER THE VISIT (complete with help of doctor):
1. Am I to return for another visit? ____Yes ____No When:_____
2. What should I do at home?
   ____Activity_____
   ____Treatments_____
   ____Precautions_____
3. Am I to phone in for reports? ____Yes ____No What type:_____
   When:_____
4. Should I report back to doctor by phone for any reason? ____Yes ____No When:__
5. Did I get my patient instruction prescription? ____Yes ____No
6. Do I need to visit Patient Education Library? ____Yes ____No
Modified from FAMILY HEALTH, 1976

---

be used on a referral or contractual basis for individual or group patient care (see Chapters 10 and 11).

Community Resources: Plan to Use Them

Human resources for patient education are not limited to the physician's staff. They include pharmacists, dietitians, hospital personnel, community health agency personnel, and patients with experience in specific areas, such as parents of deaf children or persons who are successfully living with a chronic condition. The physician should coordinate educational efforts with these outside resources and take advantage of their expertise.

Community organizational resources provide a valuable means of extending the patient education that occurs in the physician's office. Organizations may offer written or audiovisual materials, speaker and film presentations, classes, or support groups. The physician who is aware of such resources can utilize them effectively by recommending, for example, that a cancer patient join a support group, by writing an educational prescription for a patient to attend a stop-smoking class offered at the hospital, or by suggesting that another patient obtain assistance from the mental health association for stress reduction. Various agencies and organizations also may prove helpful to the physician by furnishing information on health needs and interests or by collaborating on new programs. The United Way or other community coordinating bodies usually can provide a list of voluntary associations and the services they offer.

The physician cannot and should not assume primary responsibility for patient education that can be provided by a number of different agencies and professionals. Rather, as the primary contact for health services for most patients, the physician can facilitate and reinforce the work of others (see Chapter 3).

Facilities: Plan for Effective Use of Space

Most medical offices were not designed to accommodate patient education activities; however, it is not difficult to adapt a facility for this purpose. Among family practice residency centers, this is already occurring. According to a 1982 facilities survey by the Sisters of St. Mary Regional Family Practice Residency Program, the majority of residency centers already have specific space for patient education purposes, including counseling and library facilities. Of those without space, all but a small minority expressed the desire to add these patient education facilities in the future. When a separate space is not available, creative scheduling may be necessary. Such scheduling allows for nurses to use examining rooms for teaching when the physician is elsewhere.

While the physician provides most patient education on a one to one basis in the examining room, a separate facility for patient education reinforces the importance of this activity in the practice. The patient education room serves two primary functions: A fairly private and comfortably furnished area allows the patient to receive individual education, reinforcement, and counseling from other members of the health care team. A second area, equipped as a library, enables the patient to fill an educational prescription written by the physician (for other than readily available handouts). The library includes books, pamphlets, audiovisual equipment and other teaching aids. It also should house a community resource file on health and social services.

Most patients will use the library as a resource for specific problems, such as dealing with a chronic illness, or concerns, such as parenting. However, all patients should be encouraged to browse in the library. Ideally, the patient education room will be located near the reception room, so that the library is visible and convenient for patients before and after they have seen the doctor.

The reception room can set the tone for patient education by offering a variety of materials. Copies of the office brochure can be kept at the receptionist's desk, to be handed out to new patients.

A bulletin board in the reception room should be located for maximum viewing potential. Display material might focus on a health topic pertinent to the season, such as summertime fun (avoiding sunburn, learning to swim, boating safely). Other possibilities for content are articles on health selected from popular magazines or a community spotlight on health, including all types of local classes and organizations.

A table in the reception room could be equipped with audiovisual equipment (including earphones) and cassettes on health topics. Users might be asked to note which films they view to indicate levels of interest.

If a "health-line" operates locally, a telephone and a list of available topics can be provided for use by patients.

A display rack in the reception room can offer pamphlets and selected magazines such as *American Health, America's Health,* and *Your Doctor's Rx: Being Well,* which emphasize a healthful lifestyle.

A children's corner can include educational toys, such as a doctor's kit or a hospital model, along with books and puzzles for youngsters. In the examination rooms, the walls can be used to display attractive health education posters and racks can offer a variety of reading materials: health magazines, pamphlets on topics of general interest, copies of the health-line topic list and of the office brochure, and a leaflet describing patient education services. For children, puppets or other small toys or books can be kept on hand.

The physician may want to keep anatomical models in the examination room for use in explaining conditions to patients. Similarly, with a blackboard provided on the wall, the physician can sketch parts of the anatomy.

The restroom is a useful location for emphasis of certain health topics and for specific information. Instructions can be posted on such procedures as breast self-examination and a clean catch urine sample.

In the laboratory, reading materials should be available to allow the patient to make constructive use of waiting time. Information about the purpose of laboratory tests and the meaning of results might be of particular interest in this area.

The nurses' station or other easily accessible location should be used to store the most commonly distributed handouts along with other frequently used material. Some physicians find that handouts are used more often if they are stored in each examining room.

Effective Use of Time

Although physicians recognize compelling reasons to initiate or expand patient education efforts in their practice, they often have concerns about the time and cost involved. In a group practice, the patient education program can be directed by a committee with some responsibility for budget and organization. Physician commitment remains critical, however, if the program is to succeed.

There are several aspects to the issue of time. Research has indicated that in terms of patient satisfaction, the length of visit is less important than the quality of physician-patient communication. Solutions to the time problem include effective use of office personnel and improved coordination with other resources available for patient education. The time problem will ease as more patients adopt a partnership approach to health care, and less time is wasted because of misunderstandings.

IMPLEMENTING PATIENT EDUCATION

A broad spectrum of methods exists for providing patient education. The most common methods include one-to-one discussion, provision of written materials, teaching of skills, group instruction and referral to community resources. Other methods include the use of models or illustrations, audiovisual presentations, programmed instruction, and educational prescriptions, e.g., to read a helpful book, view a television show on a pertinent health topic, or attend a class focusing on the patient's health problem. Behavioral methods include role playing and such strategies as contracts and self-monitoring.

Some types of patient education require a single method, often provided by the physician, but others necessitate a variety of methods. Many chronic care patients, for example, will benefit from the full range of common methods. It is likely that the physician and other staff will be involved as providers. In contrast, patient education concerning an office administrative matter such as insurance processing usually can be provided by one staff member with responsibility in that area.

Just as it is important to establish standard content for selected patient education priority areas, it also is necessary to determine standard methods and specific responsibilities for delivery. The one-to-one teaching by the physician is most important.

Implementing One-to-one Methods of Teaching Patients about Their Medical Problems

Perhaps the most practical assistance for the physician is an approach outlined by Ross L. Egger, who describes how effective patient education can be conducted during a 15-minute office visit. (Egger, 1980) He starts with blood pressure or medication, for example. This requires a quick check of the chart before entering the room and it identifies for the patient what the physician thinks is important.

In the second stage of the visit, the physician elicits problems by using open-ended questions. It is important to ask what the patient thinks is causing the problem and why. After listening, the physician explains to the patient what the symptoms could mean and what the physician is considering. In the third stage, the physician must be able to talk, listen and examine simultaneously. He or she tells the patient what is being checked, why, what is found, and what it means. In concluding the visit, the physician reviews the findings, the possible diagnosis, impressions of the problem and the rationale for them, possible treatment plans, the anticipated outcome, and directions for seeking help in the future.

Teaching can and will occur throughout the office visit if a tone of expectation for active patient involvement is set. This can be accomplished in part through the attitudes that personnel demonstrate as they offer explanations to patients and encourage them to ask questions and express their feelings. In addition, materials can be designed and used to encourage patient participation in learning. Self assessment aids, for example, can spur the patient's awareness of his or her health status, and patient education prescription forms can be utilized by the physician to stimulate patient learning. Finally, materials can be displayed to stir the interest of patients in health issues.

Implementing the Program for Individual Patients and Their Families

With a planned program of patient education in place, the physician must ensure that it is put into operation for individual patients. This requires assessing each patient to determine his or her needs, developing and implementing an educational plan that includes the family, then monitoring and evaluating progress and revising the plan as necessary.

There is wide agreement on the importance of assessing the individual patient in his or her particular situation before attempting to educate the patient and family. Without this understanding, patient education is likely to be ineffective. For example, presenting information that the patient already possesses is unnecessary, and counseling the patient about a treatment plan which the family does not view as helpful is a waste of time.

The assessment of a patient should include the following information: the patient's level of health care knowledge, health care skills, attitudes concerning health and experiences with the health care system, and potential for compliance and partnership. A detailed data base as shown in Table 12-1 can be collected over a period of time to aid the physician in practicing comprehensive family medicine.

EVALUATING THE PATIENT EDUCATION PROGRAM

Patient education must be evaluated to determine if it is effective. Evaluation can serve to justify a program, modify a program, or develop future learning experiences for patients (see Chapter 8).

Evaluation may focus on the individual patient, i.e., what knowledge has been learned, what skills have been mastered, what behaviors have changed. Alternatively, evaluation may examine a single patient education program or the overall patient education program (Green, Squyres, D'Altroy and Herber, 1980).

Both patients and staff should be offered opportunities to evaluate patient education. Patients can assess materials, any parts of the program in which they have participated, the instructors, and possibly the overall program. Not only can patients provide valuable information for evaluation, but they are likely to gain satisfaction from being part of the effort.

Questionnaires can be given at the end of a class, handed out in the waiting room, or included in a newsletter. Evaluation forms can be attached to the materials given to patients.

The staff can evaluate learning by patients, individual patient education programs and the overall program. Their participation also results in the likelihood that they will involve more patients.

Patient learning can be assessed informally by asking questions of the patient or by administering pre- and posttests. Mastery of skills by a patient, such as insulin injection or breast self-examination, can be assessed by the physician or other staff member. Behavioral change also may be measured, as in smoking cessation or dieting for weight loss.

Specific aspects of the teaching process can be evaluated separately to determine the effectiveness of each. For example, the communication skills used in the one-to-one interactions, the teaching materials used, and the cost of patient education should all be evaluated.

Beyond modification of the patient education program based upon evaluation, it is important to seek ideas from patients for new or different possibilities. Similarly, the staff should engage in brainstorming sessions about patient education and stay abreast of the efforts of other health care professionals. Finally, it may be effective to incorporate some variations, such as a monthly educational focus, into the patient program.

Table 12-1
Data Base for Evaluating Patient Education Potential (Collected over Time)

Age
Nationality
Religious beliefs:
   Object to or refuse blood transfusions?
   Object to or refuse any medical treatment?
Educational level
Occupation
History
   Chronic illnesses
   Illnesses of family/close friends
   Serious operations
   Hospitalizations
Knowledge
   Reading
      Newspapers
      Medical books at home
      Childhood books
      Medical magazines
      Business magazines
      Publications at library
   Classes taken
   Special interests
   Hobbies
Skills
   CPR
   Taking temperature
   Taking pulse
   Counting respirations
   Recognizing signs and symptoms of illness
Reponsibility taken for health:
   Home health diary
   Home medical records
   Home first aid kit
   Home medicine cabinet
Attitudes
   Are friends/peers health conscious?
   Are friends/peers obese, smokers, drinkers, nutrition conscious, etc.?
Assess patient's agreement with these statements:
   1. Many illnesses can be prevented.
   2. People are responsible for their own health.

   3. If you feel good, you probably have no disease.
   4. Habits like smoking influence how long you live.
   5. Poor health is largely a matter of bad luck.
   6. Doctors can do more about my health than I can.
   7. I can reduce my health risks.
Patient health improvement efforts supported by
   1. family
   2. friends
   3. community
   4. place of work
Patient interested in programs on:
   1. alcohol control
   2. blood pressure management
   3. cardiac rehabilitation
   4. diabetes management
   5. emotional problems
   6. exercise or fitness
   7. general health education
   8. human sexuality
   9. nutrition counseling
   10. smoking cessation
   11. stress management
   12. weight reduction
Patient wants educational information on:
   1. alcohol
   2. birth control
   3. diet
   4. drug abuse
   5. emotional problems
   6. exercise
   7. financial problems
   8. health hazards
   9. legal problems
   10. loneliness
   11. marital problems
   12. medical emergencies
   13. breast self-examination
   14. sexual problems
   15. smoking
   16. venereal disease

Evaluating Communications Skills

Communications skills are an important aspect of effective patient education and may require development on the part of the physician and staff (Svarstad, 1976). One area of skills is communication of medical information. For most patients, information should be provided in nontechnical terms, for example, using the phrase "too much in your blood" rather than "ketosis." Sometimes the use of an analogy will prove helpful in explaining a condition. It is also important for instructions to be specific. When a plan is developed to teach self-care skills to diabetics, for example, it is valuable to use standard terminology for communicating concepts.

A second area of communications skills involves methods of encouraging questions and assessing comprehension and adherence (Falvo, 1984). Reactions can be elicited from patients by asking open-ended questions such as, "What else would you like to know about your condition?" "What does this information mean to you?" and "What kinds of problems are you having in following this routine?"

It may be useful for the physician and others involved in patient education to tape record some of their sessions with patients and to evaluate the effectiveness of their communication. Using a voice-activated tape recorder is a nonintrusive and inexpensive method for evaluation. The physician may simply inform patients that some visits may be taped for evaluation of the physician's communication style. Many physicians are able to evaluate the effectiveness of their patient education by taping several visits and listening to themselves away from the office setting. If the physician is not comfortable with self-evaluation, he or she may enlist the assistance of a patient/health educator, social worker, or clinical psychologist.

It should be stressed that no theory of communication or behavior is applicable for all kinds of illnesses and conditions nor for all ages of patients. There are considerable differences in motivating a child, and "unsophisticated" adult, and a sophisticated adult. Table 12-2 provides a suggested checklist for evaluating one to one patient communication and education (Fass, Vahldieck, and Meyer, 1983).

Evaluate Teaching Materials

Instructional materials can be of considerable assistance in patient education; however, it is critical that they be utilized properly in a supplementary role. Materials cannot take the place of one to one patient education, but they will prove effective when they are used to reinforce information already discussed by the physician or other provider.

A second caution about materials concerns the process of selection from the vast array of electronic and printed materials available, which includes video and audio presentations; pamphlets, fact sheets and other written materials; and illustrations and models. It is essential for the physician to be involved in selecting the material to be used so that it will be consistent with the information normally given in one-to-one oral communication. Following are recommended resources for patient education handouts on health topics and on medications: *The Family Physician's Compendium of Patient Information*, 1983–84. Biomedical Information Corp., 800 Second Ave., New York, NY 10017; *Instructions for Patients* (3rd ed.), H. Winter Griffith, 1982, W. B. Saunders Co., West Washington Square, Philadelphia, PA 19105: *Patient Care* (Patient Education Aids appearing in journal), Patient Care Communications, Inc., 16 Thorndal Circle, PO Box

Table 12-2
Checklist for Evaluating One-to-one Patient Education Interactions

---

The physician-teacher

Asks the reasons for the visit
Asks about prior and ongoing treatment
Explains what he/she is doing during the exam
Explains what he/she finds in the exam
Offers a specific treatment plan
Explains and justifies the treatment plan
Discusses alternative plans of treatment
Specifies how the patient should followup
Assesses the patient's understanding of the treatment plan
Asks open-ended questions
Invites questions from the patient
Answers questions from the patient
Uses terms the patient can understand
Summarizes important points
Expresses acceptance of the patient
Provides written instructions

Adapted from Fass, M. F., Vahldieck, L. M., and Meyer, D. L., Teaching patient education skills: a curriculum for residents. Kansas City, KS: Society of Teachers of Family Medicine, 1983.

1245, Darien, CT 06820; Drug information, *1983 USP DI, Advice for the Patient* (Vol. II), United States Pharmacopeial Convention, Inc., 12601 Twinbrook Parkway, Rockville, MD 20852; *The Family Physician's Compendium of Drug Therapy*, Biomedical Information Corp., 800 Second Ave., New York, NY 10017; Patient Medication Instruction Sheets, PMI Order Dept., American Medical Association, PO Box 52, Rolling Meadows, IL 60008. When appropriate material cannot be found, it may be feasible to use an existing piece as the basis for preparing information suitable for the individual practice.

For practical purposes, materials should be selected to address the problems most frequently seen in the practice. Accumulating a large collection of materials unlikely to be used can prove costly in dollars as well as space needed for consistent use of materials. In family practice, handouts are helpful for such topics as prenatal care, child development, upper respiratory infections, fever, urinary tract infections, wounds, head injuries, low back pain, diets and hypertension. A survey of the practice will indicate the problems which require explanatory material.

Evaluation of potential patient education materials can be a fairly simple, informal process or it may develop into sophisticated methodology. In general, criteria for evaluation include content, educational level, format, and cost.

Content must be accurate, up-to-date, and sufficiently broad to cover the major areas of concern. It should be objective in point of view, and it should contain practical information for the patient. For example, if a patient is instructed to take a medication, the information should include the dosage, the frequency, etc. (see Chapter 10).

Because most physicians see patients at a variety of educational levels, there is merit in having materials available at several levels. Three different levels are recommended: a

7th–8th grade level, which requires limited reading and usually presents content in a pictoral form; a 10th–11th grade or intermediate level; a sophisticated level, appropriate for patients who are interested in and motivated to read medical material.

It has been determined that most patients read at the 6th–8th grade level, but that most patient education materials are written at a 10th–12th grade level. Readability formulas may be helpful in indicating the appropriate audience level for various materials (see Chapter 7). In general, materials for lower reading levels will have short sentences, common words and primarily one- or two-syllable words. A personal tone and a conversational style also are used.

The format of patient education materials should draw the reader into the material and aid in understanding and remembering the information. A logical presentation of information is helpful, and sections with subheadings can facilitate comprehension. Illustrations or diagrams add visual appeal and assist in clarifying information. Some physicians appreciate having space on handouts to enable them to individualize the material by writing in medicine dosages or frequencies and other instructions.

In considering the expense of a particular piece of material or equipment, it is useful to think in terms of cost per patient use and to estimate frequency of patient use. Handouts can be evaluated during actual use in the following manner.

There are various ways to utilize handouts effectively for patient education during an office visit. Three different approaches are suggested for educating a patient about a first-time diagnosis. (Brunsworth and Farrell, 1982). After providing a brief explanation of the diagnosis, the physician may (*a*) give the patient a written handout to read and return to the exam room in 5–10 minutes for questions and answers; (*b*) give the patient a written handout to take home, and check back in a week for questions, answers and re-explanations; or (*c*) have a nurse or patient educator go over the written handout with the patient and follow up with the above.

All three variations may be used, depending upon the doctor's work load and the flow of patients. The second alternative appears to lead to the most comfortable situation because the doctors can reconsider the diagnosis and evaluate the patient's response to treatment while the patient has had time to understand the disease and what can be done about it.

The patient's understanding and knowledge level should be documented in the chart upon each visit. The problem-oriented medical record is an invaluable tool for patient education. It provides a structured approach and facilitates the process of patient education as an integral, ongoing part of health care. The problem list for each patient, requiring intervention over time, comprised the physician's agenda for health care and patient education.

Patient education should be documented for several reasons: to help the physician remember what has been done; to communicate to associates and other personnel what needs to be done in their contact with the patient, and to ensure that patient education is undertaken at the proper time.

A simple method for documenting patient education is the use of progress notes which have a carbon section. After discussing the treatment plan with the patient, the physician writes an educational prescription in this section and tears off the top copy for the patient. These may be identified by subject and code number or subject and title. In addition, copies of handouts provided to the patient can be inserted into the medical record.

Evaluating Costs of Patient Education

The issue of cost merits examination. It appears that more and more third-party payers are starting to reimburse for certain types of patient education, usually physician supervised, but the reimbursement issue is not yet resolved and physicians are concerned about the costs of providing patient education.

Income for patient education should be derived from a portion of the office visit fee plus charges for any specific materials that are expensive. Contracts or grants for patient education programs are another possible income source, most likely to apply for a single component of an overall program, such as a class for diabetics. Classes are often fee-supported.

In view of the public's increasing interest in personal health maintenance, however, costs should be balanced against the benefits of patient education in attracting and retaining patients. In addition, if patient education helps to increase the patient's understanding of instructions and information, the physician benefits from fewer unnecessary callbacks and return visits. Costs also may be reduced by a decrease in broken appointments and by prevention of malpractice suits.

Teaching Patients about Their Medical Problems

Just as patient care proceeds on varied levels, so does patient education. It may be limited to giving instructions or providing information appropriate to the patient, but it can involve teaching skills, advising on alternative medical treatment and counseling on attitudes and behaviors. The specific level or taxonomy will be determined by the nature of care, by the commitment of the practice in that area, and by the patient's needs and interests (see Chapter 5).

A general understanding of learning theory is helpful background for physician and staff as they implement a program of patient education (see Chapter 6). The basic principles of adult learning developed by Malcolm Knowles have significance for the patient education setting and can be used to evaluate the education program. These principles of adult learning are summarized.

1. Environment. The physical environment for learning should be comfortable, and the psychological climate should be one of acceptance, respect, and support.
2. Needs assessment. The patient must be involved in determining learning needs (see Chapter 3).
3. Goals. The patient should be involved in formulating goals for learning experiences.
4. Problem orientation. The patient will learn best if the focus is on problem areas rather than subjects.
5. Mutual responsibility. The patient should share responsibility for learning. The role of the educator is to help the patient find the best methods of learning.
6. Practical application. It is important for the patient to be able to apply new knowledge and skills quickly.
7. Evaluation. The patient should be involved in measuring progress toward established goals and in rediagnosing learning needs.

In acute care, patient education may consist simply of a presentation of medication information to enable the patient to care for him or herself effectively. The physician discusses the purpose of the medication, informs the patient of precautions to observe while taking it, instructs on dosage and frequency, and alerts the patient to major side effects. The physician then supplements oral information with printed material on the medication, such as a patient medication instruction sheet made available by the American Medical Association. This type of patient education requires minimal planning, expense, and effort.

In contrast, patient education for a chronic condition is often quite complex and should cover a large number of content areas (see Chapter 4). These include the nature of the disability; alternative treatments, including costs, risks, benefits and likely outcomes; medication; skills for self care; living aids; safety; diet; exercise, and hygiene. In addition, education may cover sources of detailed information, the existence of myths and quackery concerning the health subject, family assistance, support groups and classes. It also is critical to assess the patient's ability to deal with problems in managing health. An overall patient education plan should be developed for chronic conditions; however, the needs and response of the individual patient will determine whether the plan is carried out in abbreviated or expanded form.

Figure 12-3 outlines the steps in patient education with emphasis on the complex issues of information transfer, skills acquisition, counseling, and environmental modification that all lend support for learning. If individuals, families, and community groups are

STEPS IN PATIENT EDUCATION

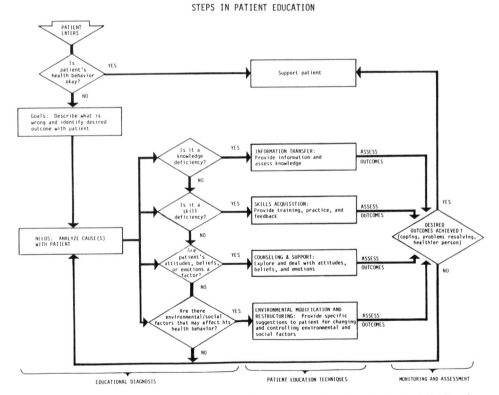

Figure 12-3. Steps in patient education. Taken from Patient Education: A Handbook for Teachers, Society of Teachers of Family Medicine, 1979, p. 43. Used with permission of the Society for Teachers of Family Medicine Kansas City, Missouri.

to partake in the partnerships that patient education offers, then each health care professional must develop these skills essential to teaching.

The teaching plan that illustrates the content of this chapter is based on the notion that patient education is a process in which many health care professionals are involved. The quality of patient care and the rewards professionals obtain from the teaching interaction with individuals, families or community groups is apparent in the partnership that develops when people are educated about their health care problems.

ACKNOWLEDGMENT

The source of the material for this chapter is taken from D. Robertson and E. H. Estes, Jr. (eds.): TEXTBOOK OF FAMILY PRACTICE. Copyrighted by Year Book Medical Publishers, Inc., Chicago (In press).

TEACHING PLAN FOR THE PATIENT WITH ARTHRITIS AND FAMILY

By Carol E. Smith

Patients coping with arthritis need teaching in several areas such as rest, exercise, pacing, pain control, nutritional counseling and medication management, joint protection, body image changes, occupational-environmental hazards, and social-emotional responses to this life-altering disease. The physician will teach on many of these topics as will the nurse, physical therapist, and pharmacist (Currie, 1984). It is hoped that patients who learn about this medical problem will manage their medications and diet appropriately, routinely follow precautions for protecting their joints, continue prescribed exercise programs, develop coping mechanisms for dealing with pain, immobility, or depression (Currie, 1982).

There are several successful approaches to teaching patients with arthritis and their families that range from outpatient instruction (Knudson, Spiegel, and Furst, 1981) to group therapy (Udelman and Udelman, 1978). Currently self-help–oriented education programs using lay-taught groups or individual instruction via audiotape are being evaluated. Tentative outcomes of such programs are encouraging. Physicians and their colleagues who are establishing patient education programs for arthritis thus have several models from which they may select. The choice will depend, as this chapter illustrates, on the needs of the patients and resources available in that practice setting (McGinty, Kratz, and Bachman, 1983).

Assessment

The staff in the medical practice initially would need to assess their own philosophy of patient education as it relates to patients with arthritis. For example, if the nurse in this practice has seen the positive outcomes of education programs taught by individuals who have the disease, she or he may encourage the counseling-oriented methods (Ferguson and Bole, 1979). The physician may express interest in the use of a contract to accomplish the teaching and increase compliance, while the receptionist may state beliefs that some computerized-assisted instruction or other audiovisual methods of teaching should be employed right in the reception room, clinic, or on a take home basis.

Gathering input from the patients and their families as to the information, skills, and attitudes they perceive as necessary for coping with their illness would be helpful, and because so much work has been done in this area of patient education, a review of current literature on this topic would be a vital component of the assessment steps.

Planning

Once the assessment is completed and the behavioral objectives of the program written, planning for incorporation of all available resources for the program begins. Pharmacists may be called upon to develop materials for handouts on steroids and other frequently used medications. Organizations such as the National Arthritis Foundation, Atlanta, GA can be contacted for materials and teaching plans they recommend (Lorig, 1981).

Planning for physical resources should also be undertaken at this time. Possibly scheduling of office or reception room space during non-office hours would be the best way to accommodate group teaching where both patient and family are present.

Implementing

Through the assessment step of this process it may be determined that a group teaching approach best suits the patient's needs, resources of the practice, and philosophical leanings of the staff. However, this does not mean that other teaching strategies would not be implemented along with the group counseling type sessions. Availability of take-home self-instruction materials (handouts, audiovisual aids, or computer-assisted instruction) could be used to augment the cognitive and psychomotor education. Follow-up telephone interaction by the nurse could be used to reinforce the attitudinal or affective aspects of the teaching program. Naturally, during each office visit with the patient, the physician institutes one-to-one patient education and provides an "instruction prescription."

Evaluating

Evaluating the outcomes of the arthritic education program would include measurements of disease progression, patient and family attitudes towards their medical regimen, and their use of the coping mechanisms taught. Evaluation also takes into account the physician's and staff's judgments about the quality of teaching provided. The nurse in the practice might sit in on the group sessions to evaluate the instruction; the physician could use the checklist for evaluating one-to-one interactions; and the health educator in the practice could review the handouts or audiovisual materials for reading level and appropriateness for adult learning. The office manager would evaluate use of personal and physical resources and calculate the cost-effectiveness of the program. The total staff would discuss and judge the benefits of the program and determine their "paybacks" in terms of patient welfare, staff satisfaction, and recruitment of new patients into the practice.

The teaching plan that follows (Tables 12-3, 12-4, and 12-5) illustrates a group program for patients and their family, developed by the staff of a medical practice.

Table 12-3
Teaching Plan for Patients with Arthritis

Assessment	Plan/learning objectives	Interventions	Evaluation
		Affective	
Ask the patient/family "What are your greatest concerns or fears about arthritis?"	Patient will develop skills for coping with their perceived limitations/fears, etc.	Utilize a coping methods scale to identify patients' strengths and discuss other ways to cope.	Patient/family state new coping mechanism they will use.
Use empathic/reflective statements when patient reveals feelings about pain/immobility/body image changes, etc.	Patient will ventilate feelings about illness.	Tell the patient that others with the illness experience similar feelings and find it helpful to ventilate.	Patient continues to communicate. Does not appear withdrawn.
	Patient/family will attend group session with other patients and families with this medical problem.	Use follow-up telephone calls to reinforce use of coping mechanisms.	Patient/family interact readily at each office visit with the physician.

Table 12-4
Teaching Plan for Patients with Arthritis

Assessment	Plan/learning objectives	Interventions	Evaluation
		Cognitive	
Ask the patient/family what they know about steroid therapy. Ask pharmacists about content of medications.	Patient/family lists the therapeutic effect of steroids.	Give patient/family medication facts pamphlet on steroids.	Ask patient to tell you the reason steroids administered.
	Patient/family describe side effects they would report.	Show patient/family the pills as they are given, discuss schedule.	Ask patient to show you how many pills he or she would take.
	Patient/family states schedule and dosage of medication.	Have patient give own medications from bedside supply before leaving hospital.	Observe patient's self-medication schedule.
	Patient/family verbalizes that medication cannot be abruptly discontinued.		

Table 12-5
Teaching Plan for Patients with Arthritis

Assessment	Plan/learning objectives	Interventions	Evaluation
		Psychomotor	
Observe/record patient's joint pain and mobility limitations. Determine if national organizations or community resources have materials available on this topic.	Patient demonstrates active range of motion (ROM). Patient applies splinting/bracing devices correctly. Patient demonstrates safe use of heat for pain. Patient demonstrates correct body mechanics for occupational requirements. Patient/family demonstrate joint protection principles.	Refer to physical therapist for ROM/brace/pain instruction. Refer to occupational health or public health nurse for followup.	Observe patient: ROM exercises Application of brace/splint Body mechanics Use of joint protection principles

REFERENCES

Brunworth, D., and Farrell, M. E. Starting a patient education program in a small town: what does it take? In M. N. Currie (Ed.). *Patient education in the primary care setting. Proceedings of the fifth annual conference.* Kansas City, MO: St. Mary's Hospital of Kansas City Family Practice Residency, 1982.

Currie, B. E., and Beasley, J. W. *Health promotion: principles and clinical applications.* New York: Appleton-Century-Crofts, 1982.

Currie, M. N. (Ed.). *Patient education in the primary care setting. Proceedings of the sixth annual conference.* Kansas City, MO: The Project for Patient Education in Family Practice, St. Mary's Hospital, 1984.

Egger, R. L. Patient education in the private physician's office—1. In J. H. Zurhellen (ed.). *Patient education in the primary care setting. Proceedings of the fourth annual conference.* Memphis, TN: The University of Tennessee Center for the Health Sciences Department of Family Medicine, 1980.

Evans, E. E., and Haynes, R. B. Patient compliance. In R. E. Rakel (Ed.). *Textbook of family practice,* (3rd ed.). Philadelphia: W. B. Saunders Company, 1984.

Falvo, D. R. *Effective communication in patient education: A guide to increased compliance.* Rockville, MD: Aspen System Corp., 1984.

Fass, M. F., Vahldieck, L. M., and Meyer, D. L. *Teaching patient education skills: A curriculum for residents.* Kansas City, MO: Society of Teachers of Family Medicine, 1983.

Ferguson, K., and Bole, G. G. Family support, health beliefs, therapeutic compliance, in patients with rheumatoid arthritis. *Patient Counsel Health Education,* 1979, *1,* 101–105.

Green, L. W., Squyres, W. D., D'Altroy, L. H., and Herber, B. What do recent evaluations of patient education tell us? W. D. Squyres (Ed.). New York: Springer Publishing Co., 1980.

Griffith, H. W., Attarian, P., and Harrison, W. T. Patient health education. In R. B. Taylor (Ed.). *Family medicine: principles and practice* (2nd ed.). New York: Springer-Verlag, 1983.

Knudson, K. G., Spiegel, T. M., and Furst, D. E. Outpatient education program for rheumatoid arthritis patients. *Patient Counsel and Health Education,* 1981, *3,* 77–82.

Levine, D. M., Bone, L. R., Steinwachs, D. M., Parry, R. E., Morisky, P., Sadler, J. The physician's role in improving patient outcome in high blood pressure control. *Maryland State Medical Journal,* 1983, *32,* 291–293.

Lorig, K. Arthritis self-help course leader's manual. Atlanta. GA: Arthritis Foundation, 1981.

McGinty, D. L., Kratz, C. A., and Bachman, I. Starting a patient education program in the private practice primary care setting. In M. N. Currie (Ed.). *Patient education in the primary care setting. Proceedings of the sixth annual conference.* Kansas City, MO: The project for patient education in family practice, St. Mary's Hospital, 1983.

Miller, L. V., and Goldstein, J. More efficient care of diabetic patients in a county hospital setting. *New England Journal of Medicine,* 1972, *286,* 1388–1391.

Mumford, E., Schlesinger, H. J., and Glass, G. V. The effects of psychological intervention on recovery from surgery and heart attacks: An analysis of the literature. *American Journal of Public Health,* 1982, *72,* 141–52.

National Task Force on Training Family Physicians in Patient Education. *Patient education: a handbook for teachers.* Kansas City, MO: Society of Teachers of Family Medicine, 1979.

Robertson, D., and Estes, E. H., Jr. (Eds.). Textbook of family practice. Chicago, IL: Year Book Medical. In press.

Rosenberg, S. G. Patient education leads to better care for heart patients, H.S.M.H.A. *Health Report,* 1971, *86,* 793–802.

Svarstad, B. L. Physician-patient communication and patient conformity with medical advice. In D. Mechanic (Ed.). *The growth of bureaucratic medicine: an inquiry into the dynamics of patient behavior and the organization of medical care.* New York: John Wiley and Sons, Incorporated, 1976.

Udelman, H., and Udelman, D. Group therapy with rheumatoid arthritis patients. *American Journal of Psychotherapy,* 1978, *32,* 288.

Wechsler, H., Levine, S., and Idelson, R. K. The physician's role in health promotion—a survey of primary care practitioners. *New England Journal of Medicine,* 1983, *308,* 97–100.

Index

Page numbers followed by *t* indicate tables.